PROSTHODONTICS IN CLINICAL PRACTICE

PROSTHODONTICS IN CLINICAL PRACTICE

Robert S Klugman, DDS

Former Senior Clinical Lecturer
Department of Prosthodontics
Hebrew University-Hadassah School of Dental Medicine
Private practice
Jerusalem, Israel

Contributions by

Harold Preiskel, MDS, MSc, FDS RCS

Consultant in Prosthetic Dentistry
Guy's Hospital
Private practice
London, UK

and

Avinoam Yaffe, DMD

Professor, Department of Prosthodontics
Director, Graduate Training Program
Hebrew University-Hadassah School of Dental Medicine
Jerusalem, Israel

informa
healthcare

© 2002 Informa UK Ltd

First published in the United Kingdom in 2002 by Martin Dunitz, now part of Informa Healthcare.

Reprinted in 2008 by Informa Healthcare, Telephone House, 69-77 Paul Street, London EC2A 4LQ. Informa Healthcare is a trading division of Informa UK Ltd. Registered Office: 37/41 Mortimer Street, London W1T 3JH. Registered in England and Wales number 1072954.

Tel: +44 (0)20 7017 5000
Fax: +44 (0)20 7017 6699
Website: www.informahealthcare.com

A CIP record for this book is available from the British Library.
Library of Congress Cataloging-in-Publication Data

Data available on application

ISBN-10: 1-85317-817-9
ISBN-13: 978-1-85317-817-7

Distributed in the United States and Canada by
Thieme New York
333 Seventh Avenue
New York, NY 10001

Book orders in the rest of the world

Paul Abrahams
Tel: +44 (0)20 7017 4036
Email: bookorders@informa.com

Composition by Scribe Design, Ashford, UK
Printed and bound in India by Replika Press Pvt. Ltd

CONTENTS

FOREWORD

It has been a pleasure and privilege to make a contribution to this project. The book represents the fruits of a lifetime's experience of the principal author; within it you will find pearls of wisdom and a great deal of common sense. The work represents more than a series of case reports and far more than a technique-oriented clinical manual: it is all about the treatment of patients and adapting prosthodontic techniques to the individual situation, rather than the other way round. So often overlooked is the fact that patients who have suffered severe tooth loss do not usuallly arrive for treatment with a mouth in pristine condition. Yet Dr Klugman and his graduate students take patients, establish rapport, and motivate them. This is a book about the real world, and one for all who are interested in prosthodontics; it illustrates how relatively inexperienced colleagues can carry out involved procedures provided they are set out in a step-by-step logical process. Make no mistake that there is anything simple about some of the plans of treatment: adult orthodontics, site preparation for implants and implant prosthodontics, together with complex fixed and removable prostheses, all feature within the text. Some of the techniques employed have been available for many years, but techniques, after all, are only means to an end. Dr Klugman has been able to take advantage of his clinical experience to adapt these well-tried methods to present-day prosthodontics, and in this he has succeeded admirably.

Harold Preiskel

PREFACE

The idea for writing this book came while sitting in one of the seminars of our graduate program in Prosthodontics.

One of our students was presenting a progress report of his patient, discussing the diagnosis, and the possible treatment plans. Finally, he showed his treatment and explained its rationale. As I sat there, the thought came to me, what a waste of information this is; the student is presenting a beautifully documented treatment for a very difficult patient with superb radiographs and slides. What a shame that only the 12 or so people in the room are viewing it.

The purpose of the book is to share our treatment modalities and rationale of treatment with as many dentists as possible.

Our seminars provide at least one hour of case presentation time with a continuation possible the following week. During the presentation, the instructors and other students question the diagnosis and treatment plan, volunteering their opinions and alternative treatment strategies. It's a give and take situation. It is our conviction, that this is one of the best learning processes for a graduate student.

The Graduate Program in Oral Rehabilitation was initiated in 1978 when the Israeli Parliament passed a law recognizing dental specialties. Until that year, the only specialization recognized by the Ministry of Health was Oral and Maxillofacial Surgery, which was a 5-year program. In 1979, the Department of Oral Rehabilitation set up a program to teach Graduate Prosthodontics.

The program is of 3½ years duration and includes certain clinical and basic science requirements. Successful completion of the program enables the student to be eligible for the specialty licensing examination administered by the Ministry of Health in order to qualify as a specialist in Oral Rehabilitation. In the first years, one or two students were accepted to the program and, as time went on, the program was expanded to include up to four students per year. This gave a core group of between 12 and 16 students to participate in seminars and treat patients.

Today the program encompasses four days a week, in which the students spend 4 hours in seminars each week. These consist of case presentations, literature reviews, and research on prosthetic subjects, and additional full day seminars as needed. The students spend 3 days a week treating clinical patients under the supervision of board certified instructors. The remainder of their time is spent in clinical or original research. Many of the students carry out basic research projects leading to a Masters degree or Doctorate.

The program is integrated with other specialty programs at the Dental School, including Periodontics, Orthodontics, Oral Surgery, and Endodontics. The graduate students treat implant patients. They plan and oversee the surgical phase, but do not perform the surgical procedures. Most periodontal surgery, endodontic, oral surgical, and orthodontic procedures are referred to graduate students or specialists in the other disciplines.

The philosophy of treatment in the program is based on the clinical and learning experiences of the faculty, who have themselves been trained in Prosthodontics at The University of Pennsylvania, New York University, and The University of Toronto, in the 1960s and 1970s. Thus their diverse backgrounds mean that the faculty members bring to the program varied ideas of treatment. We have tried to incorporate the best aspects of each of these programs for our own syllabus. Some of the methods we use have been developed here in Israel.

I would like to personally thank all the graduate students, former and present, especially those who contributed to the book, the faculty of the program, Professor Jacob Ehrlich, Professor Avinoam Yaffe (Program Director), Dr Israel Tamari, and Dr Erez Mann. Special thanks go to Professor Harold Preiskel and Professor Avinoam Yaffe who provided editorial commentaries, who made great efforts in helping me, and without whose aid I doubt that the book would have been written.

INTRODUCTION

The book is divided into four parts according to the primary problem of the patient: Periodontal breakdown, Dysfunctional habit patterns, Extensive loss of teeth, and Congenital disorders. Naturally, most patients overlap and fall into more than one category.

The basis for all our prosthodontic treatment, is a healthy periodontium. The main goal of our treatment is to identify the causative factors of the patient's dental problem, and thus be able to control them. Therefore a prerequisite of all treatment is for us to determine these causative factors and, together with the patient, control them. This is done by initiating meticulous oral hygiene and controlling dietary habits and food consumption. At the beginning of treatment, the patient undergoes initial preparation until they prove that they will cooperate completely in their own treatment, by executing excellent oral hygiene. Techniques include flossing, correct toothbrushing, use of stimulators and all periodontal aids necessary to maintain a healthy periodontium. For patients with caries, a dietary analysis is made and the patient is carefully checked to see that they adhere to their new diet. The initial therapy permits us to check the individual patient's biological response and determine whether the disease activity can be controlled. In some cases, due to genetic factors or the patient's personality, the biological response cannot be controlled, and this will naturally alter the treatment plan. Unless otherwise noted, all patients were non-smokers.

A speech therapist provides ancillary treatment, if needed. All past medical histories are carefully evaluated and, if necessary, consultations with the patient's physician are conducted prior to any dental procedures.

One of the philosophies of our treatment is to give the anterior teeth the added function of supporting the vertical dimension of occlusion. The anterior teeth are customarily only used for incising food, speech, esthetics, and anterior guidance in eccentric movements of the mandible. By utilizing the proprioceptive properties of the anterior teeth to provide biological feedback, the occlusal forces applied to the teeth are reduced. This is especially important for patients with mutilated dentitions, where the vertical dimension of occlusion has to be changed. It is also important for patients whose treatment requires increasing the vertical dimension for biomechanical reasons, in order to make space available for restorations.

It is our experience over many years that opening vertical dimension using the anterior teeth, especially the cuspid teeth, will reduce biting force and prevent intrusion of the other teeth. In fact, in most patients, we are most probably restoring vertical dimension that was lost rather than increasing the vertical dimension. These patients now usually close in a more retruded jaw position than their previous acquired one. In patients with a full complement of teeth where change in the vertical dimension of occlusion is required, we prefer using a 'canine platform',[1-3] a modified method for posterior tooth eruption as opposed to a removable appliance (Hawley). We have found that this approach minimizes the need for a full mouth reconstruction and the necessity of restoring otherwise healthy teeth.

In periodontally involved dentitions, and in patients where the overbite is reduced and the overjet increased due to opening of the vertical dimension, we strive on one end and are imposed by the other to diminish lateral forces that are applied to the teeth by decreasing cuspal angles. This then requires flattening of cuspal height in the posterior teeth.

In patients where the remaining teeth do not have the ability to support and guide the occlusion, due to advanced periodontal disease and alveolar bone loss, implants are utilized to give additional occlusal support. Nevertheless, when using implants for occlusal support, we prefer that all lateral and protrusive movements of the mandible be guided by the remaining natural teeth.[4–6]

In those patients where the vertical dimension is altered, the determining factors are usually biomechanical, to acquire enough gingival occlusal space for the restorations. In these cases, we try and limit the amount of change to the minimum that is necessary. Since an increase in vertical dimension of occlusion in patients with advanced adult periodontitis worsens the crown-to-root ratio, we utilize orthodontic treatment of passive or active eruption of the teeth to improve this ratio. Using these treatment modalities demands meticulous oral hygiene and constant scaling and curettage to attain eruption of the teeth, accompanied by healthy supporting tissues.

All treatment is fully documented by photographs and radiographs, thus providing the source for most of the material for this book. The patient follow-up is usually done by the graduate student in their own private practice after completion of the treatment.

Although there are two other systems (the American and the International) in use today, the classification system used in this book to describe tooth position is Palmer's. Palmer's classification divides the mouth into four quadrants: the upper (maxillary) teeth are noted above a horizontal line; the lower (mandibular) teeth are noted below the horizontal line; the right side of the mouth is noted to the left of a vertical line, and the left side of the mouth is noted to the right of the vertical line; teeth are numbered from 1 to 8 in each quadrant, starting at the center of the mouth.

This gives a grid as follows:

(Upper)
Right side 8 7 6 5 4 3 2 1 | 1 2 3 4 5 6 7 8 Left side
_____|_____
(Lower) |
Right side 8 7 6 5 4 3 2 1 | 1 2 3 4 5 6 7 8 Left side

Thus, in discussion of the maxillary right first premolar in this book, it will be noted like this:

(In the American classification the tooth would be number 5 and in the International classification it would be number 14.)

REFERENCES

1   Yaffe A, Ehrlich J, The canine platform a modified method for posterior tooth eruption, *Compend Cont Education* (1985) **6**:382–5.
2   Abrams L, Occlusal adjustment by selective grinding. In: Goldman HM, Cohen DW, eds, *Periodontal Therapy*, 6th edn (CV Mosby: St Louis, 1980).
3   Amsterdam M, Peridontal prosthesis. Twenty-five years in retrospect, *Alpha Omegan* (scientific issue) (1974) December.
4   Hannam AG, Matthews B, Reflex jaw opening in response to stimulation of periodontal mechanoreceptors in the cat, *Arch Oral Biol* (1969) **14**:415.
5   Wood WW, Tobias DL, EMG response to alteration of tooth contacts on occlusal splints during maximal clenching, *J Prosthet Dent* (1984) **51**(3):394–6.
6   Storey AT, Neurophysiological aspects of TMD, presented at the American Dental Association, Chicago, 1982.

TECHNICAL INFORMATION

In patients receiving fixed partial prostheses, the graduate students prepare the teeth which will be used as abutments for the prosthesis. The preparation of choice in mature and periodontally compromised patients is the knife edge preparation. We feel that complete shoulder or chamfer preparations are not suitable in these situations since they require too much root structure reduction. The students then usually make either single copper band elastomeric impressions to impression the prepared teeth or elastomeric complete arch impressions. Due to the many problems associated with elastomeric complete arch impressions, such as retraction cord displacement, microhemorrhage, errant air bubbles (usually at the finishing line), etc, we have found it to be more accurate to use single copper band elastomeric impressions.[1] This is especially true in periodontally involved teeth and whenever a knife edge preparation is indicated.

The graduate students prepare all the teeth to be utilized for the prosthesis and temporize them in as many visits as necessary—this will naturally vary with each patient. After all the teeth have been fully prepared for the fixed prosthesis and checked for proper tooth reduction by measuring the thickness of the provisional restoration, and proper finishing lines, each tooth is impressioned individually and, if incorrect, it can be easily repeated until a satisfactory result is achieved. Again, we would like to emphasize that in our experience, when we have used full arch elastomeric impressions, we find that it is very difficult to get an accurate impression of all the prepared teeth in one impression, especially in periodontally involved patients where there are long clinical crowns and multiple preparations.[1] In the laboratory phase, it is also difficult to achieve an undistorted wax pattern on withdrawal for multiple abutment cases. One of the advantages of a full arch elastomeric impression is that it permits a single casting with accuracy and eliminates the need for soldering; however, in periodontally involved teeth with long clinical crowns it is extremely difficult to achieve an undistorted wax pattern removal for a single casting. This usually leads to additional treatment, which is both time consuming and traumatic to the patient.

A copper band is measured and trimmed to fit the prepared tooth, and then annealed in an ethyl alcohol 70% solution. This produces a softer, more pliable band with a clean polished surface which will not have a rebound effect after the acrylic resin is placed. The band is lined with soft, quick-setting methyl methacrylate resin and allowed to set on the prepared tooth.

The band is removed, and the resin is internally relieved to a depth of 0.5 mm. An escape hole is drilled in the occlusal or incisal area to prevent air bubbles and then the impression is relined using a blue or green Xantropen wash technique. The impressions are cast immediately in die stone; the dies are removed and trimmed after 1 hour. The dies are hardened with a drop of cyanoacrylate (Super Glue-5: Loctite International, Welwyn Garden City, UK) to give a very fine protective layer, and coated with a thin layer of petroleum jelly.

Duralay (Reliance Dental Manufacturing Company, Worth, IL, USA) or Pattern resin copings (GC Company: Kasugai Aichi, Japan) are then made on the prepared dies using a Neylon paintbrush technique. The Neylon technique is a brush-on technique that uses a fine brush dipped in monomer and then in resin powder to pick up a small ball of resin which is then placed on the prepared tooth, starting at the occlusal or incisal surfaces and working towards the gingival margins. A hole is cut in the labial occlusal or incisal corner of the coping to ensure that the coping is fully seated on the prepared tooth during try-in. Pattern resin copings are individually fitted on the prepared teeth and checked clinically for fit and the accuracy of their margins. The copings are also used for centric relation recording and vertical dimension registration. The resin copings are then picked up with a full arch elastomeric impression (Impregum) material. The individual dies are then placed into their respective copings in the impression and a master working model is fabricated.[2,3] A centric relation record is then recorded, usually at the vertical dimension of occlusion, and the models placed in an articulator and the individual elements of the prosthesis are waxed and cast.

Once the metal framework of the prosthesis is returned by the laboratory, the individual metal elements are checked in the mouth, and joined together using resin. The metal framework prosthesis is then sent to the laboratory for soldering. On return, the prosthesis is then checked in the mouth again and another centric relation record made. The soldered copings are then picked up with a full arch elastomeric impression (Impregum) material to capture soft tissue detail.

At this stage, the individual dies are not needed and the laboratory technician places reinforced resin into the lubricated (petroleum jelly) metal framework in the impression, and dental stone for the remainder of the model. This is the final master working model. This technique gives not only fine tissue detail but also a reproducible positive seat for the castings whenever they are removed from the model, thus avoiding damage to the model by constant removal and placement.

The master working models are articulated to the semi-adjustable articulator (Hanau: Teledyne Hanau, Buffalo, NY, USA) by means of a face bow registration and centric relation records performed at the vertical dimension of occlusion as determined by the provisional restorations. Since the working models are articulated at the vertical dimension of occlusion, it is felt that a fully adjustable articulator is not necessary.[4]

The porcelain is then baked and fitted in the patient's mouth, with special attention paid to fit and occlusion. If necessary, the occlusion is adjusted using small round diamond stones until the articulating paper shows that there is uniform and even contact in centric relation (coincident to centric occlusion) between all the posterior teeth and that the anterior teeth are in light contact only. The prostheses are then returned to the laboratory where the final glaze of the porcelain is done.

At the insertion appointment, the prostheses are 'cemented' with a paste of petroleum jelly and zinc oxide ointment (only) for 24–72 hours. The patient then returns and the occlusion is rechecked and adjusted if necessary. The restorations are then cemented with a mixture of zinc oxide and eugenol cement (Temp-Bond: Romulus, MI, USA) and petroleum jelly for a further 72 hours. If there is no washout after 72 hours, the restorations are cemented with just Temp-Bond for a 3-week period. They are then carefully removed and checked for wash-out, and adjusted if necessary.

The patient is questioned at each visit after the initial insertion as to comfort and whether there is any sensitivity with the new restorations. Only after everything is to the patient's and our satisfaction, are the restorations permanently cemented with zincoxyphosphate cement. The prepared teeth are first dried and only then are the restorations cemented. The restorations are cemented in the smallest individual units possible, one at a time, with the remaining teeth in occlusion and provide the correct seating forces during cementation. After cementation, the occlusion is checked again to verify its accuracy.

ACKNOWLEDGEMENT

I would like to thank Ardent Dental Laboratory who did most of the laboratory work pictured in the book.

REFERENCES

1   Gelbard S, Aoskar Y, Zelkind M, Stern N, Effect of impression materials and techniques on the marginal fit of metal castings, *J Prosthet Dent* (1994) **71**(1):1–6.
2   Azizogli MA, Catania EM, Weiner S, Comparison of the accuracy of working casts made by direct and transfer coping procedures, *J Prosthet Dent* (1999) **81**(4):392–8.
3   Lin CC, Ziebert GJ, Donegan SJ, Dhuru VB, Accuracy of impression materials for complete-arch fixed partial dentures, *J Prosthet Dent* (1988) **59**(3):288–91.
4   Weinberg L, *Atlas of Crown and Bridge Prosthodontics* (Mosby: St Louis, 1965).

I   DYSFUNCTIONAL HABIT PATTERNS

PATIENT 1   RETROGRADE WEAR

Treatment by Mordehai Katz

THE PATIENT

The patient, a 56-year-old self-employed building contractor, came to the clinic for dental treatment. His chief complaints were (Figures 1.1–1.3):

'I can't eat.'
'My lower front tooth is shaky.'
'Sometimes my side teeth hurt me.'

PAST MEDICAL HISTORY

The patient's medical history was un-remarkable; he had no allergies, and was not taking any medication.

PAST DENTAL HISTORY

The patient had never visited a dentist regularly. The last visit to a dentist was at

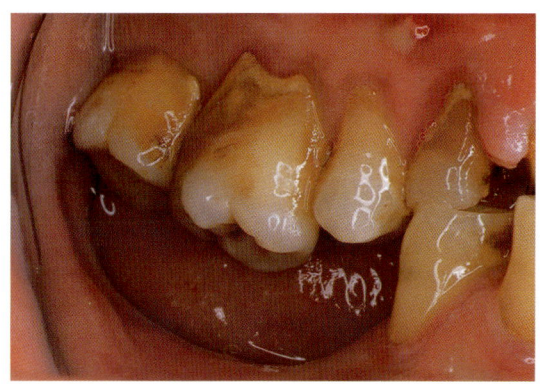

Figure 1.2

Posterior teeth—right side.

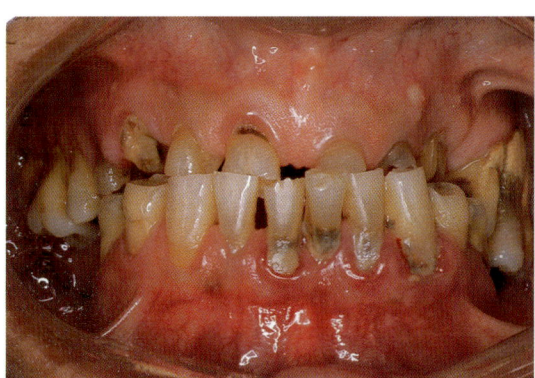

Figure 1.1

Front view of anterior teeth.

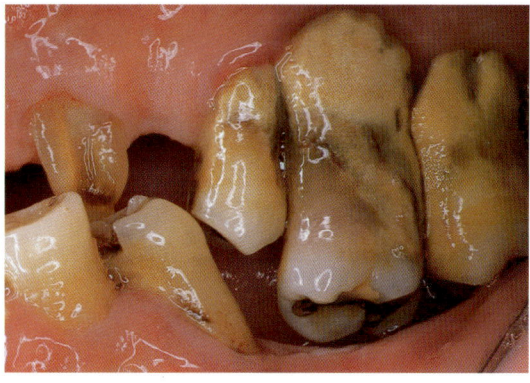

Figure 1.3

Posterior teeth—left side.

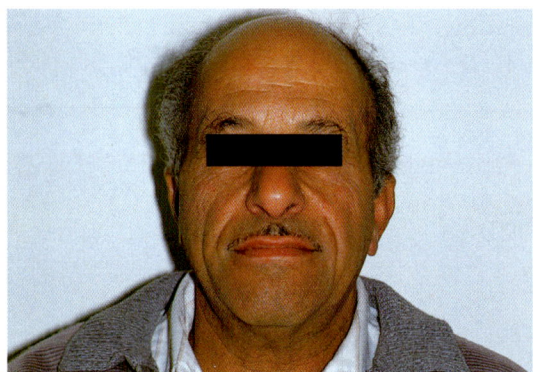

Figure 1.4

Face—frontal view.

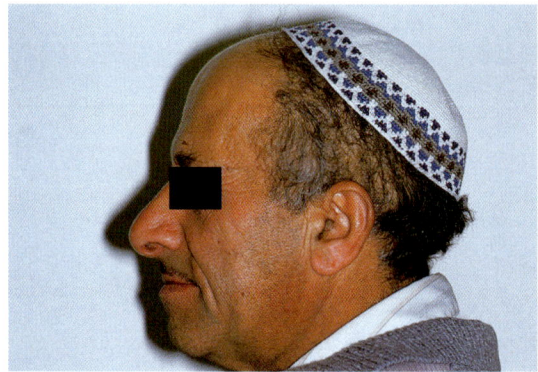

Figure 1.5

Face—side view.

the age of 16 at which time his mandibular molars were extracted. He claimed that he always had the spaces between his front teeth, but he felt that they were getting wider. He brushed his teeth twice a day, morning and evening; he did not use any toothpaste, only a toothbrush.

EXTRA-ORAL EXAMINATION
(Figures 1.4 and 1.5)

- Symmetrical face
- Profile—straight to convex
- Normal temporomandibular joint
- Normal facial musculature
- Maximum opening of 40 mm
- Mandibular movements—slight deviation to the left upon opening and the reverse upon closing
- Slight midline discrepancy

INTRA-ORAL AND FULL-MOUTH PERIAPICAL RADIOGRAPH EXAMINATION

Maxilla (Figure 1.6):

- Very poor oral hygiene
- Parabolic arch

- Caries
- Spacing between the anterior teeth
- Missing right third molar, and left first premolar teeth
- Amalgam restorations on the left and right premolars and molars
- Retrograde wear
- Spacing due to the extraction of the left first premolar and subsequent drifting of the left cuspid distally
- Left cuspid—pulp exposure
- Fistulas in the buccal vestibulum of the area of the right first premolar and left lateral incisor teeth

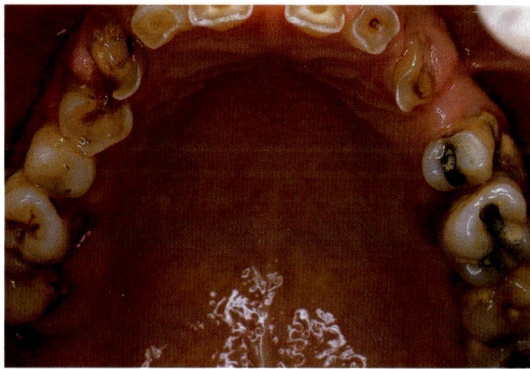

Figure 1.6

Maxillary arch—palatal view.

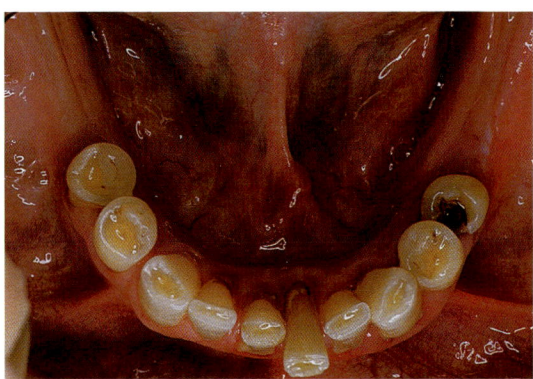

Figure 1.7

Mandibular arch.

- Overeruption of the first premolars and molars on both sides

Mandible (Figure 1.7):

- Parabolic arch
- Residual ridges are thin and extremely resorbed:

$$\frac{}{|5}$$

- Caries
- Missing teeth:

$$\frac{}{8\,7\,6\ |\ 6\,7\,8}$$

- Left central incisor labially tipped

Occlusal examination (Figures 1.1–1.3) revealed that the patient was Angle class III with anterior cross-bite. The interocclusal rest space was 5.0 mm. Overjet was –1.0 mm and overbite was 3.0 mm. The difference between centric relation and centric occlusion was 1.0 mm anterio-posteriorly.

- Mobility class 2 on the maxillary left first molar, class 1 on the maxillary left second molar, and ½ on the maxillary left lateral incisor teeth.
- Mobility class 3 on the mandibular left central incisor, class 2 on the mandibular right central incisor, class 1 on the mandibular lateral incisor, and class ½ on the right mandibular cuspid.
- Fremitus in closing movements on maxillary right first premolar and incisor teeth.
- Non-working side interferences in left lateral movements between the maxillary right lateral incisor and the mandibular first premolar, and the maxillary right central incisor and the mandibular cuspid.
- Non-working side interferences in right lateral movements between the maxillary left central incisor and the left mandibular cuspid and left lateral incisor.
- Anterior guidance at the beginning of protrusive movements, including the mandibular right premolars and at the end of the protrusive movement, the left first premolar also participates.

There was working side contact in right lateral movements between the right maxillary second premolar and the right mandibular second premolar, and in left lateral movements between the maxillary left second premolar and the mandibular left second premolar.

Periodontal examination (Figures 1.8 and 1.9) revealed large amounts of calculus and plaque, probing depths of up to 6.0 mm on some of the mandibular teeth and up to 7.0 mm on some of the maxillary teeth. There was bleeding on probing (BOP) on most of the teeth. There was gingival recession around some of the teeth (Figures 1.1–1.3).

The maxillary right first molar had class 2 furcation involvement on the buccal surface, and class 1 furcation on the mesial surface, and the maxillary left first molar had class 3 furcation involvement on buccal, mesial and distal surfaces. The

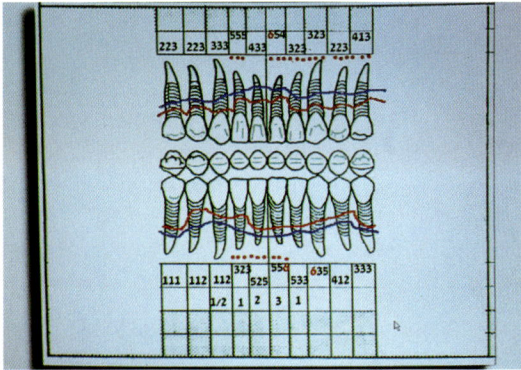

Figure 1.8

Periodontal chart—mandible.

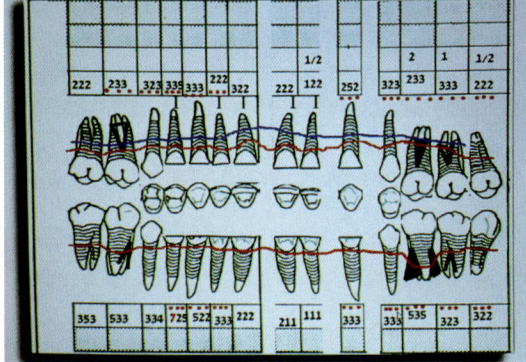

Figure 1.9

Periodontal chart—maxilla.

second left molar had class 1 furcation involvement on the buccal and mesial surfaces.

FULL-MOUTH PERIAPICAL SURVEY (Figure 1.10)

- Periapical lesions:

$$\frac{6\ 4\ 3\ \ |\ \ 2\ 3}{}$$

- Caries: $\dfrac{}{\ \ 5}$

- Extensive horizontal and vertical bone loss around most of the remaining teeth
- Less than ⅓ bone support:

$$\frac{4\ \ |\ \ 3\ 6\ 8}{2\ 1\ \ |\ \ 1\ 2}$$

- Less than ⅔ bone support:

$$\frac{7\ 6\ 2\ 1\ \ |\ \ 5\ 7}{5\ 4\ 3\ \ |\ \ 3\ 4\ 5}$$

- Over ⅔ bone support:

$$\frac{5\ 3\ \ |\ \ 1\ 2}{}$$

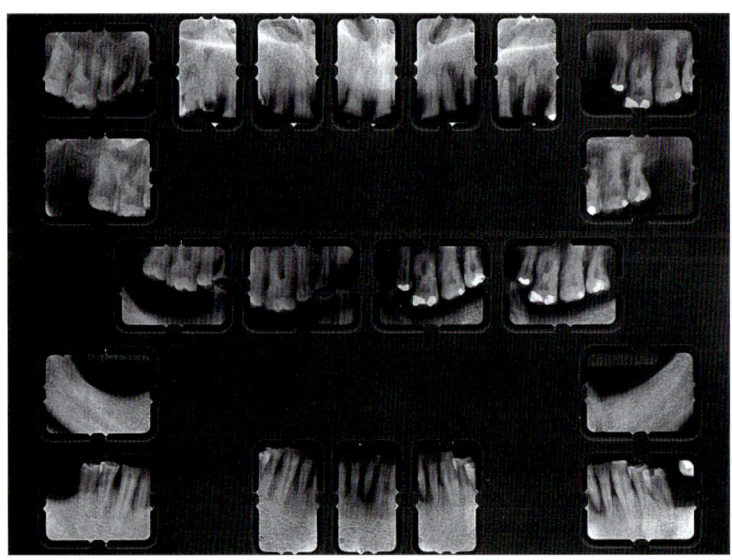

Figure 1.10

Radiographs of maxilla and mandible—pre-treatment.

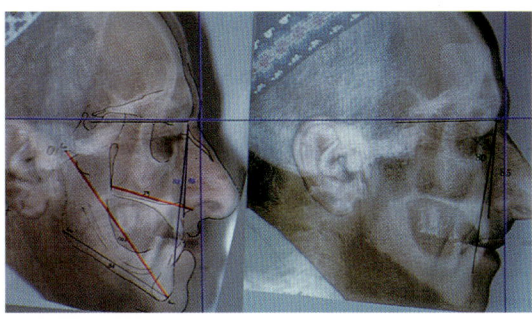

Figure 1.11

Cephalometric analysis.

CEPHALOMETRIC ANALYSIS

The cephalometric analysis (Figure 1.11) was done to evaluate the following relationships:

- Relation of the maxilla to the skull
- Relation of the mandible to the skull
- Relation of the maxilla to the mandible

Determined values:

	Measurement	Average
Go—Gn	82	84
Co—Gn	125	122.5
Palatal plane point A	59	59

(Go, gonial; Gn, gnathion; Co, condyle.)

Interarch relationships:

SNA   85
SNB   83
ANB   2   2
(SNA, sela nasion point A; SNB, sela nasion point B; ANB, difference between A and B.)

INDIVIDUAL TOOTH PROGNOSIS

- Hopeless:

$$\frac{4\ |\ 6}{1\ |\ 1}$$

- Questionable:

$$\frac{3\ |\ 2\ 3\ 7}{2\ |\ 2}$$

- Poor:

$$\frac{6\ |}{\ \ |\ 5}$$

- Fair:

$$\frac{7\ 2\ 1\ |\ 1\ 5}{5\ 4\ 3\ |\ 3\ 4}$$

- Good: none

DIAGNOSIS

- Pseudo-Angle class III
- Advanced adult periodontitis
- Reduced posterior occlusal support
- Missing teeth accompanied by shifting of teeth
- Extreme wear due to occupational involvement
- Caries
- Reduced vertical dimension
- Faulty occlusal plane with extrusion and tipping of teeth
- Secondary occlusal trauma with primary origins
- Periapical lesions

ABOUT THE PATIENT

The patient was very pleasant and willing to do what was necessary to have treatment. He was cooperative and had no preference for a fixed or removable restoration.

POTENTIAL TREATMENT PROBLEMS

- Many missing teeth accompanied by extensive resorption of the residual alveolar ridges, extrusion, and shifting of teeth

- Extensive loss of tooth structure due to intense wear as well as periodontal and periapical pathologies
- Many of the remaining teeth had severe periodontal problems and their prognosis was guarded
- Loss of vertical dimension and extrusion causing a faulty occlusal plane

TREATMENT PLAN

PHASE 1: INITIAL PREPARATION

- Initial periodontal therapy including:
    oral hygiene instruction
    scaling and root planing
- Extraction of hopeless teeth
- Caries excavation and endodontic treatment where necessary
- Evaluation of patient cooperation
- Provisional fixed prosthesis restoring lost vertical dimension and providing occlusal support in the new vertical dimension

Re-evaluation led to the second phase of the treatment plan.

PHASE 2: TREATMENT OPTIONS

Maxilla:

- Fixed and partial removable prostheses
- Fixed prosthesis supported by natural teeth and implants
- Fixed partial prosthesis supported by natural teeth

Mandible:

- Fixed and partial removable prostheses
- Fixed prosthesis supported by natural teeth and implants

TREATMENT

Initial treatment consisted of oral hygiene instruction, scaling and root planing (Figures 1.12–1.14) The hopeless teeth, maxillary right first premolar, cuspid, left cuspid and left first molar, were then extracted. Endodontic therapy was carried out on the maxillary right first molar, left lateral incisor, left second premolar and the left second and third molars. These teeth were then restored with composite resin restorations to replace the material removed in the endodontic preparation.

After ruling out an abrasive diet, erosive components, and day and night bruxism, it was concluded that the retrograde wear of the patient's remaining teeth was due to the fact that he had lost many teeth over the years and the remaining teeth were required to take over all masticatory function. In addition, his professional occupation as a builder, where he was constantly involved in an environment of dust, was also a contributing factor to the retrograde wear.

In order to restore the loss of coronal tooth structure over the years, the remaining maxillary teeth were then prepared and provisional restorations placed at a new vertical dimension of occlusion, thus providing cross-arch splinting. This new vertical dimension was determined by the functional and biomechanical requirements for treatment.

The provisional restorations in the new vertical dimension and occlusal scheme provided the following:

- Maximum occlusal contacts
- Lateral jaw movements without balancing side prematurities
- Separation of the teeth during lateral movement of less than 1.0 mm

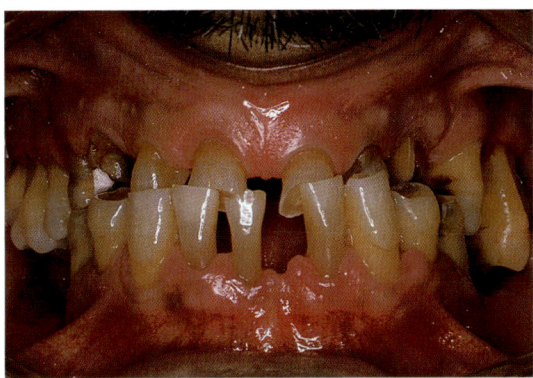

Figure 1.12

After initial preparation—front view.

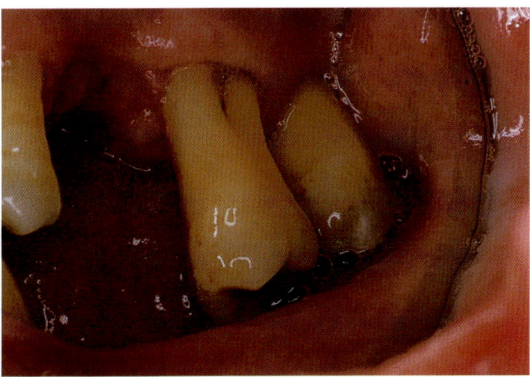

Figure 1.13

After initial preparation—left side.

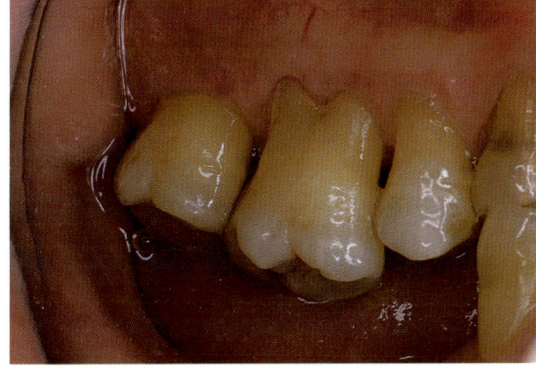

Figure 1.14

After initial preparation—right side.

- Change of vertical dimension to enable maximum contact in centric relation with the anterior teeth
- Better overbite and overjet relationships for protrusive movement disclusion (these can be seen clinically and also on the cephalometric radiograph done after the insertion of the transitional restorations)
- SNB (after treatment with provisonals) 80
- ANB (after treatment with provisonals)   5

A CT (computerized tomography) radiograph was then done to determine the possibility of implant placement in the mandible. The radiograph revealed lack of bone for implants due to the severe resorption of the alveolar ridge over many years, most probably due to the early loss of teeth.

Endodontic therapy was also carried out on the mandibular left second premolar. To improve its prognosis the tooth was shortened, changing its poor crown-to-root ratio, and then restored with a coping thus enabling it to be used as an abutment for a removable partial denture. The mandibular removable partial denture would replace the missing molar teeth as well as the missing left central incisor and second premolar.

There was a dramatic improvement in the patient's periodontal condition due to his improved oral hygiene and cooperation, and it was decided to complete the patient's treatment with replacing the transitional restorations in the permanent prostheses and duplicating both the vertical dimension and occlusal scheme of the transitional restorations.

In the maxilla, copper band elastomeric impressions were made of all the prepared teeth and pattern resin copings made to fit the stone dies. A polyether full arch impression was then taken of the maxilla and the

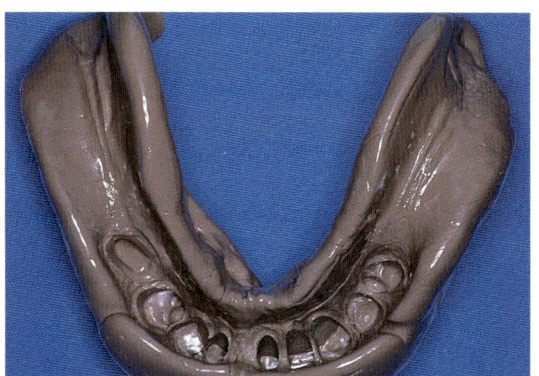

Figure 1.15

Mandible, final impression, Mercaptan rubber

master model poured. Mesio-occlusal rest preparations were prepared in the mandible on the left first premolar and right second premolar teeth.

A mercaptan rubber base impression was then made using a border molded custom tray (Figure 1.15). The mandibular metal framework was fitted and adjusted in the mouth. An acrylic resin bite tray was constructed on the metal framework. This tray and the pattern resin copings of the maxillary teeth were used to record the centric relation at the same vertical dimension of occlusion as

the transitional restorations. A facebow registration was taken and the models mounted on a Hanau articulator. The maxillary metal copings were fitted and connected with pattern resin for soldering. The soldered prosthesis was then checked in the mouth, and a polyether impression (Figure 1.16) was then made for tissue detail and a pick-up of the fixed prosthesis in order to make a final master model.

This was mounted on a Hanau articulator by means of a facebow registration and the pattern resin registration on the soldered metal prosthesis. The shade was chosen and porcelain baked to the metal. The bisque bake maxillary prosthesis was fitted in the mouth and the occlusion checked and adjusted with the missing mandibular teeth that had been set up on the partial denture. The porcelain was glazed and the mandibular prosthesis processed. The denture teeth were made of porcelain in order to match the material in the fixed prosthesis in the maxilla.

The maxillary prosthesis was cemented temporarily and the mandibular prosthesis inserted and adjusted. After 2 weeks, the

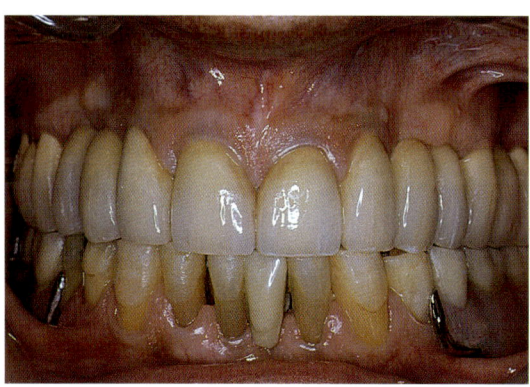

Figure 1.16

Treatment completed—fixed prosthesis, anterior view.

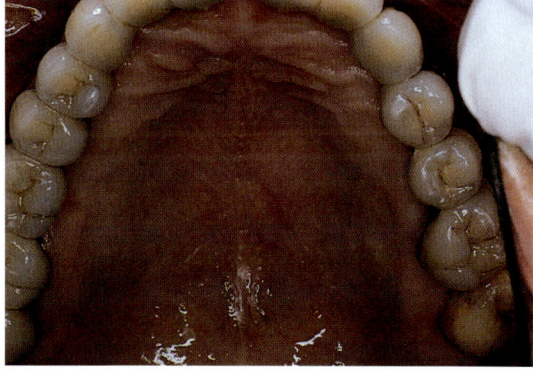

Figure 1.17

Treatment completed—restorations, maxilla.

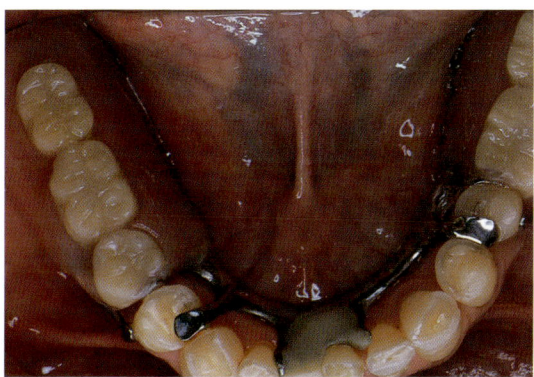

Figure 1.18

Treatment completed—restorations, mandible.

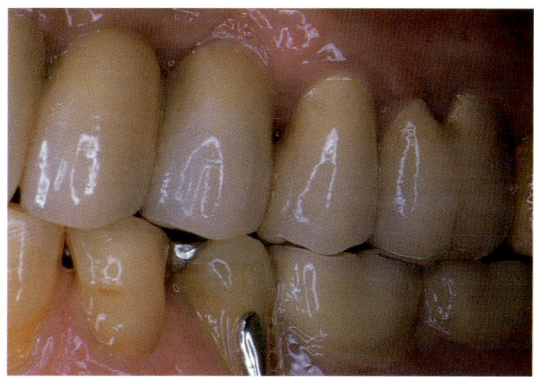

Figure 1.19

Treatment completed—restorations, left side.

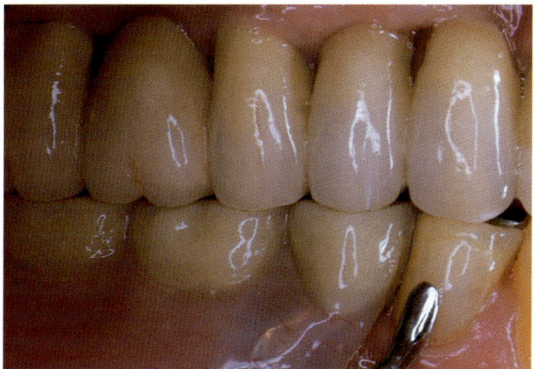

Figure 1.20

Treatment completed—restorations, right side.

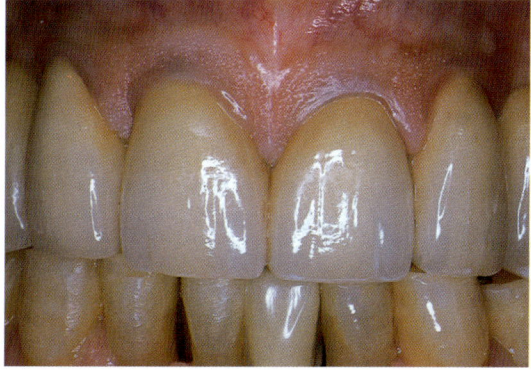

Figure 1.21

Treatment completed—restorations, anterior teeth, close-up.

maxillary prosthesis was cemented with a permanent cement (zinc oxyphosphate) (Figures 1.17–1.21).

SUMMARY

The patient came to the clinic for dental treatment complaining of pain, a loose tooth, and difficulty in eating. He had not visited a dentist for 40 years and thought that by brushing his teeth twice daily, it was sufficient. He suffered from very poor oral hygiene, and advanced periodontal disease. He had many missing teeth and some of the remaining teeth were mobile with fremitus and periapical pathology. There was extensive wear, severe extrusion of teeth, midline discrepancy, poor occlusal relationships, anterior cross-bite, spacing in the maxilla, and caries. Radiographs ruled out the use of implants in the mandible without pre-prosthetic surgery. Through increased awareness of the importance of oral hygiene, extensive periodontal, endodontic and prosthetic treatment, a functional and esthetic result was attained.

CASE DISCUSSION
AVINOAM YAFFE

This 56-year-old person presented to the graduate clinic with the complaint of difficulty in eating, pain, and mobile teeth. It was the purpose of our treatment to include the anterior teeth in occlusal support for several reasons: many posterior teeth were missing, thus occlusal support was lacking; secondly it was intended to achieve anterior guidance in order to disocclude whatever posterior teeth were left, and to allow freedom in lateral excursions. In order to accomplish this, we took advantage of the IC–RC (intercuspal position–retruded cuspal position) discrepancy; and made a slight change in vertical dimension along with minor adjunctive orthodontics to close the anterior diastema. These three factors enabled us to change a pathologic, malfunctioning, unesthetic occlusion into a physiologic, esthetic, long-lasting occlusal scheme, that included the anterior teeth in support, along with all the other functions of anterior teeth, to the patient's satisfaction.

CASE DISCUSSION
HAROLD PREISKEL

This sensible plan of treatment involved extensive reconstruction of both jaws, establishing a new occlusal plane and table. Whether or not there was an erosive component to the loss of tooth substance is largely irrevelant. There was almost certainly a significant forward mandibular posture.

The decision to use porcelain artificial teeth on the removable prosthesis is understandable, although this requires vertical space to allow for the diatoric design to retain the porcelain. In fact, what really matters is not so much the hardness of the occlusal surface, but the coefficient of friction between the upper and lower surfaces. Provided the glaze of the opposing porcelain is not disturbed, modern cross-linked resin teeth will function perfectly well, and if they should need to be changed after 5 to 8 years, it is not such a disaster. Furthermore, if an incorrect assessment of the maxillo/mandibular relations had been made at the outset, which is quite likely in long-term cases of forward mandibular posture, then resetting or replacing, or even adjusting resin teeth would be considerably easier. I would expect this restoration to function well for many years.

PATIENT 2 BRUXISM

Treatment by Doron Bar-Hen

THE PATIENT

A 57-year-old woman, employed as a laboratory technician, presented herself for treatment at our clinic. She had no specific complaints but her private dentist brought to her attention that she was bruxing her teeth so strongly that in a short period of time she would expose the pulps in her teeth (see Figures 2.4 and 2.6).

PAST MEDICAL HISTORY

For the past 4 years she had been under treatment for high blood pressure and was now stabilized, with her blood pressure being 130/90. She was taking 75 mg of Normiten (altenolol), 20 mg of Convertin (enalapril maleate), and 100 mg of aspirin daily. She has also been receiving hormonal therapy of Astrogil and Ortogestin since ceasing her menstrual cycle a few years ago.

PAST DENTAL HISTORY

The patient had been treated by her private dentist until 2 months previous to his referral of her to the graduate program of the Department of Oral Rehabilitation at Hadassah. The reason for the referral was the severe wear of her anterior teeth and his fear that she would grind away all the coronal tooth structure in the near future (Figure 2.1).

EXTRA-ORAL EXAMINATION
(Figures 2.1 and 2.2)

- Normal facial symmetry
- Straight profile
- Normally functioning muscles of mastication and well developed masseter muscles
- Temporomandibular joints were normal without crepitus
- No deviation or pain on opening or closing movements
- Function and phonetics were normal

INTRA-ORAL AND FULL-MOUTH PERIAPICAL RADIOGRAPH EXAMINATION

- Soft tissues, tongue, floor of the mouth, and palate were all normal (Figure 2.3)
- Extreme wear of the teeth with exposed dentine, prominent more on the anterior than the posterior teeth (Figure 2.4)
- Deep overbite with reduced interocclusal space, and tissue impingement of the palatal maxillary tissue due to contact with the mandibular anterior teeth (Figure 2.5)
- Maxillary right second and third molars were missing and the maxillary left third molar was impacted (Figures 2.6 and 2.10)
- Spaced dentition between the maxillary left lateral incisor, cuspid and first

13

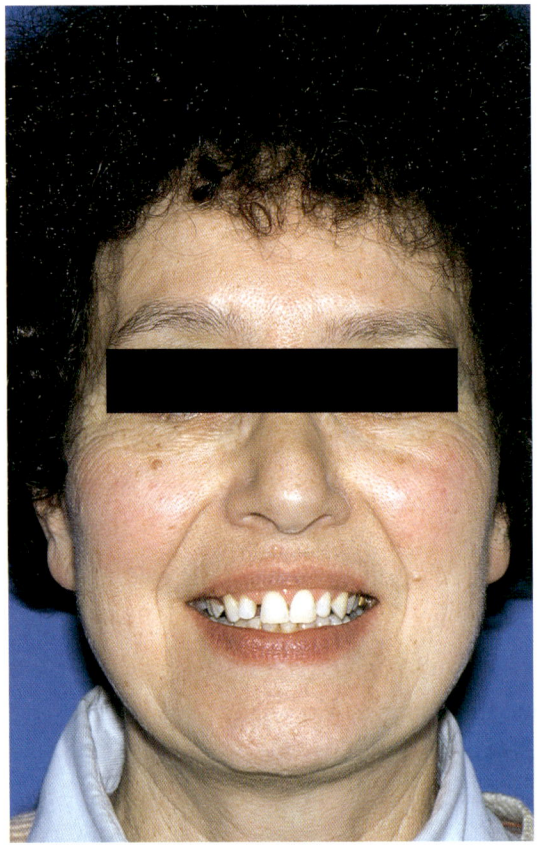

Figure 2.1

Face—frontal view.

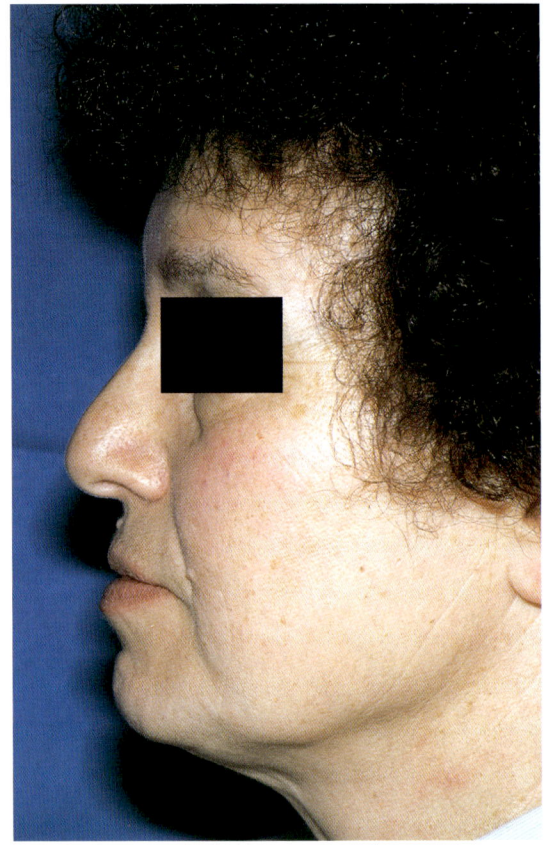

Figure 2.2

Face—profile view.

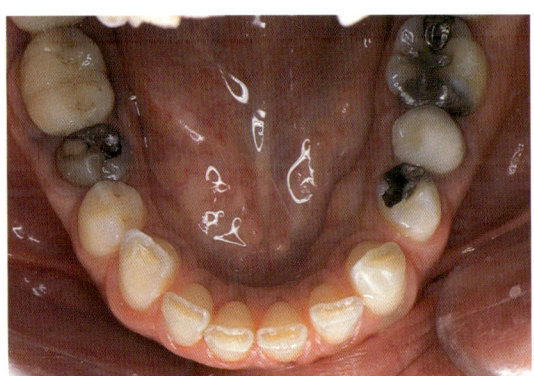

Figure 2.3

Mandibular arch—lingual view.

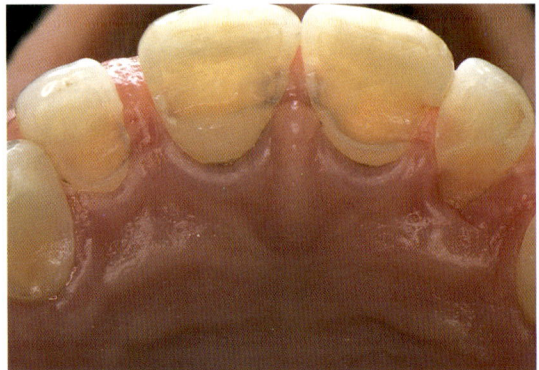

Figure 2.4

Anterior maxillary teeth—palatal view, showing extensive wear.

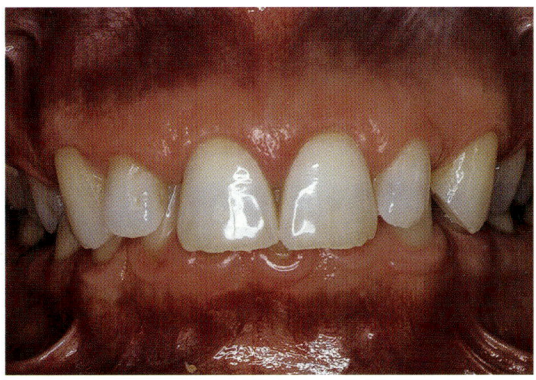

Figure 2.5

Anterior teeth—labial view, showing deep overbite.

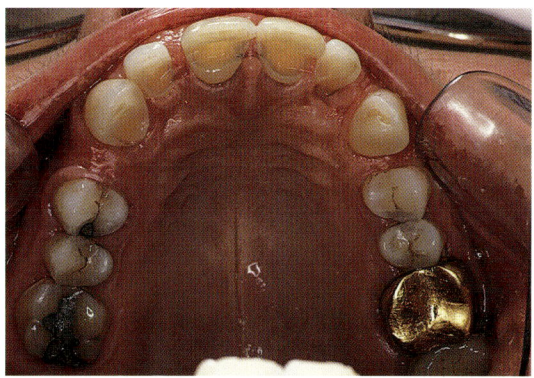

Figure 2.6

Maxillary arch—palatal view.

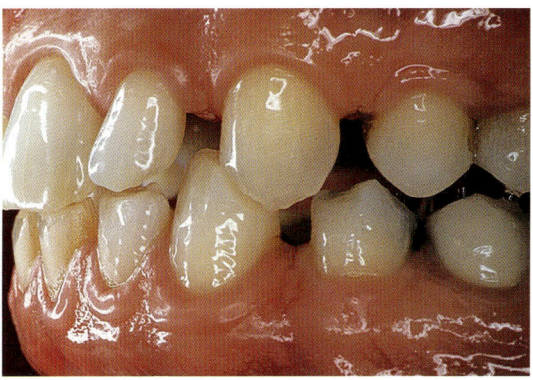

Figure 2.7

Occlusion—left side.

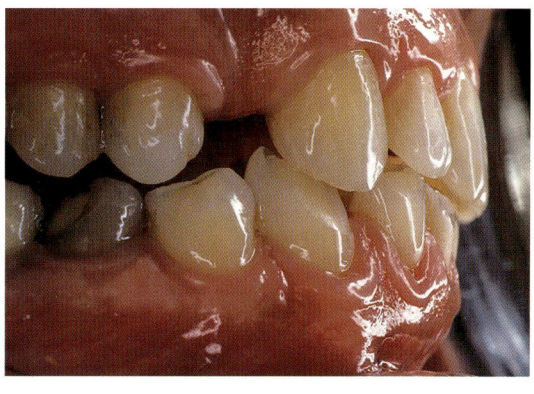

Figure 2.8

Occlusion—right side.

premolar, as well as that between the maxillary right cuspid and first premolar. According to the patient, these spaces always existed and did not bother her
- Mandibular right third molar was missing (Figure 2.10).

Occlusal analysis (Figures 2.7 and 2.8) revealed that the patient was Angle class 1 with a vertical overbite of 6.0 mm and a horizontal overjet of 3.0 mm.

In addition, she has Fremitus class 1 on the maxillary right cuspid, right central incisor, left central incisor, and left cuspid and fremitus class 2 on the maxillary left lateral incisor. The maximum opening was 42.0 mm and the interocclusal rest space was 3.0 mm. There was palatal impingement of the anterior mandibular teeth onto the gingiva of the right maxillary central incisor and both lateral incisor teeth.

Periodontal examination revealed moderate with localized advanced periodontitis with probing depths up to 5–6 mm on the mandibular molars and bleeding on probing on some teeth (Figure 2.9).

Radiographic examination (Figure 2.10) revealed:

- Shortened roots
- Secondary caries

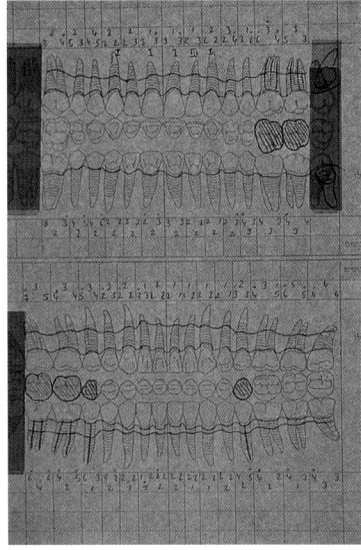

Figure 2.9

Periodontal chart—maxilla and mandible.

- Adequate endodontic therapy with some localized periapical rarefying osteitis (mandibular right first molar)
- Remnants of an old amalgam restoration around the mandibular second premolar and first molar
- Widened periodontal ligament around maxillary right first premolar
- Overhanging margins on mandibular left first premolar and left second molar
- Minimal generalized horizontal bone loss

INDIVIDUAL TOOTH PROGNOSIS

The prognosis for all the remaining teeth was good.

DIAGNOSIS

- Bruxism and severe wear of the anterior teeth
- Possible loss of vertical dimension
- Deep overbite
- Primary occlusal trauma
- Moderate with localized advanced adult periodontitis

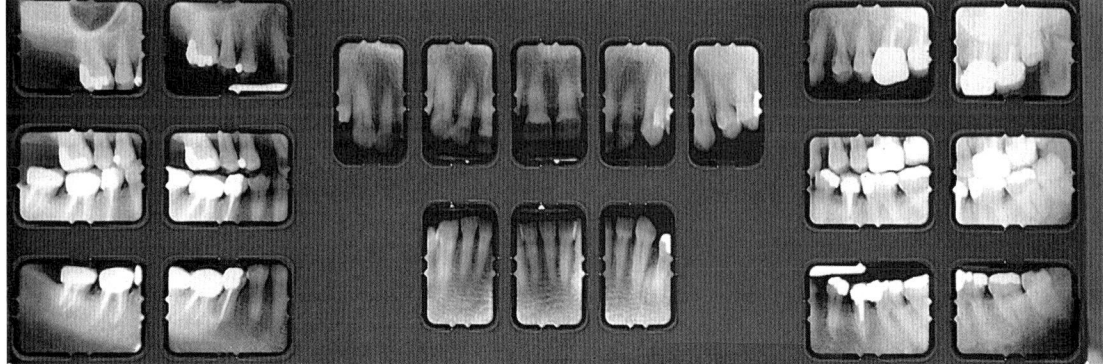

Figure 2.10

Radiographs of maxilla and mandible—pre-treatment.

- Secondary caries
- Chronic periapical area
- Faulty restoration (secondary caries)
- Spaced dentition
- High blood pressure
- Hormonal imbalance

ABOUT THE PATIENT

The patient was punctual for her appointments, cooperated in her treatment, and understood the reasons for her treatment even though she had no subjective complaints.

POTENTIAL DIFFICULTIES INVOLVED IN THE TREATMENT

The traumatic deep overbite, coupled with the great amount of tooth structure lost, jeopardized the maxillary anterior teeth, thus requiring a quick solution. Another difficulty would be the adaptation of the patient to the required changes in her daytime habit patterns (avoiding bruxism) which, at the age of 57, is not easy. Any possible restoration would require change in the vertical dimension of occlusion in order to restore the anterior teeth and adaptation of the patient to this procedure could not be forecast. Another possible problem with multiple restorations might be the unfavorable change in the crown-to-root ratio and the possibility that tooth eruption would not succeed. After discussion with the patient, it was concluded that the patient was not a 'night grinder' but rather, bruxed her teeth during the day while working in the laboratory and peering through a microscope, concentrating on her work.

TREATMENT PLAN

PHASE 1

- Scaling, root planing and oral hygiene instruction
- Conservative dentistry to replace faulty restoration and restore carious teeth
- Explanation of the bruxing problem to the patient and making her aware of the harm that it causes in order to convince her that she should stop bruxing of her own volition
- Changing the vertical dimension of occlusion by the use of a canine platform to allow eruption of the posterior teeth

PHASE 2

Conservative dentistry to restore the teeth in the new vertical dimension, after passive eruption.

PHASE 3

If passive eruption did not take place, restoration of the teeth with fixed prosthodontics to the new vertical dimension.

TREATMENT

PHASE 1

The treatment included scaling, root planing, oral hygiene instruction, and restoration of teeth with faulty restorations and caries. The daytime bruxing problem and the resultant harm that it causes was stressed in discussions with

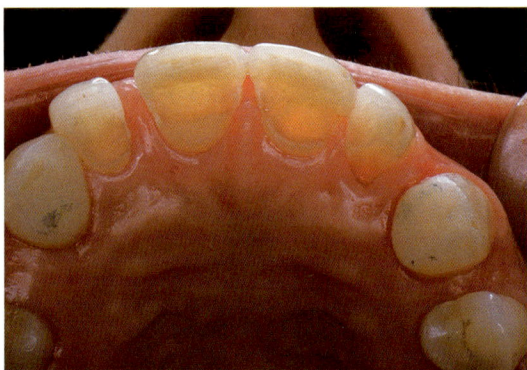

Figure 2.11

Anterior maxillary teeth—palatal view, showing canine platform.

the patient. The patient on her own volition, by concentrating on not bruxing during her working hours, was able to cease bruxing. A new vertical dimension of occlusion was established by the use of a canine platform to enable passive eruption of the posterior teeth (Figure 2.11). The canine platform increased the vertical dimension by about 3.0 mm, as measured at the maxillary and mandibular central incisors, and 1.0 mm in the molar areas.

PHASE 2

After one month when the patient appeared to have adapted to this new vertical dimension of occlusion without any problems, the maxillary central and lateral incisor teeth were bonded with composite resin to contact the mandibular incisor teeth (Figures 2.12 and 2.13).

After three more months, when the posterior teeth failed to erupt into occlusion, it was thought that the tongue occupied the opened existing space and prevented the eruption of the posterior teeth (Figures 2.14 and 2.15). At that time, the lingual surfaces of the mandibular premolar and molar teeth were built up by bonding composite resin material to create an overbite between the mandibular lingual cusps and the maxillary lingual cusps, in order to prevent the tongue from entering the space between the teeth, and interfering with the passive eruption process (Figures 2.16 and 2.17).

One month later, the posterior maxillary and mandibular teeth erupted into occlusal contact and the lingual additions to the mandibular teeth were removed and the surfaces polished (Figures 2.18 and 2.19).

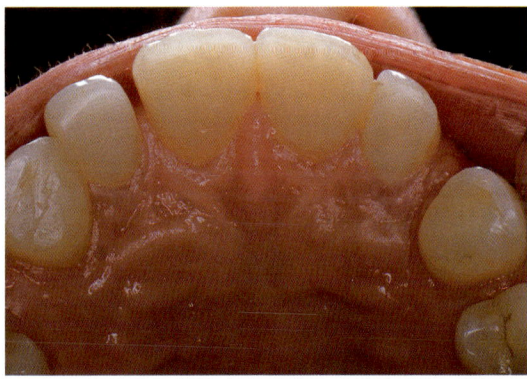

Figure 2.12

Anterior maxillary teeth—palatal view, showing composite buildup.

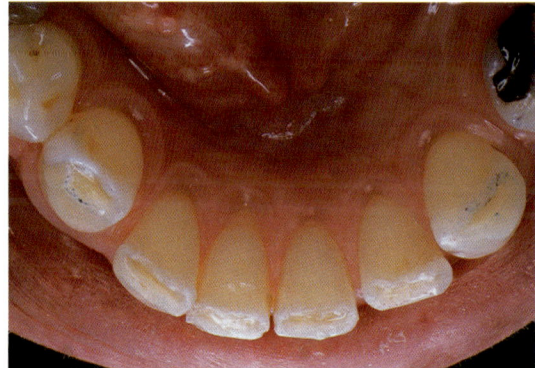

Figure 2.13

Anterior mandibular teeth—lingual view, showing composite buildup.

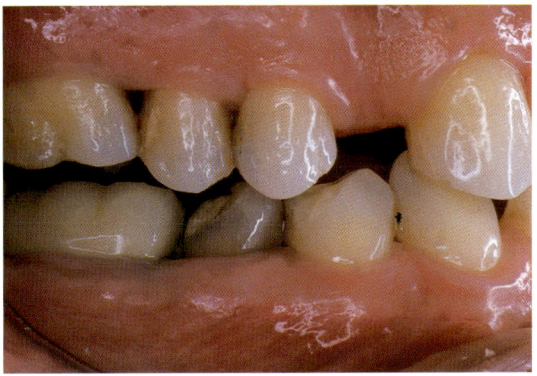

Figure 2.14

Right side, showing failure of teeth to passively erupt.

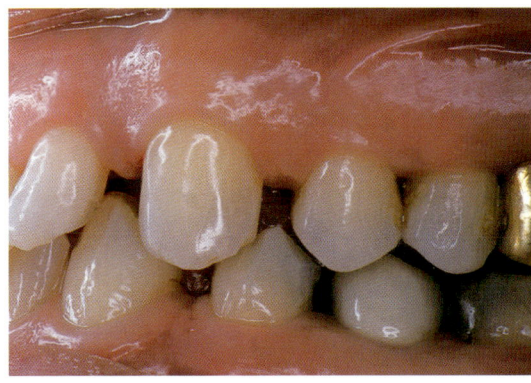

Figure 2.15

Left side, showing failure of teeth to passively erupt.

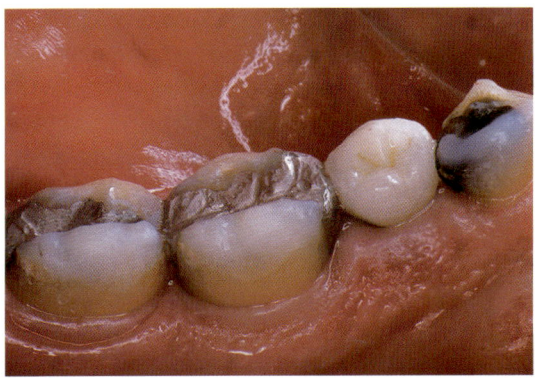

Figure 2.16

Mandibular left posterior segment, showing lingual cusp composite buildup.

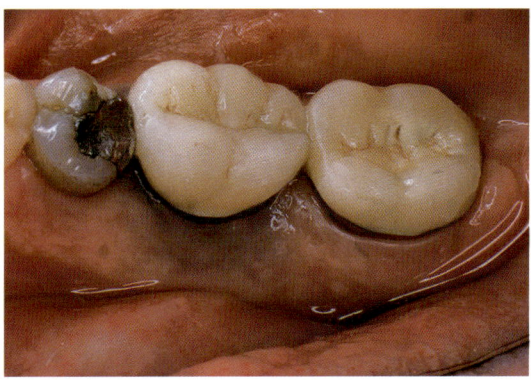

Figure 2.17

Mandibular right posterior segment, showing lingual cusp composite buildup.

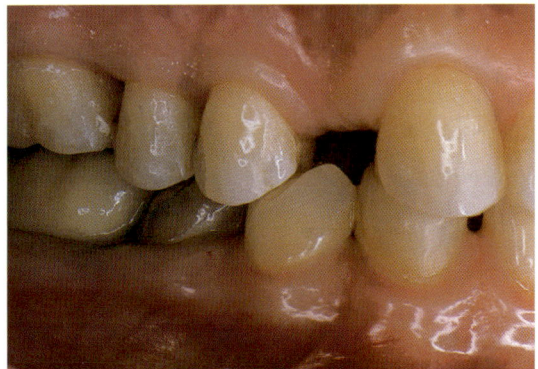

Figure 2.18

Right side, showing teeth passively erupted to contact.

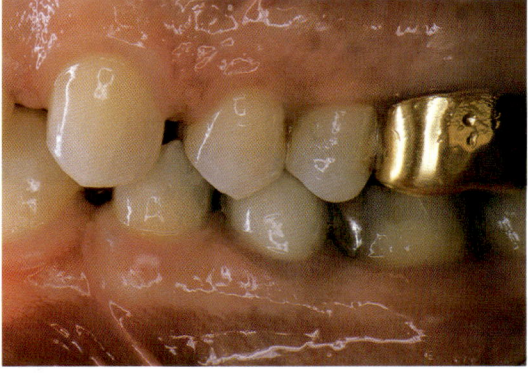

Figure 2.19

Left side, showing teeth passively erupted to contact.

A hard night guard to be worn only at night was made for the patient as a protective device to prevent continuing tooth structure loss. This was done to prevent wear of the composite material that had been placed on the anterior teeth.

The patient has been followed for one and a half years and there has been no abnormal lose of tooth structure in this time.

PHASE 3

This was not required.

SUMMARY

The patient, a 57-year-old female laboratory technician, presented with a severe problem of abnormal tooth wear due to bruxism. After scaling, curettage and oral hygiene instruction, and restoration of teeth with faulty restorations and caries, a conservative method of treatment was attempted that involved the use of a canine platform to increase the vertical dimension of occlusion. The anterior teeth were then restored to occlusal contact with bonding and composite resin restorations.

When the posterior teeth failed to erupt passively into occlusion as anticipated, due to tongue interference, an attempt to eliminate this interference by building up the lingual cusps of the mandibular posterior teeth (through bonding and composite resin) was made. This succeeded, and within 3 months the posterior teeth were in contact. The patient has maintained this new vertical dimension of occlusion for over 18 months.

CASE DISCUSSION
AVINOAM YAFFE

A 57-year-old woman presented herself to the graduate program with traumatic deep overbite accompanied by severe wear with loss of tooth structure aggravated by impingement and laceration of the interdental papillae in the anterior maxilla. At that stage no restoration could be done due to the deep overbite. An increase in vertical dimension was mandatory in order to solve the problem. The change in vertical dimension could be accomplished by complete mouth restoration of at least two quadrants, either in the maxilla or mandible.

A conservative approach was taken to solve the problem. Instead of increasing the vertical dimension by the use of restorations, thus increasing the crown-to-root ratio, a platform was added to the maxillary cuspid teeth using composite resin material. This created a space between the maxillary and mandibular teeth, enabling these teeth to erupt towards each other until contact was established. At that new vertical dimension, composite resin was added to the severely worn anterior teeth, thus restoring the teeth with minimal expense, and keeping the crown-to-root ratio the same as that before the increase in vertical dimension. Thus a complicated situation was solved by a simple, cost-effective and esthetic restoration.

CASE DISCUSSION
HAROLD PREISKEL

This patient's treatment represents an example of sensible planning. Instead of leading with the air turbine, a mistake that is so easily made in these circumstances, the operators chose to make occlusal stops on the canines to allow the molar teeth to erupt. Once this had been achieved, it was a relatively straightforward process to rebuild the dentition. It is interesting to note that the original problem worried the patient's dentist more than the patient herself, yet the team were able to motivate their patient to undergo a time-consuming, if not invasive, course of treatment. Equally important in this case is the maintenance therapy.

PATIENT 3 EXTENSIVE TOOTH WEAR

Treatment by Yehuda Shahal

THE PATIENT

A 43-year-old retired army officer presented himself for examination and consultation with the following complaints:

'I have small and worn teeth and they are ugly' (Figure 3.1).
'If I don't have them treated now, I am afraid that I will lose my teeth.'

During his military service, he served as a tank mechanic and at the time of his treatment had his own garage.

PAST MEDICAL HISTORY

His medical history was negative with no unusual findings.

PAST DENTAL HISTORY

His dental history was uneventful. He only went to the dentist when he had pain.

EXTRA-ORAL EXAMINATION
(Figures 3.2 and 3.3)

- Normal facial symmetry
- Slightly square facial outline
- Straight profile with competent lips
- Lower third of the face was slightly smaller than the other two thirds
- Accentuated labio-mental fold
- Maximum opening was 46 mm
- No deviation in either opening or closing movements
- No muscle sensitivity was noted
- Jaw movements were normal

INTRA-ORAL AND FULL-MOUTH PERIAPICAL EXAMINATION

Maxilla (Figures 3.4 and 3.5):

- Wide, symmetrical, and oval shape jaw, with a class 1 hard palate
- Shallow vestibulum
- Missing teeth:

$$\frac{8\,5 \mid 8}{}$$

- Soft tissue was normal

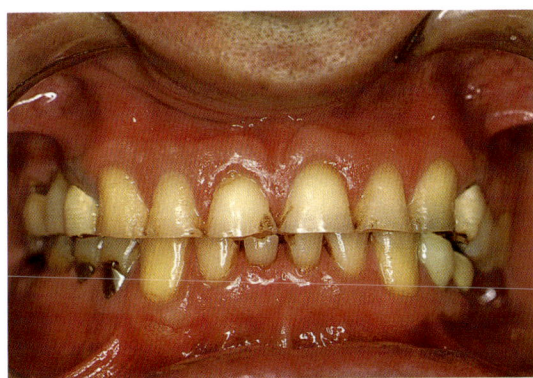

Figure 3.1

Front view of anterior teeth.

23

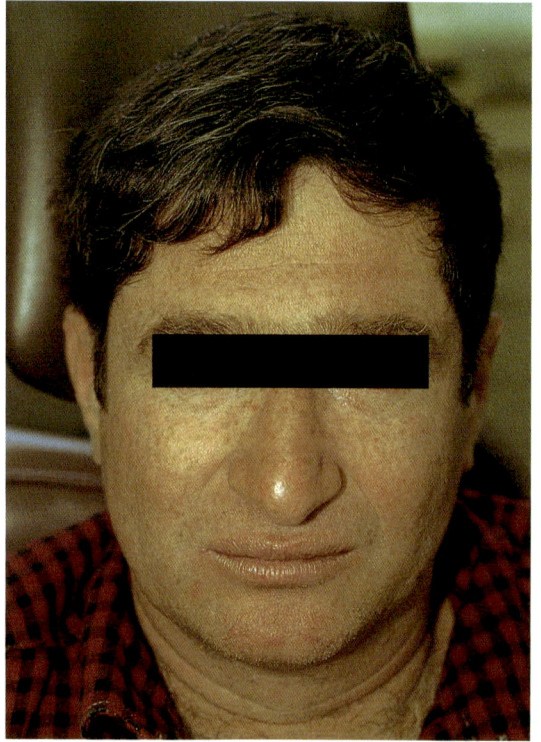

Figure 3.2

Frontal facial view.

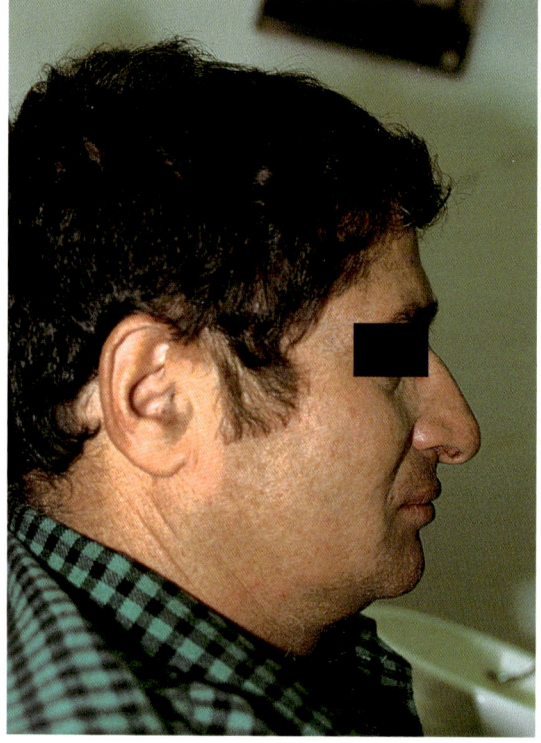

Figure 3.3

Side face view.

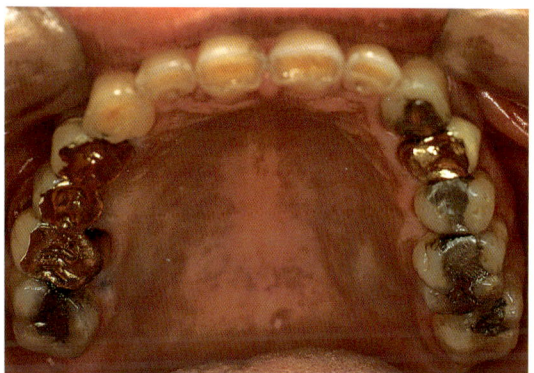

Figure 3.4

Maxillary arch.

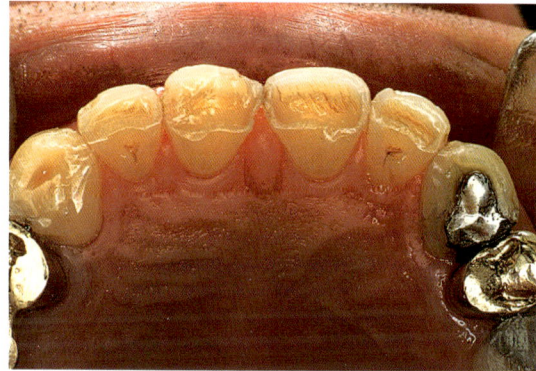

Figure 3.5

Lingual view of maxillary anterior teeth.

- Caries:

$$\frac{7\ \big|\ 3}{}$$

- Extrusion of the right second molar

- Veneer crowns and amalgam restorations on some of the teeth
- Large amounts of wear on the anterior teeth accompanied by chipping of

the enamel and cupping of the dentine

• Wear facets on the left maxillary premolars were noted, but not on the left maxillary molars

• Absence of wear facets on the left maxillary second molar tooth

• There were wear facets on the surfaces of the guiding cusps of the fixed maxillary prosthesis on the right side and the veneer crown on the left first premolar tooth (Figures 3.4 and 3.6):

$$\frac{6\text{-}X\text{-}4 \mid 4}{}$$

• The first left maxillary premolar had a 10-year-old veneer crown with inflamed soft tissue around it.

Mandible (Figure 3.7):

• Missing teeth:

$$\frac{ \mid }{8 \mid 6\ 7\ 8}$$

• Ovoid jaw shape

• High floor of the mouth with wide and broad muscle attachments

• Shallow vestibulum

• Edentulous areas of the jaw showed resorption in the both the vertical and bucco-lingual dimensions

• Right first molar had a broken amalgam restoration with overhang

• Right second premolar had a faulty disto-occlusal amalgam restoration with marginal overhang and wear facets

• Veneer crowns on the left premolar teeth with slight inflammation around the crowns

• Left premolars had gingival class V amalgam restorations

• Severe wear patterns on the anterior teeth with open contact points due to the wear (Figure 3.8)

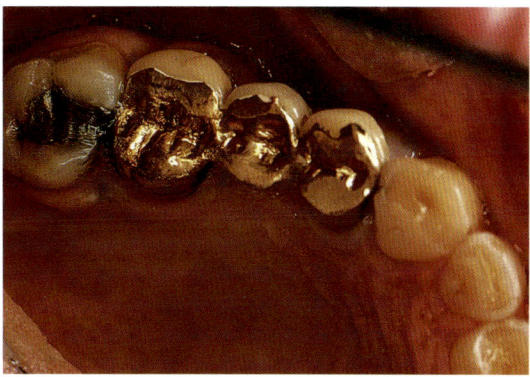

Figure 3.6

Maxillary right posterior quadrant.

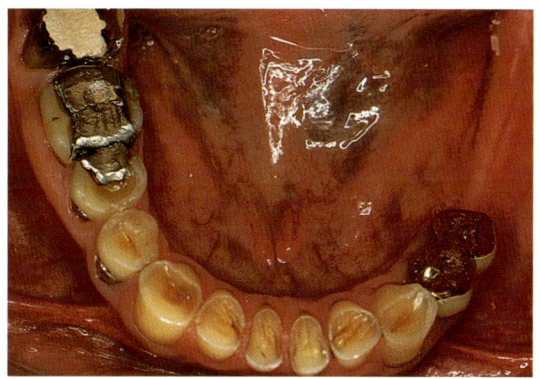

Figure 3.7

Mandibular arch.

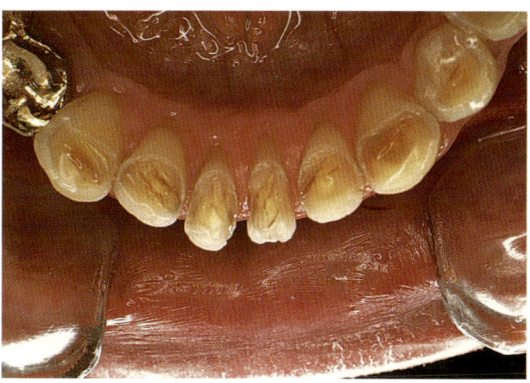

Figure 3.8

Lingual view of mandibular anterior teeth.

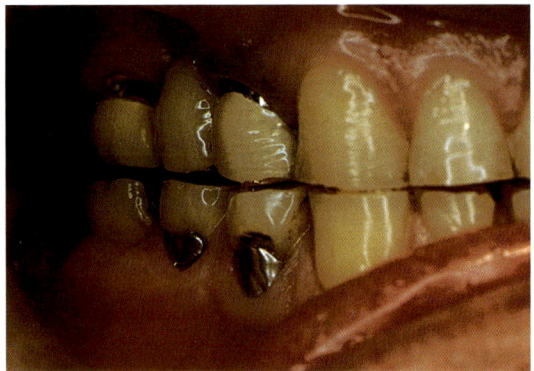

Figure 3.9

Right lateral jaw movement.

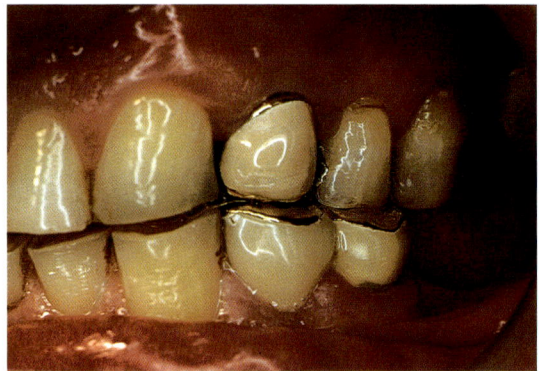

Figure 3.10

Left lateral jaw movement.

An occlusal examination revealed that the patient was Angle class 1 classification, with 0.0 mm overbite and an overjet of 2.0 mm (Figure 3.1). The interocclusal rest space was 4.0 mm and the maximum opening was 46 mm, without deviation in opening or closing movements. The mandibular midline was slightly left of the center of the face.

There was a 1.0 mm discrepancy between centric occlusion (IC) and centric relation (CR). Lateral jaw movements were group function on both sides—this in spite of the amount of wear of the anterior teeth

(Figures 3.9 and 3.10). There were no balancing side contacts. In protrusive movements, there was disarticulation by the anterior teeth and the premolars on the right side, and on the left side the posterior teeth were in contact. There was no fremitus or mobility of any of the teeth. The patient had a removable partial mandibular denture, which he felt was unsatisfactory and did not use.

The periodontal examination (Figures 3.11 and 3.12) revealed probing depths of up to 3.0 mm on the maxillary teeth and up to

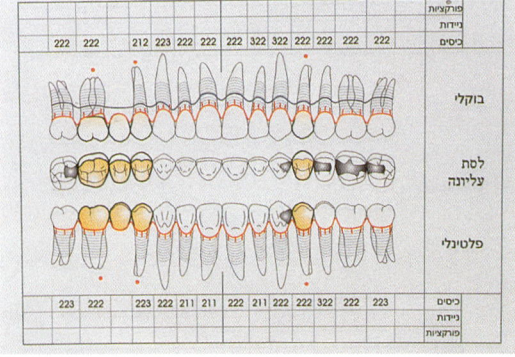

Figure 3.11

Maxillary periodontal chart.

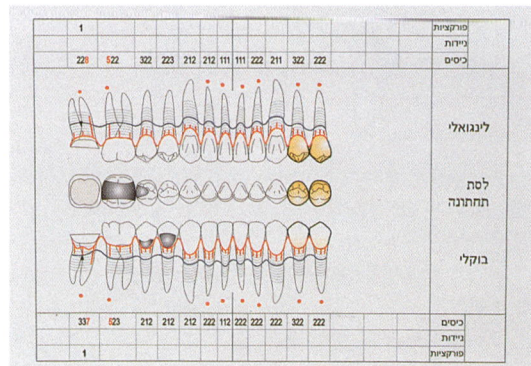

Figure 3.12

Mandibular periodontal chart.

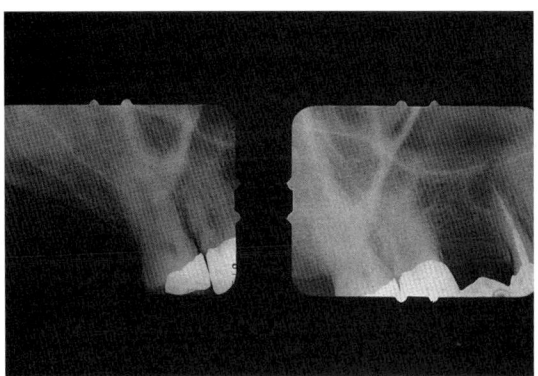

Figure 3.13

Radiographs of right maxillary posterior quadrant.

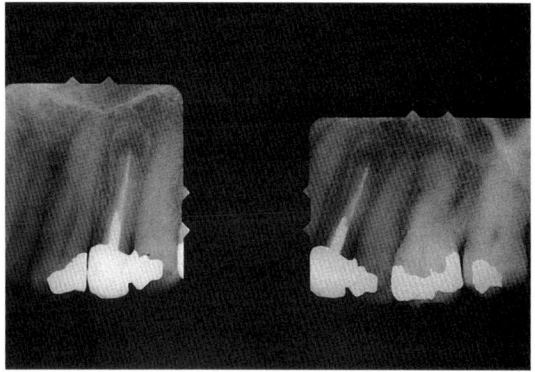

Figure 3.14

Radiographs of left maxillary posterior quadrant.

3.0 mm on most of the mandibular teeth, with slight bleeding on probing (BOP) on some of the teeth with restorations. There was inflammation around the fixed bridge in the right posterior maxilla. The right mandibular molars had probing depths of 5.0–8.0 mm, and furcation involvement class I was found on the right second molar, both in the buccal as well as the lingual furcas. There was a boney defect on the mesial surface of the right second molar.

RADIOGRAPH EXAMINATION
(Figures 3.13 and 3.14)

The right first maxillary premolar had narrow roots, an old root canal restoration, a dentatus type post, and an asymptomatic periapical lesion. The left maxillary first premolar had narrow roots, an old root canal filling, a dentatus type post, and an asymptomatic periapical lesion. There was extended root trunk in the left maxillary first and second molars. The right mandibular second molar had a temporary restoration following root canal therapy.

INDIVIDUAL TOOTH PROGNOSIS

- Hopeless: none
- Poor:

$$\frac{4 \mid 4}{7 \mid}$$

- Fair:

$$\frac{\mid}{6 \mid}$$

- Good: the remaining teeth

Note: The first maxillary premolar teeth had existing root canals with periapical lesions that, although asymptomatic, would require removal of the posts and renewal of the root canal therapy should new restorations be required. The roots were also very thin, making the removal of the existing posts very difficult without fracturing the teeth. Therefore these teeth were considered to have a poor prognosis. The second right mandibular molar tooth had an infraboney pocket on the mesial and also a furcation involvement and a very broken down coronal portion, leaving a very doubtful prognosis for the long term for this tooth.

DIAGNOSIS

- Gingivitis with localized periodontitis
- Excessive tooth wear
- Missing teeth
- Faulty restorations
- Poor esthetics
- Decreased vertical dimension
- Periapical lesions

PATIENT DISPOSITION AND EXPECTATION

The patient was introverted, hardly ever speaking or smiling, but with a strong motivation for dental treatment. In spite of the distances involved for him to get to the clinic, he was prepared to come at any time for treatment. He wanted to save as many teeth as possible and to improve the esthetic appearance of his mouth. He also preferred to have a fixed rather than a removable restoration.

POTENTIAL TREATMENT PROBLEMS

- The patient was a relatively young man with extensive tooth wear
- The many existing restorations were very large and faulty
- Some of the teeth had old endodontic treatments with periapical lesions
- Many of the teeth had calcification of the pulp chambers and some of the canals
- The patient expressed his desire not to have a removable mandibular partial denture

DISCUSSION OF THE CAUSES OF WEAR IN THIS PATIENT

Considering that this patient exhibited extreme wear in some of his teeth, it was felt that before proceeding with treatment, it would be wise to discern the cause of the extreme wear. The dental literature refers to the causative agents in extreme wear as that of multiple factors. Mohl describes the causes of dental tooth wear as 'contributing factors' rather than 'etiologic factors'.[1] The factors generally mentioned in the literature are: parafunction, diet, salivary secretions, excessive biting force, and occupational hazards. As for parafunction, the patient informed us that he had never bruxed his teeth, and was aware what bruxism meant. He also lacked any of the other symptoms of bruxism, had a normal maximum jaw opening and free lateral excursions without tenderness in his muscles. In order to examine whether diet was a contributory factor, the patient was asked to record in writing all food and beverages that he consumed during the day for a period of 2 weeks. This revealed that he did not have an abrasive or erosive diet. With regard to salivary function, the patient was examined for three different factors: the rate of excretion, the pH of the saliva, and the buffer capacity of the saliva. The results showed that there were no contributing factors in his saliva to cause the extreme wear that was evidenced on his anterior teeth.

All these findings led to the conclusion that the wear of the patient's teeth was probably a result of the fact that he was a tank driver and mechanic for 20 years in an army field unit that involved testing and driving tanks many hours a day in a dusty environment. This was in the era when tanks were not air-conditioned and the mixture of dust and vibration encountered during his many hours in the open tank thus caused the excessive wear of his front teeth. The contributing facts for this theory were that in

[1] Mohl ND, Zarb GA, Carlsson GE, Rugh JD, *Textbook of Occlusion* (Quintessence: London, 1988).

the posterior maxillary teeth, there was no wear of the teeth. This was due to the fact that the opposing mandibular posterior teeth were extracted early in his army career and therefore could not cause wear of the opposing maxillary teeth. These teeth showed no signs of wear, even though they were present for 26 years prior to the period when he worked as a mechanic on tanks. Further proof of this theory could be found in the fact that the greatest amount of wear was found mostly in the anterior teeth. This was due to the fact that the amplitude of jaw movements during vibrations of the body encountered while driving the tank is greater in the anterior region than in the posterior region. Therefore, it was felt that as the patient had retired from the army, and was not involved in testing and repairing heavy tanks any more, the wear would not be a factor. This was also proven by the fact that during the transitional phase of treatment, the restorations did not undergo any wear.

TREATMENT ALTERNATIVES

Maxilla:

- Fixed anterior partial prosthesis

Mandible:

- Fixed partial prosthesis with a shortened arch form
- Fixed partial prosthesis with implant support
- Fixed partial prosthesis with cantilever
- Fixed and removable partial prostheses

TREATMENT

Initial preparation included scaling, curettage, root planing, and oral hygiene instruction. At the end of this stage, an obvious improvement in the periodontal supporting tissue could be seen and at the periodontal recharting it was observed that the pocket depths had diminished greatly and that the bleeding on probing had disappeared.

Existing restorations that contributed to the periodontal problems were removed early in treatment. The crown on the maxillary left first premolar was removed, and since there was a periapical lesion on the tooth, the root canal therapy was redone after removal of the two dentatus type posts (Figures 3.15 and 3.16). The tooth was followed up for 1 year, during which the periapical lesion remained the

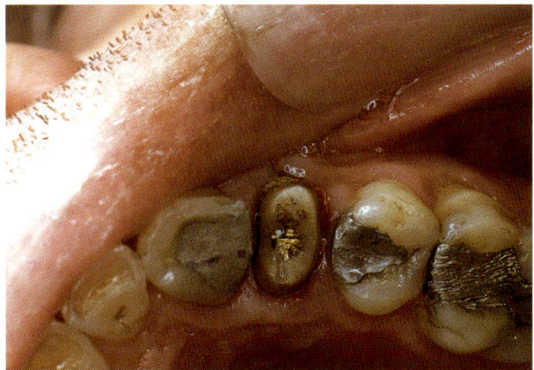

Figure 3.15

Clinical view of left maxillary first premolar, pre-treatment.

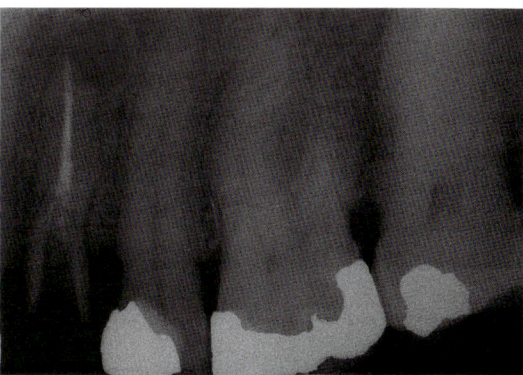

Figure 3.16

Radiograph of post-treatment left maxillary first premolar.

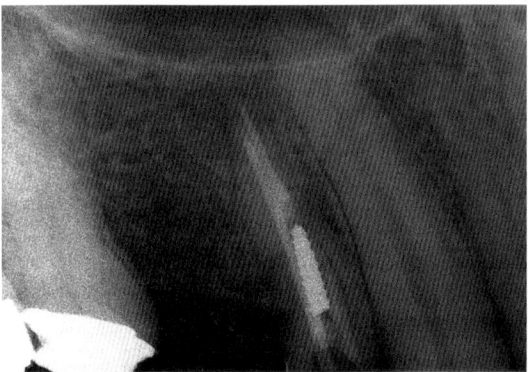

Figure 3.17

Radiograph of right maxillary first premolar, pre-treatment.

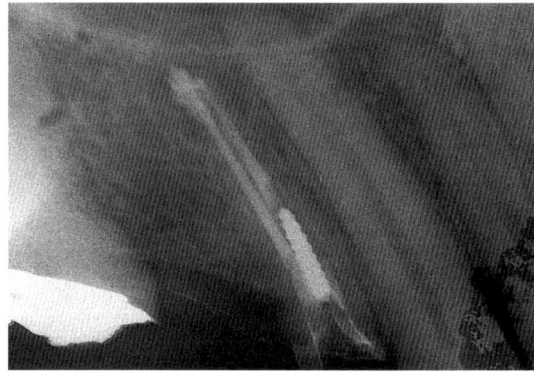

Figure 3.18

Radiograph of right maxillary first premolar, post-treatment.

same size and there was no evidence of healing, and since the walls of the roots of the tooth were very thin, it was decided to extract the tooth. The root canal filling was redone on the maxillary right first premolar and the tooth was followed up for 1 year (Figures 3.17 and 3.18). Caries was excavated on the mandibular left premolars and, due to the extensive caries into the pulp chamber, these teeth were also treated endodontically (Figure 3.19). The mandibular right second premolar and first molar were also treated endodontically due to the extensive caries extending into the pulp chamber (Figures 3.20 and 3.21). These teeth then received transitional restorations. Upon excavation, the mandibular right second molar was found to have a cracked mesial root and the root was removed.

In order to satisfy the patient's desire for improved esthetics, the vertical dimension of occlusion was increased and esthetic transitional restorations were done on the anterior maxillary and mandibular teeth (Figures 3.22 and 3.23). Due to the short clinical crown in the mandibular incisor teeth, and the mandibular left first premolar, crown lengthening procedures were done on those teeth.

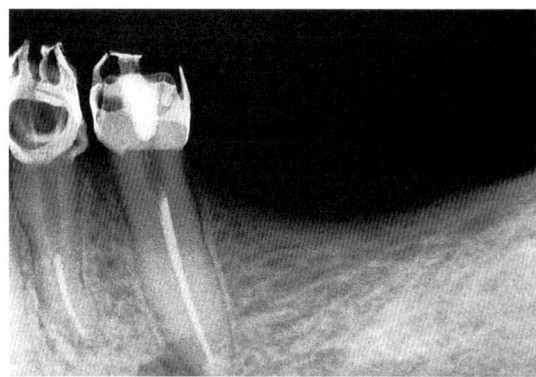

Figure 3.19

Radiograph post-treatment of left mandibular premolars.

The orthodontic phase of treatment was started using a coil spring to separate the right mandibular first molar in order to eliminate root proximity and ensure maximum embrasure space for periodontal maintenance.Upon completion of the orthodontic treatment, followed by periodontal re-evaluation (Figures 3.24 and 3.25), cast posts were placed in the endodontically treated teeth. As the patient had no problems with the increased vertical dimension, and the periodontal tissues reacted favorably to the treatment, and the patient was very satisfied with his new esthetic

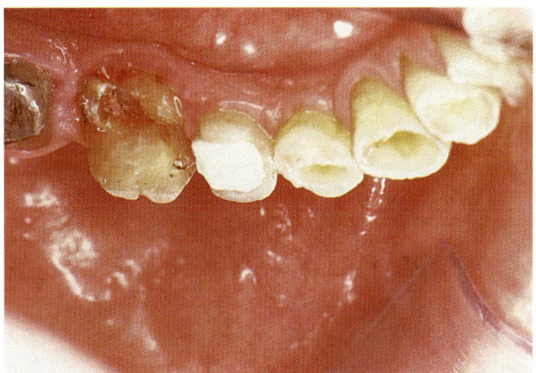

Figure 3.20

Clinical view of right mandibular premolars and molar area, pre-treatment.

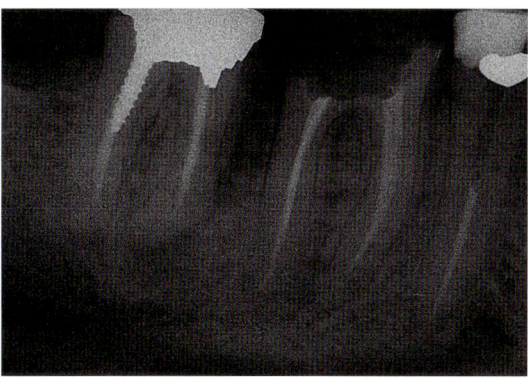

Figure 3.21

Radiograph post-treatment of right mandibular premolar and molar area.

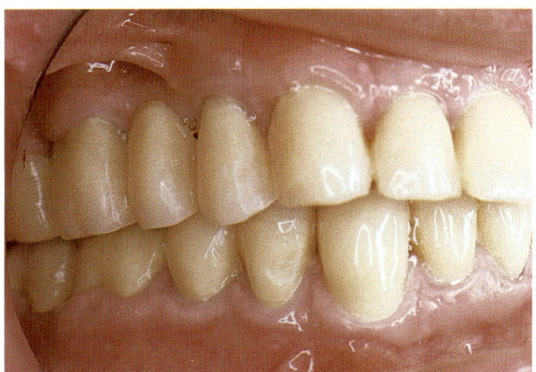

Figure 3.22

Transitional restorations right side.

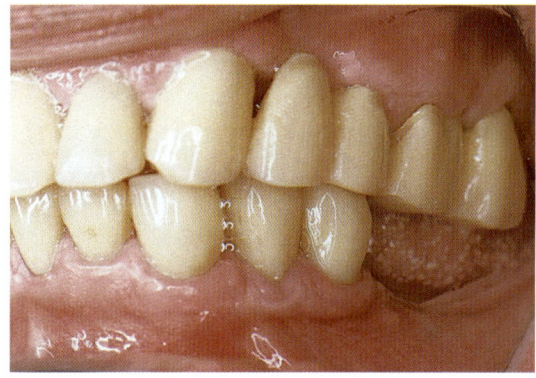

Figure 3.23

Transitional restorations left side.

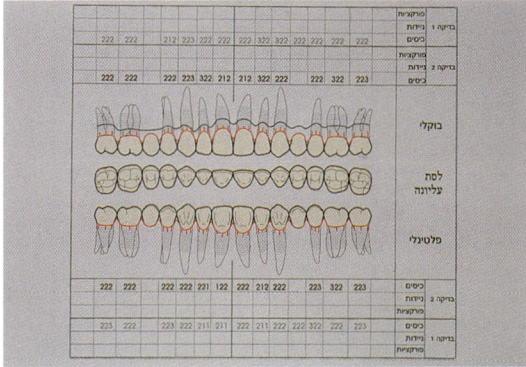

Figure 3.24

Periodontal chart at re-evaluation—maxilla.

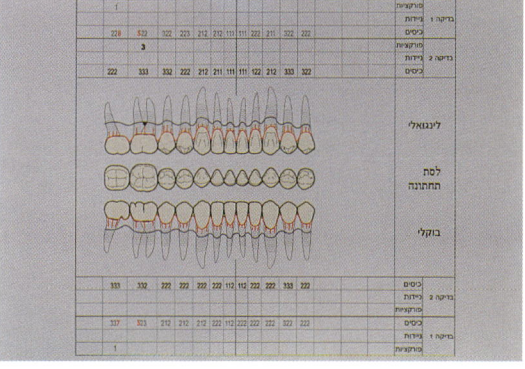

Figure 3.25

Periodontal chart at re-evaluation—mandible.

appearance, the final treatment plan was then carried out.

It was decided to restore the mandible with a premolar occlusion on the left side for the following reasons:

- Since implants could not be done with the amount of remaining bone—to place implants would require additional surgical procedures to add bone
- The lack of posterior teeth in the mandibular left quadrant did not bother the patient
- He very much desired a fixed prosthesis
- The removable partial denture would only replace two teeth, and the patient would most probably not use it
- It would then require splinting the maxillary molars on that side in order to prevent overeruption

Due to the extensive period of time involved in the initial treatment phases and the periodontal surgery and orthodontic treatment, the transitional restorations were then replaced by new prostheses. These were built to the new established vertical dimension dictated by the plane of occlusion and the esthetic demands of the patient as well as the biomechanical considerations (Figures 3.26 and 3.27).

After a period of time it was clear that the patient adapted very well to his new restorations. Copper band impressions were then taken of all the prepared teeth and Duralay resin copings were made. These copings were used to record centric relation at the vertical dimension of the temporary restorations and for the final impression for the master model (Figures 3.28–3.32). The metal copings were then fitted (Figures 3.33 and 3.34) and soldered, and after try-in of the soldered metal framework another elastomeric impression was done for tissue detail. These models were mounted on a semi-adjustable Hanau articulator utilizing a facebow registration and centric records taken at the vertical dimension of occlusion utilizing Duralay with a Neylon technique.

At this point the porcelain was baked and the occlusion checked in the mouth at the biscuit bake stage and all adjustments

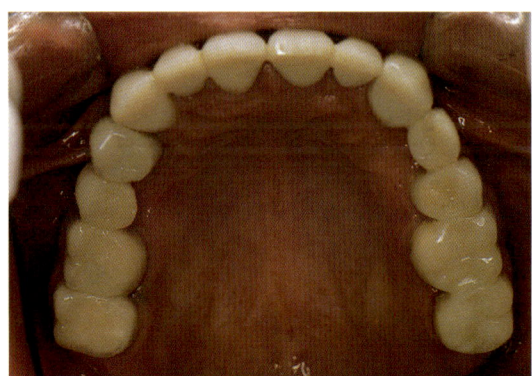

Figure 3.26

New transitional restorations—maxilla.

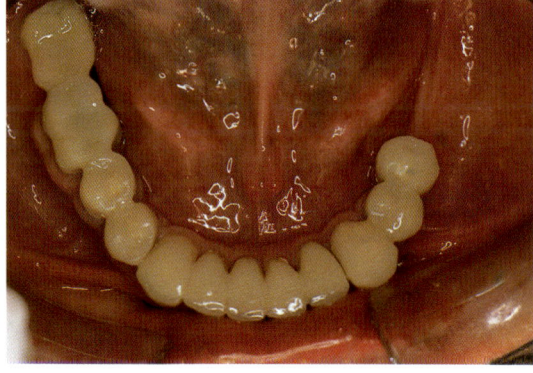

Figure 3.27

New transitional restorations—mandible.

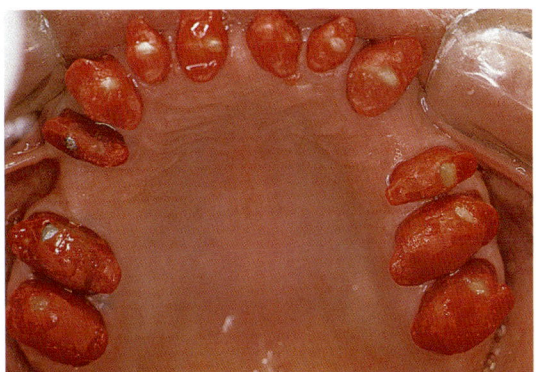

Figure 3.28

Duralay copings fitted—maxilla.

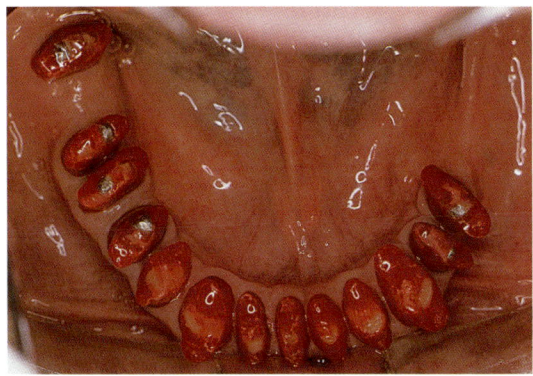

Figure 3.29

Duralay copings fitted—mandible.

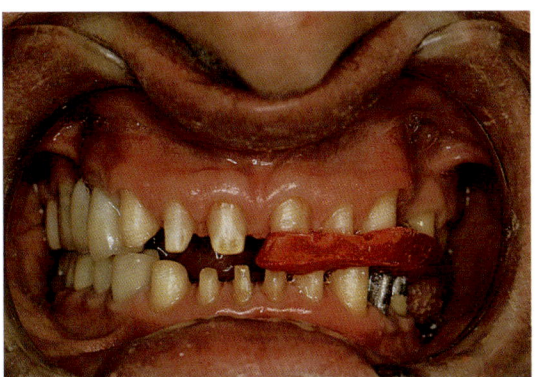

Figure 3.30

Centric relation record—left side.

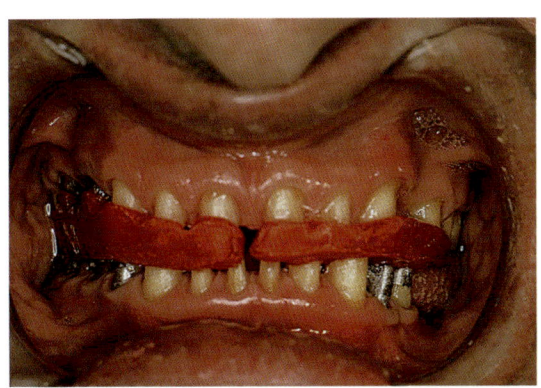

Figure 3.31

Centric relation record—completed.

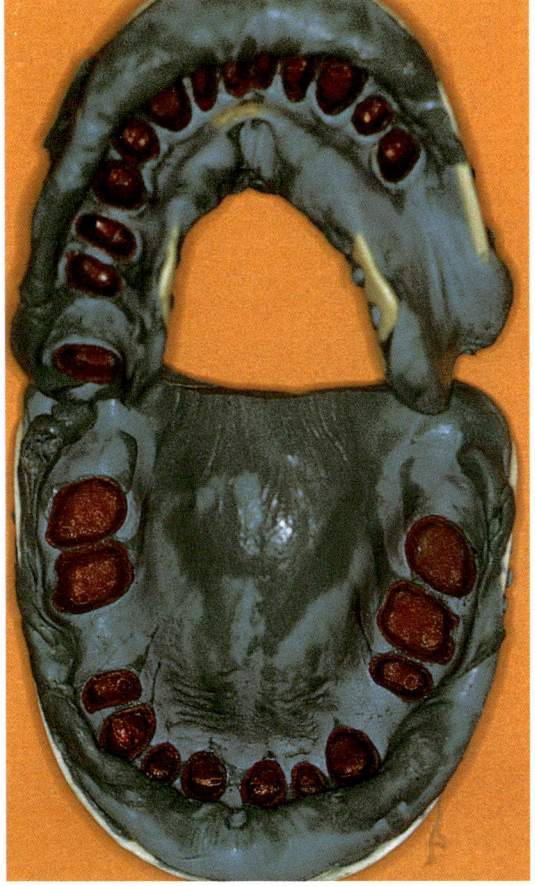

Figure 3.32

Elastomeric pick-up impressions of Duralay copings—maxilla and mandible.

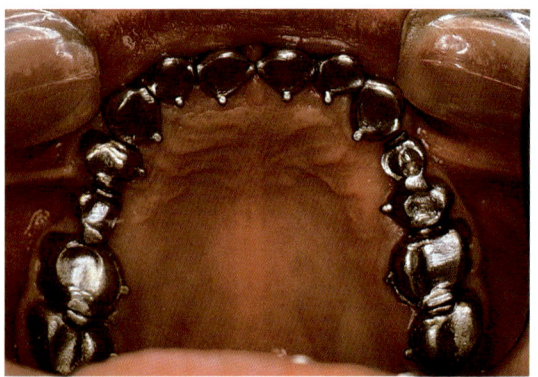

Figure 3.33

Metal copings fitted—maxilla.

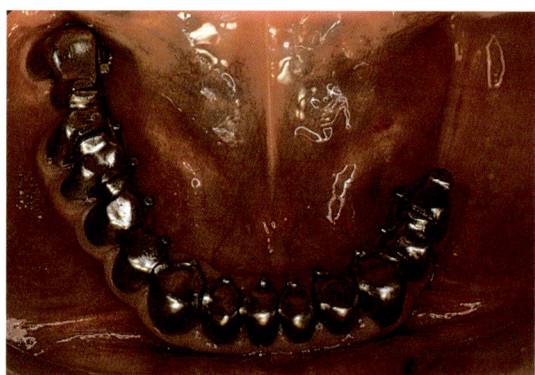

Figure 3.34

Metal copings fitted—mandible.

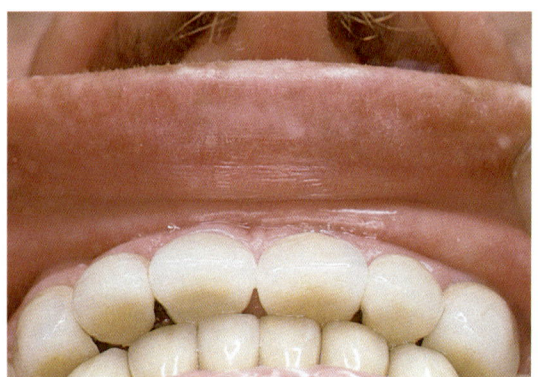

Figure 3.35

Incisal platform incorporated into anterior maxillary teeth.

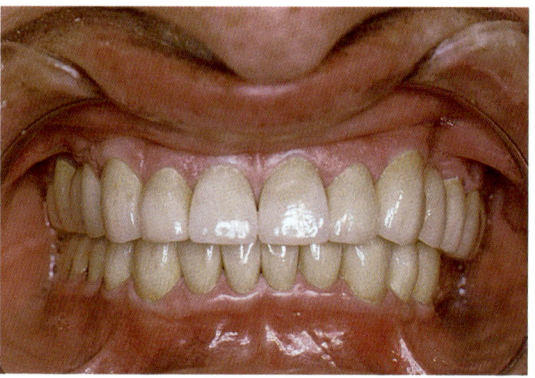

Figure 3.36

Case cemented, post-treatment.

needed were then made. The anterior maxillary teeth incorporated an incisal platform (Figure 3.35) to enable continuous contact during jaw movement and to bring the incisal forces as close as possible to the long axis of the teeth. The crowns and bridges were cemented with Temp-Bond for a period of 1 month. The crowns and bridges were then cemented with zinc oxyphosphate cement for permanent cementation (Figures 3.36–3.38).

The patient has been returning for follow-up and maintenance twice a year for three years and has had no problems.

SUMMARY

The patient presented with a severe problem of extreme wear on many of his teeth and a reduced vertical dimension of occlusion. He also had furcation involvements and periapical lesions. The wear was correctly diagnosed as due to occupational hazards, which were no longer a factor in deciding his treatment. With endodontic, orthodontic and periodontal treatment accompanied by occlusal therapy, the patient received a physiological occlusion at the optimum vertical dimension of occlusion.

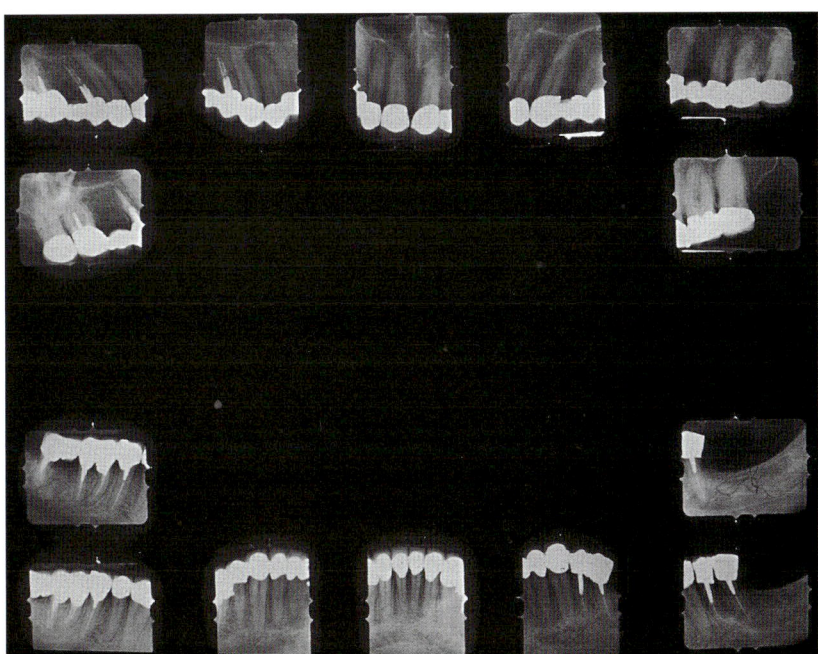

Figure 3.37

Radiographs of case, post-treatment.

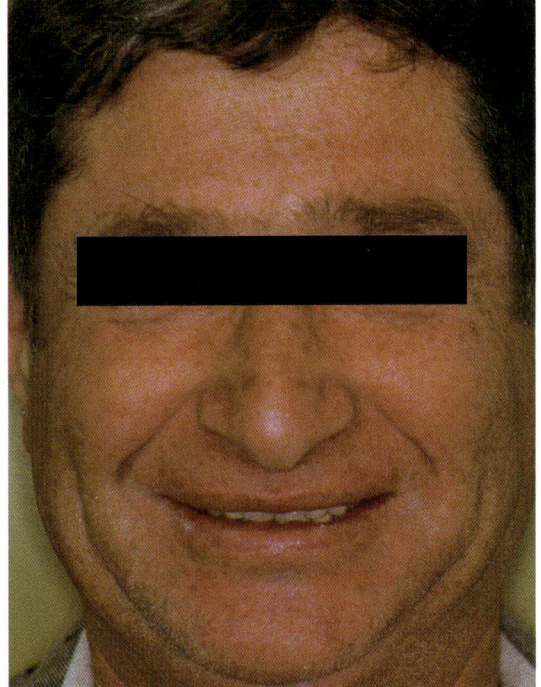

Figure 3.38

Frontal face view of patient, post-treatment.

CASE DISCUSSION
AVINOAM YAFFE

This patient represented a severe case of tooth wear accompanied by reduced vertical dimension and a faulty occlusal plane, further aggravated by missing teeth, caries, and faulty endodontic treatment. The severe wear required periodontal surgery for crown lengthening procedures, thus jeopardizing the crown-to-root ratio. The existence of a free end saddle in the mandible further reduced occlusal support. The case was handled with caution by increasing the vertical dimension and the crown lengthening procedures to the minimum required. In order to make up for the missing posterior support, the anterior teeth were restored and the incisal areas were modified to participate in support in addition to their role in esthetics, speech, and disarticulation of the posterior teeth in jaw movements. The cuspal guiding planes were built to a minimum to reduce lateral forces in order to improve the overall prognosis of the case.

CASE DISCUSSION
HAROLD PREISKEL

While patients who have spent many years driving tanks in dusty environments must be a rare breed, those who are suffering extensive tooth wear are abundant. Indeed, with the increasing life span of our population and the reduced incidence of caries, the treatment of worn down dentitions may be one of the most difficult situations to confront us in the early part of the new century. In this particular instance, the operators have presented tooth substance loss, but this will not apply to many other patients.

The sensibly chosen staged approach produced the occasional surprise that all of us find in a long course of treatment. A split root can be difficult to detect at the outset. While increasing the vertical dimension of occlusion seemed reasonable, it is not clear whether the operators deliberately increased this measurement beyond the level they estimated had existed before the tooth wear occurred. There was little alternative to making a change if a good looking outcome was to be achieved. An excellent result was obtained.

II PERIODONTAL BREAKDOWN

PATIENT 4 NEGLECTED DENTITION

Treatment by Tzachi Lehr

THE PATIENT

A 50-year-old woman, employed as a senior secretary, came to the clinic for dental treatment. Her chief complaints were (Figures 4.1 and 4.2):

'My teeth look awful.'
'My front tooth is loose.'
'My front teeth stick out.'
'Lately, my speech seems to be changing.'
'I know that I have no choice and need lots of work done on my teeth.'

PAST MEDICAL HISTORY

The patient's medical history was unremarkable.

PAST DENTAL HISTORY

The patient had never gone regularly to a dentist. The last visit to a dentist was 10 years ago, and she could not recall what treatment she received then. Recently she found it difficult to chew her food. She had

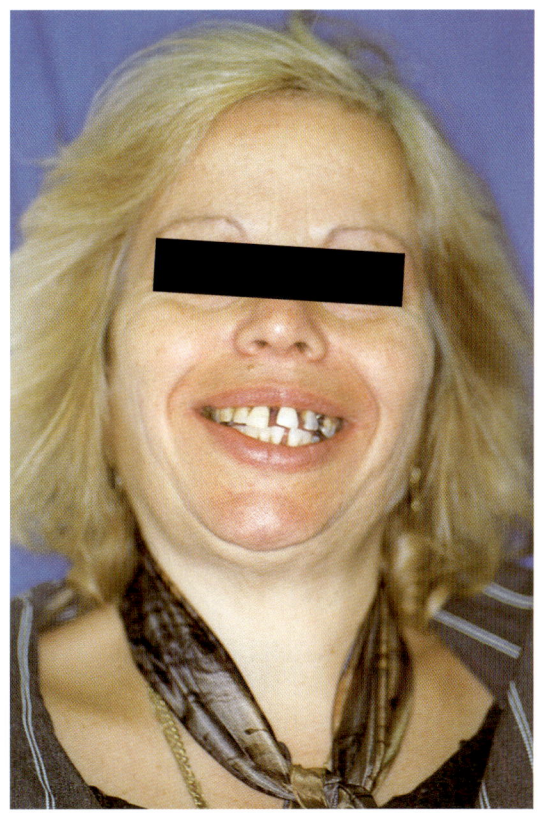

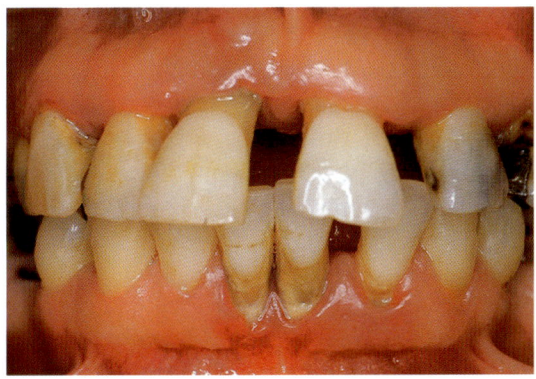

Figure 4.1

Anterior teeth—labial view.

Figure 4.2

Face—frontal view.

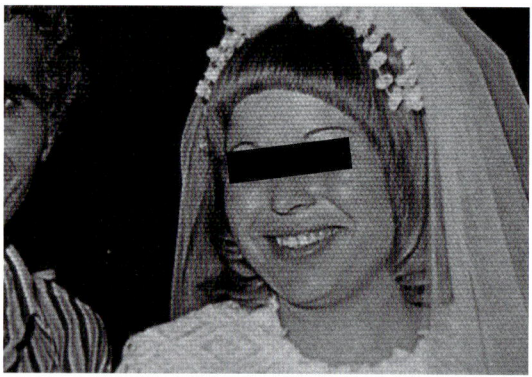

Figure 4.3

Face—frontal view (from 27 years ago).

no habits that she was aware of, but was very conscious of her poor appearance. She compared her current appearance with that of herself almost 30 years ago, showing a large smile and healthy teeth (Figure 4.3).

EXTRA-ORAL EXAMINATION
(Figures 4.2 and 4.4)

- Symmetrical face
- Profile—slight tendency to bi-maxillary protrusion
- Temporomandibular joint was normal
- Normal facial musculature
- Maximum opening of 50 mm
- Mandibular movements were within normal limits
- Trapped lower lip

INTRA-ORAL AND FULL-MOUTH PERIAPICAL RADIOGRAPH EXAMINATION

Maxilla (Figure 4.5):

- Parabolic arch
- Caries

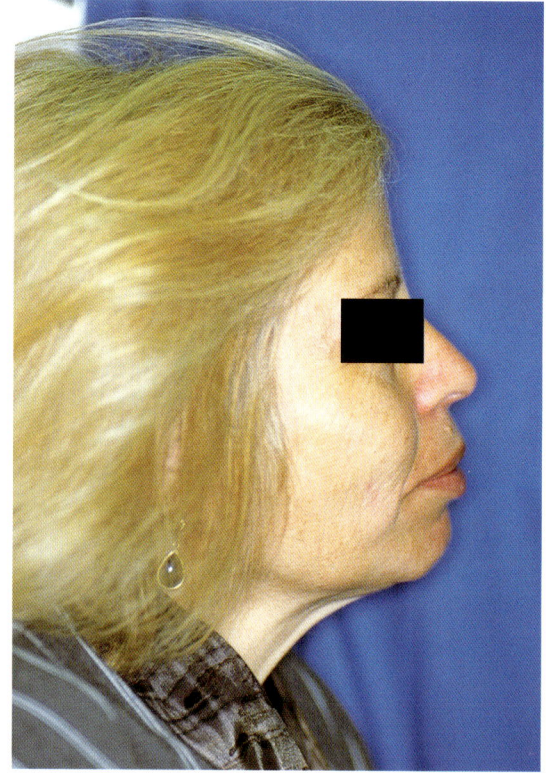

Figure 4.4

Face—side view.

- Spacing between the anterior teeth (see Figure 4.1)
- Missing right and left third molar, and left second molar teeth
- Right and left first molars—residual roots
- Exudate around right central incisor
- Large amalgam restorations on the left and right premolars
- Left cuspid with large caries in the coronal section, extending into the root

Mandible (Figure 4.6):

- Parabolic arch
- Amalgam restorations on the posterior teeth
- Right second premolar—residual root

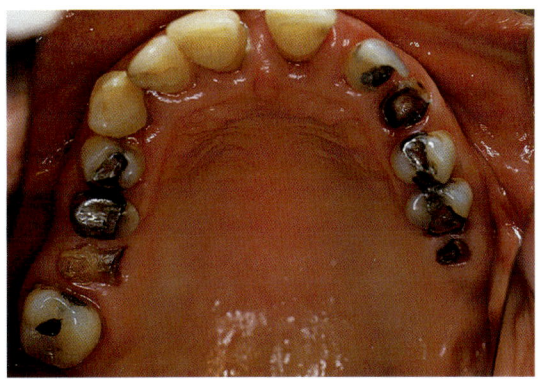

Figure 4.5

Maxillary arch—palatal view.

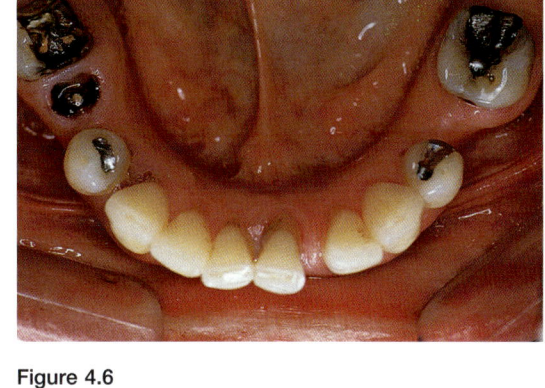

Figure 4.6

Mandibular arch—lingual view.

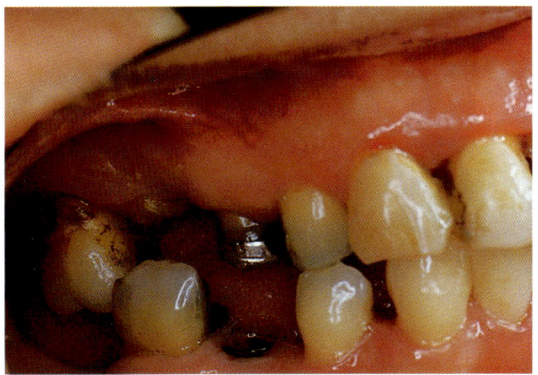

Figure 4.7

Occlusion—right side.

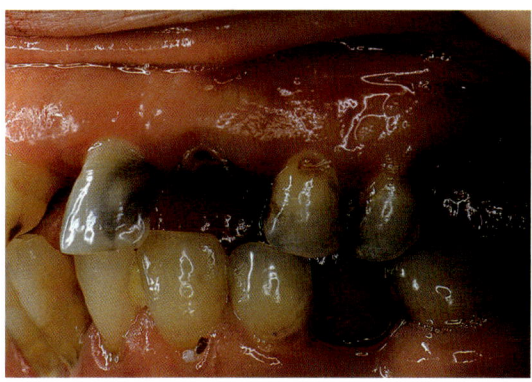

Figure 4.8

Occlusion—left side.

- Missing teeth: right and left second and third molars, and left second premolar
- Exudate around right cuspid
- Caries:

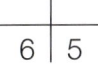

Occlusal examination (Figures 4.7 and 4.8) revealed that the patient was Angle class I. The interocclusal rest space was 4.0 mm. Overjet was 7.0 mm and overbite was 2.0 mm. There was a difference between centric relation and centric occlusion of less than 1.0 mm. There was a midline discrepancy. There was spacing between the maxillary incisor teeth and the left lateral incisor and left cuspid, and drifting of teeth.

Fremitus:

- Maxillary right central incisor—grade III in closing and protrusive movements
- Maxillary right lateral incisor—grade II in closing and protrusive movements
- Maxillary right first premolar—grade I in closing movements
- Maxillary left central and lateral incisors—grade II in protrusive movement

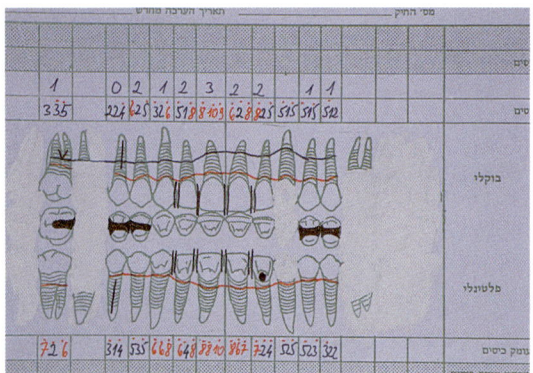

Figure 4.9

Periodontal chart—pre-treatment, maxilla.

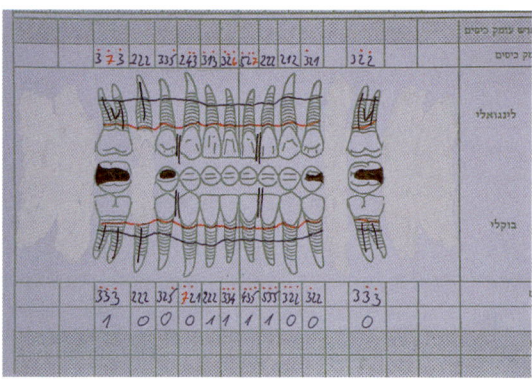

Figure 4.10

Periodontal chart—pre-treatment, mandible.

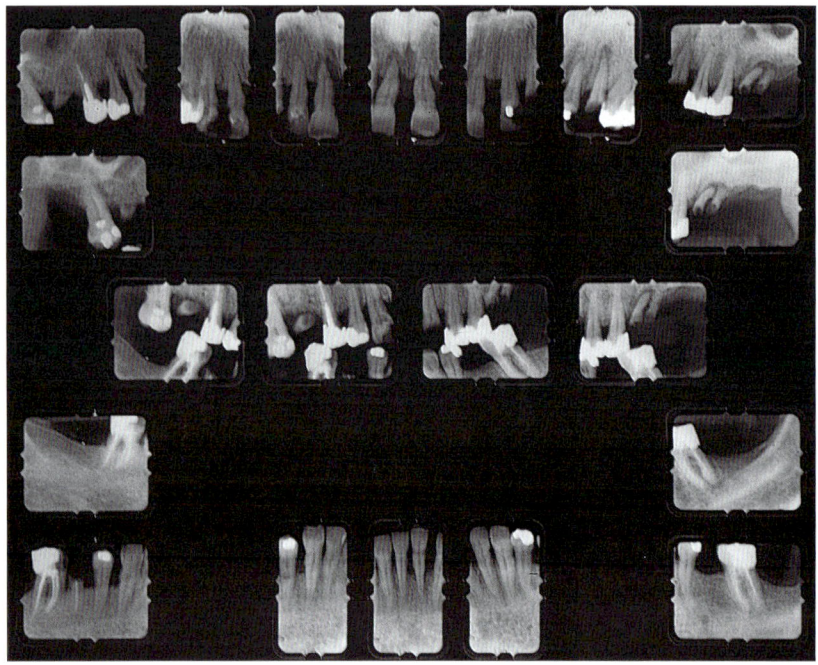

Figure 4.11

Radiographs of maxilla and mandible—pre-treatment.

Periodontal examination (Figures 4.9 and 4.10) revealed calculus and plaque, probing depths of up to 8.0 mm on most of the maxillary teeth and up to 7.0 mm on some of the mandibular teeth. There was bleeding of the gingiva on probing (BOP) on most of the teeth. There was slight gingival recession around some of the teeth. Class 1 and 2 mobility was observed on many of the maxillary teeth and class 3 on the maxillary right central incisor and the maxillary right first premolar. The mandibular molars had class 1 furcation involvement on the buccal and lingual surfaces. The maxillary right second molar had class 1 furcation involvement on the buccal surfaces.

FULL-MOUTH PERIAPICAL SURVEY (Figure 4.11)

- Endodontic treatment:

$$\frac{5\ |\ 5}{6\ 5\ |\ 6}$$

- Perio-endo lesion around the right maxillary central incisor
- Periapical lesions around the left maxillary cuspid and residual roots of the first maxillary molars, and mandibular right second premolar
- Rampant caries and secondary caries
- Extensive horizontal and vertical bone loss around most of the remaining teeth

INDIVIDUAL TOOTH PROGNOSIS

- Hopeless:

$$\frac{6\ 1\ |\ 3\ 6}{5\ |\ }$$

- Questionable:

$$\frac{\ |\ 1}{6\ |\ }$$

- Poor:

$$\frac{7\ 4\ 2\ |\ 4}{1\ |\ 1}$$

- Fair:

$$\frac{5\ 3\ |\ 5}{4\ 3\ 2\ |\ 2\ 3\ 4\ 6}$$

- Good: none

SUMMARY OF FINDINGS

A 50-year-old patient, in good health, came to the clinic complaining of poor esthetics, and mobility of a front tooth. She had poor oral hygiene, plaque and calculus, and severe inflammation accompanied by deep probing depths, reduced alveolar bone support and furcation involvements. Some of the teeth were mobile and had undergone shifting. There was anterior flaring and spacing in the maxilla and mandible, residual roots, and deep caries in many teeth.

DIAGNOSIS

- Advanced adult periodontitis
- Missing teeth accompanied by shifting and drifting of teeth
- Reduced posterior occlusal support
- Reduced vertical dimension
- Secondary occlusal trauma
- Trapped lower lip
- Faulty esthetics
- Faulty restorations
- Rampant caries
- Periapical lesions
- Faulty occlusal plane

ABOUT THE PATIENT

The patient was highly motivated for treatment. She was aware of her condition. She requested a fixed rather than a removable restoration and would be willing to have implants if they were necessary for a fixed prosthesis.

POTENTIAL TREATMENT PROBLEMS

- Many missing teeth
- The distribution of the remaining teeth was unfavorable

- Many of the remaining teeth had severe periodontal problems and their prognosis was guarded
- Treatment would possibly include opening the vertical dimension of occlusion in order to retract the maxillary anterior teeth, which would cause an unfavorable crown-to-root ratio on periodontally involved teeth

TREATMENT PLAN

PHASE 1: INITIAL PREPARATION

- Initial periodontal therapy including:
  oral hygiene instruction
  scaling and root planing
- Extraction of the hopeless teeth except for the maxillary right central incisor
- Endodontic treatment for the maxillary left lateral incisor tooth
- Provisional restoration for the maxillary left lateral incisor tooth
- Caries excavation
- Evaluation of patient cooperation
- Retraction of the mandibular anterior teeth and temporary fixation
- Retraction of the maxillary anterior teeth, extraction of the right central incisor, and fixation by means of a provisional fixed prosthesis

Re-evaluation of the first phase of the treatment plan.

PHASE 2: TREATMENT OPTIONS

Maxilla:

- Fixed prosthesis, with premolar occlusion in maxilla on left side
- Fixed prosthesis supported by teeth and implants

- Fixed and partial removable prostheses
- Overdenture

Mandible:

- Fixed prosthesis supported by natural teeth
- Fixed and partial removable prostheses
- Fixed prosthesis supported by natural teeth and implants

TREATMENT

Initial treatment consisted of oral hygiene instruction, scaling and root planing. The maxillary left lateral incisor was reprepared, the caries excavated, and a provisional crown made. Provisional crown restorations were made on the mandibular right first molar and left first molar. Due to the patient's improved oral hygiene and cooperation there was a dramatic improvement in her periodontal condition (Figure 4.12).

These teeth as well as the mandibular right first and mandibular left first premolars were utilized as anchorage for orthodontic retraction of the mandibular anterior teeth by means of elastics (Figures 4.13 and 4.14). The maxillary premolars were prepared for full coverage and transitional crowns were placed. Then, with lingual buttons used on these teeth for retention, the maxillary anterior teeth were retracted to close the spaces (Figures 4.15 and 4.16). The retracted mandibular teeth were splinted with orthodontic wiring, and the remaining maxillary teeth were prepared for full coverage and provisionally restored (Figure 4.17). At this time the maxillary central incisor was extracted.

In the mandible it was decided to make a fixed prosthesis, and thus a computerized tomography (CT) radiograph was made to

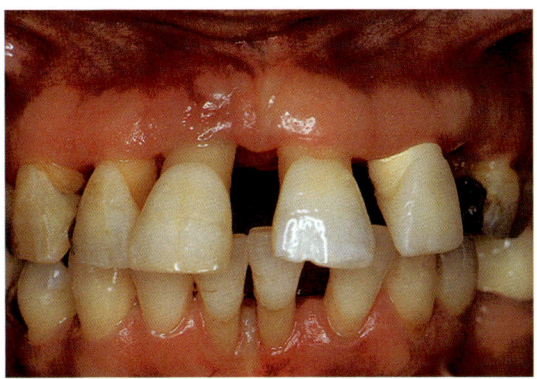

Figure 4.12

Anterior teeth—labial view, after initial preparation.

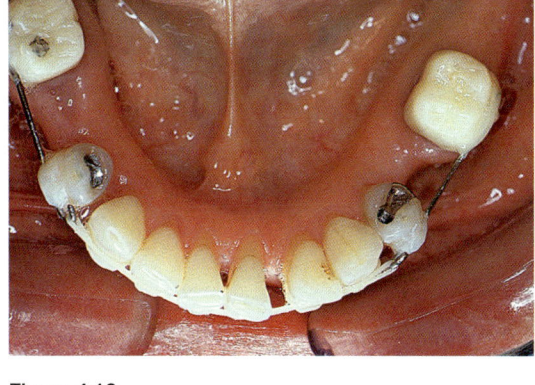

Figure 4.13

Anterior teeth—orthodontic treatment to close spaces and retract teeth: mandible, start.

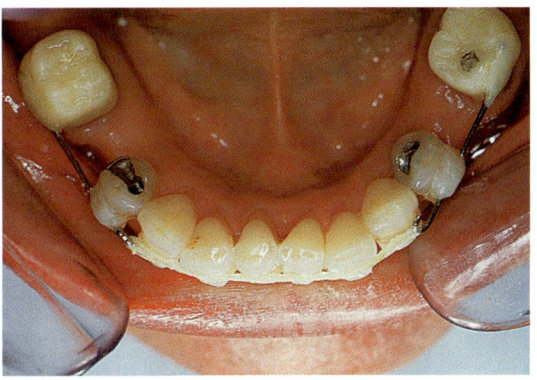

Figure 4.14

Orthodontic treatment, mandible, finish.

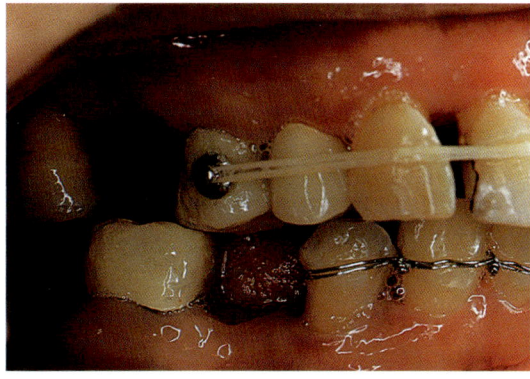

Figure 4.15

Orthodontic treatment, retraction of anterior maxillary teeth, right side.

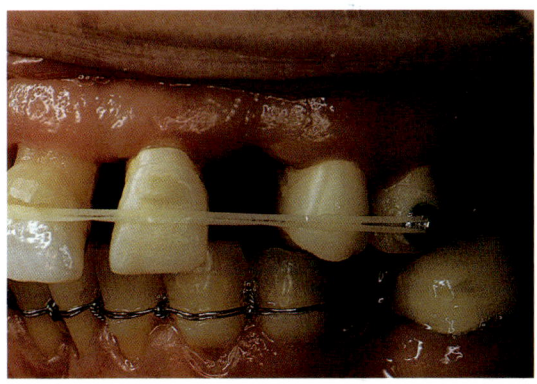

Figure 4.16

Orthodontic treatment, retraction of anterior maxillary teeth, left side.

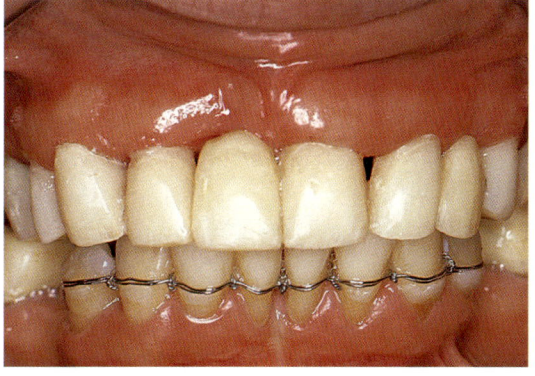

Figure 4.17

Maxillary teeth showing provisional splints.

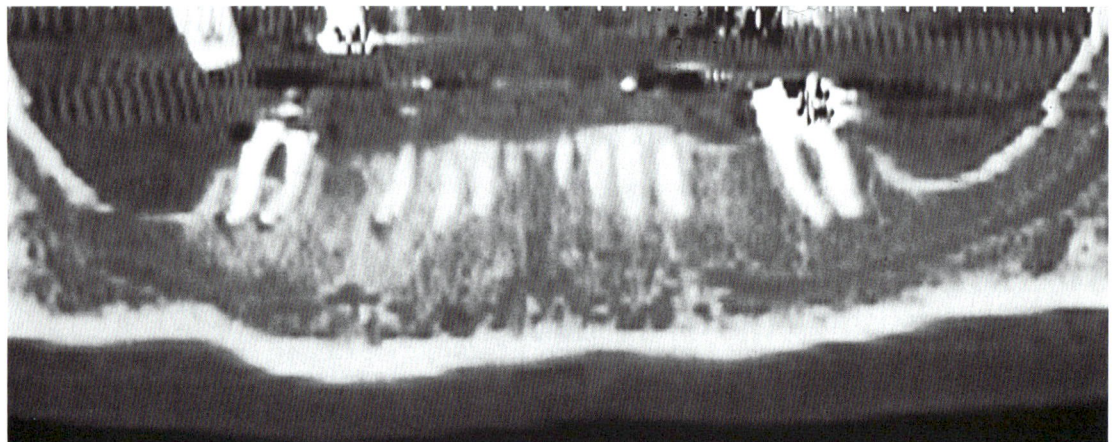

Figure 4.18

CT radiograph of mandible.

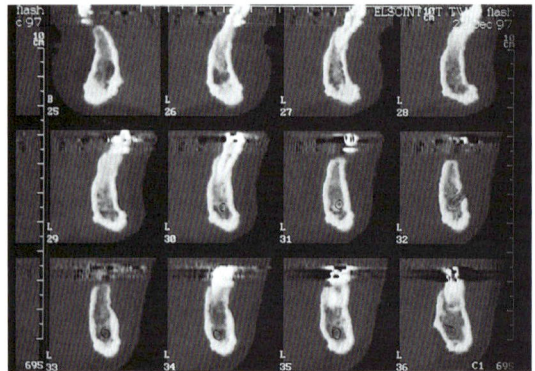

Figure 4.19

CT radiograph of mandible, left side.

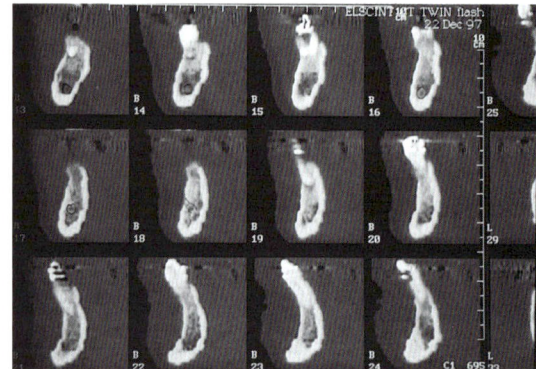

Figure 4.20

CT radiograph of mandible, right side.

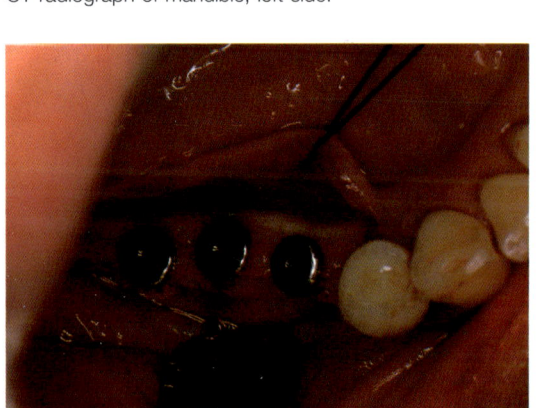

Figure 4.21

Implant placement, right side.

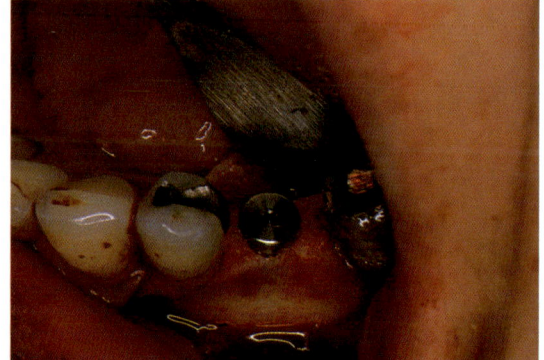

Figure 4.22

Implant placement, left side.

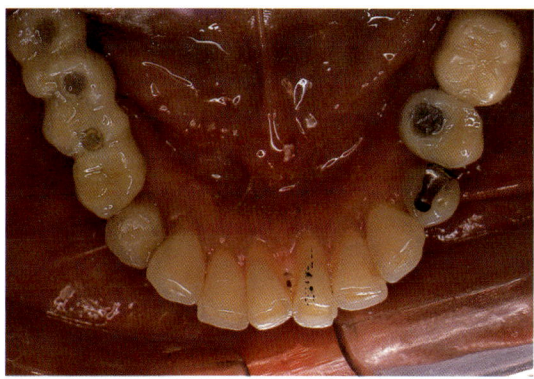

Figure 4.23

Mandible with provisional restorations on implants.

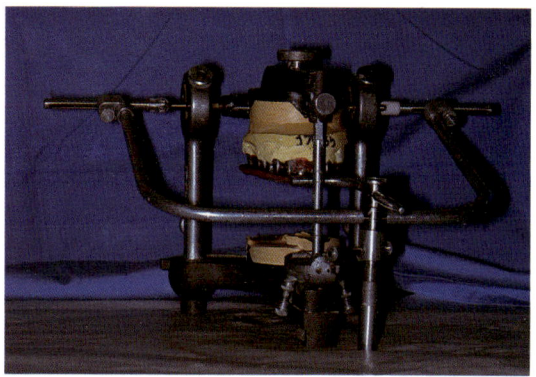

Figure 4.24

Mounting of maxillary model on Hanau articulator with facebow registration.

check the quality and quantity of bone and the possibility of implant therapy. The radiograph showed that it would be possible to place three implants on the right side, distal to the first premolar, and a single implant on the left side in the area of the second premolar (Figures 4.18–4.20). An acrylic resin surgical stent was prepared and used during the implant placement, and three Branemark implants were placed in the right posterior region of the mandible and one between the left first premolar and the left first molar (Figures 4.21 and 4.22). After 3 months, the implants were exposed and abutments placed. New provisional restorations were made for the implants (Figure 4.23).

Copper band elastomeric impressions were made of all the prepared teeth and pattern resin copings made to fit the stone dies. These copings and transfer copings for the implants were fitted in the mouth and used to record centric relation at the vertical dimension of occlusion of the provisional restorations. A polyether full arch impression was then taken of the maxilla and the master model poured and mounted to the mandibular model of the transitional removable partial denture by means of the Pattern resin centric record.

Metal copings for the natural teeth and gold copings were then cast and fitted in the mouth and connected by Pattern resin for soldering. These were soldered together, refitted and a new centric relation record made. A polyether impression was then taken for tissue detail and a pick-up of the fixed prosthesis in the maxilla in order to make a final master model. This was mounted on a Hanau articulator by means of a facebow registration (Figure 4.24) and the Pattern resin registration on the soldered metal prosthesis. The shade was chosen and porcelain baked to the metal. This was fitted in the mouth and the occlusion adjusted to the lower jaw. The porcelain was then glazed and the prostheses on the natural teeth cemented with Temp-Bond for 2 weeks. The implant supported prostheses were screw retained (Figures 4.25–4.29).

SUMMARY

This patient presented with a very severe case of adult periodontitis. She also had

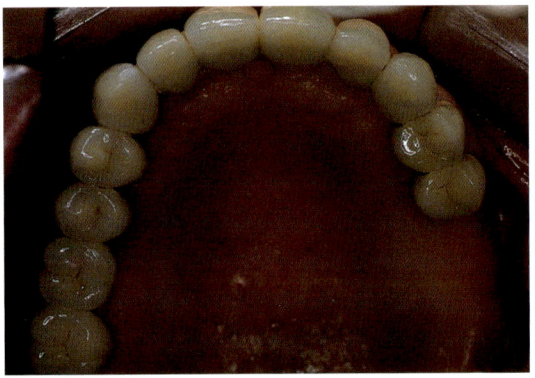

Figure 4.25

Mandible—polyether impression for coping pick-up.

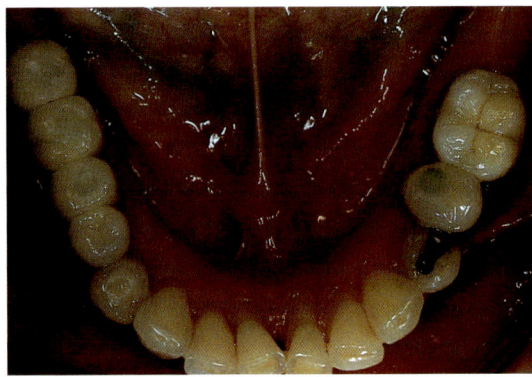

Figure 4.26

Maxilla—polyether impression for coping pick-up.

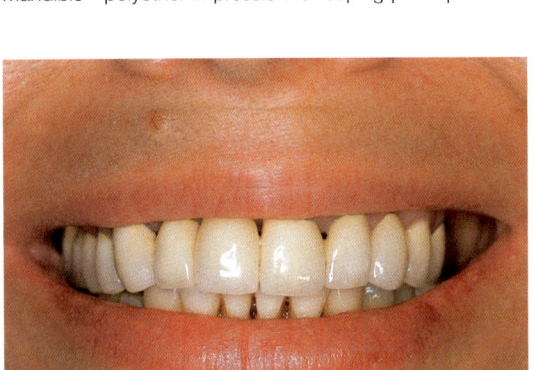

Figure 4.27

Treatment completed—permanent restorations, anterior view.

rampant caries and several hopeless teeth, many missing teeth, and severe bone loss. There were tipped, malpositioned, and extruded teeth. The patient wanted fixed prostheses and was willing to change her oral hygiene habits and cooperate in her treatment. However, one of the potential problems with the treatment plan was that by increasing vertical dimension, the crown-to-root ratio would increase the lever forces on the teeth. This was avoided by first retracting the mandibular anterior teeth, and then the maxillary anterior teeth, and then leveling the mandibular anterior

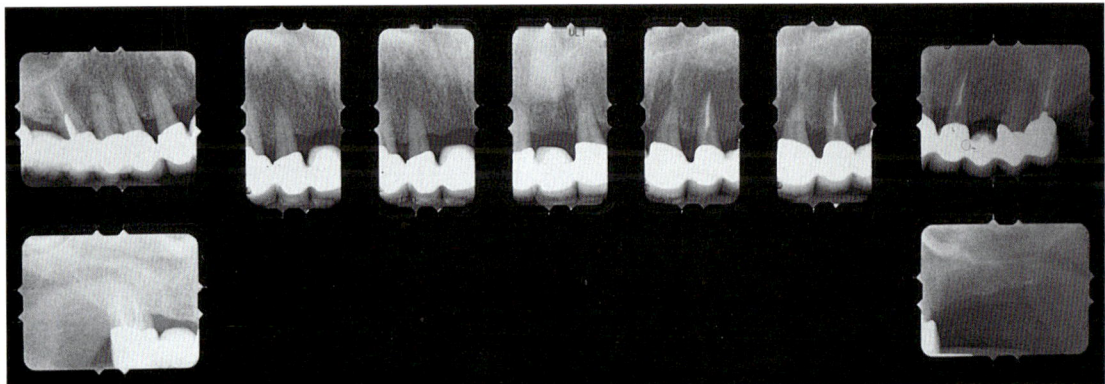

Figure 4.28

Treatment completed—permanent restorations, maxilla.

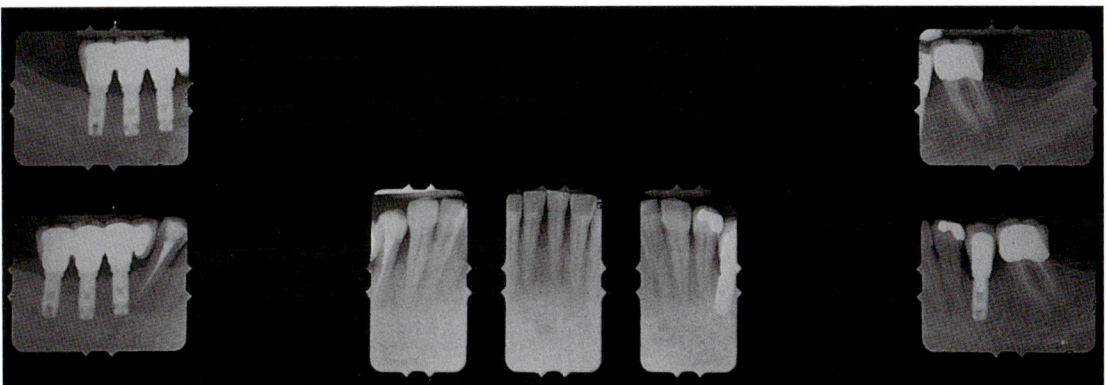

Figure 4.29

Treatment completed—permanent restorations, mandible.

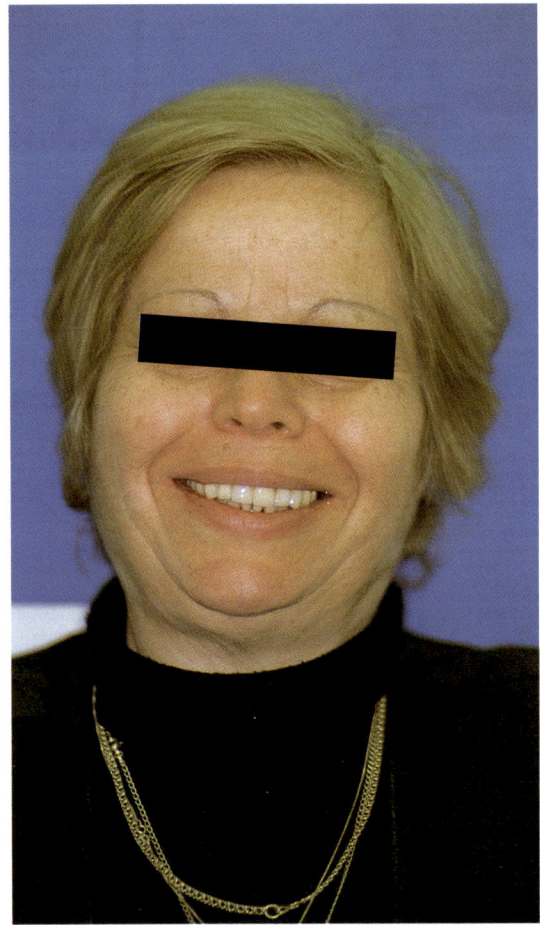

Figure 4.30

Treatment completed—face, frontal view

teeth, thus bringing the patient from inter-cuspal position (IC) to retruded cuspal position (RC): this enabled retraction of these without a change in vertical dimension. It was thus possible to restore the maxilla with a fixed prosthesis in spite of the poor prognosis of the teeth when the patient initially presented, by means of the biomechanical changes that occurred during treatment. These included improvement of the patient's periodontal condition not only due to her improved oral hygiene, but also by the new position of the teeth in the alveolar bone, which directed the occlusal forces in the long axis of the tooth. All the teeth, including the anterior teeth, were now utilized for occlusal support and also reducing lateral forces to a minimum. With periodontal, endodontic, orthodontic, implant therapy, an esthetic and functional result was achieved.

CASE DISCUSSION
AVINOAM YAFFE

In the case presented above, we have improved the remaining teeth prognosis by periodontal and orthodontic treatment, along with a carefully planned occlusal scheme.

The orthodontic retraction of the lower anterior teeth improved the periodontal condition of the teeth, redirected the occlusal forces in a more favorable direction, and the leveling of the teeth that followed their retraction improved the crown-to-root ratio. The same can be claimed for the upper remaining anterior teeth. Additional support was gained by implants that are carefully protected from lateral forces by the occlusal scheme that was applied in this case. It can be concluded that by utilizing a multidisciplinary approach, we maximized tooth potential and provided a functional, physiologic and esthetic restoration to the patient with minimal surgical intervention.

CASE DISCUSSION
HAROLD PREISKEL

Many prosthodontists dread a patient with a neglected dentition who presents with a photograph taken three decades previously and expects the clock turned back with a magic wand. Although no such device was available to the operators, they have achieved an excellent result with sensibly planned periodontal and orthodontic treatment. Retracting the mandibular anterior teeth at an early stage avoided the hazards of increasing the crown-to-root ratio of the maxillary teeth that had such poor bone support. The timing and the placement of the mandibular implants was sensible and allowed the restoration of a full arcade of teeth.

PATIENT 5

UNNOTICED PERIODONTAL DETERIORATION

Treatment by Tzachi Lehr

THE PATIENT

The patient, a 47-year-old woman, employed as a secretary, came to the clinic for dental treatment. Her chief complaints were (Figures 5.1 and 5.2):

'My teeth are moving.'
'I am getting spaces between my teeth which I didn't have when I was younger.' (see Figure 5.3)
'My mouth has an odor.'
'When I chew, it hurts.'

PAST MEDICAL HISTORY

The patient suffered from pulmonary valve regurgitation and an allergy to penicillin,

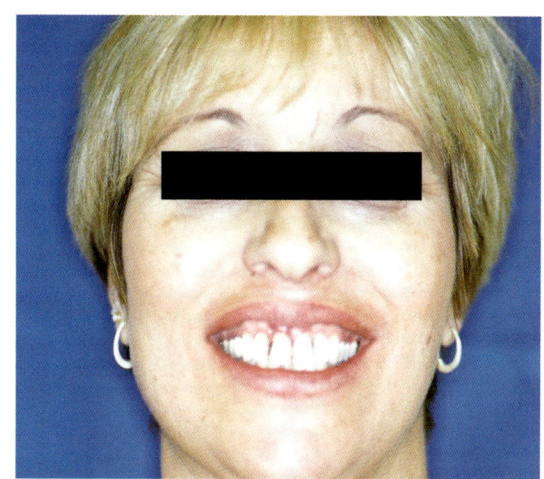

Figure 5.2

Face—frontal view (forced smile).

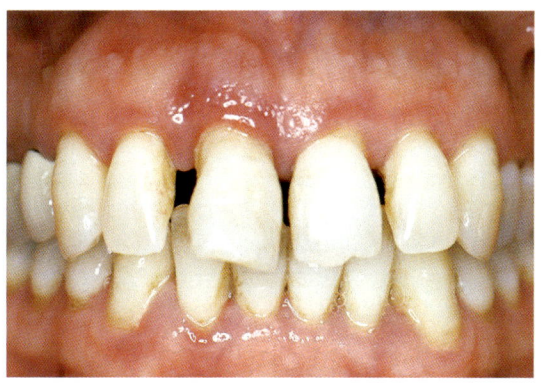

Figure 5.1

Anterior teeth—labial view.

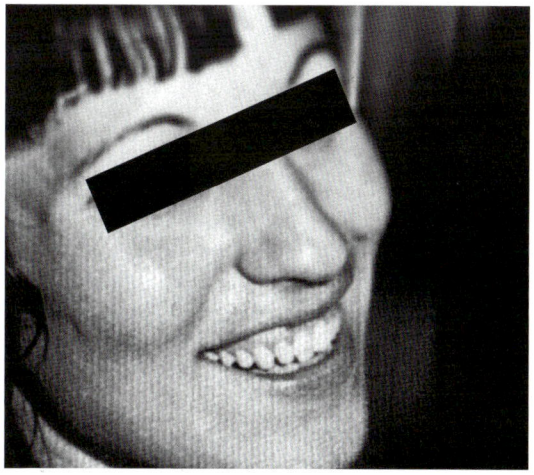

Figure 5.3

Face—frontal view (from 23 years ago).

thus, would require prophylaxsis with ERIC (erythromycin capsules) prior to dental treatment.

The patient underwent periodontal surgery 2 years ago. She also disclosed that she had a habit of cracking nuts.

EXTRA-ORAL EXAMINATION
(Figures 5.2 and 5.4)

- Symmetrical face, although the right masseter muscle was more developed than the left one
- In profile, she had a tendency to bi-maxillary protrusion

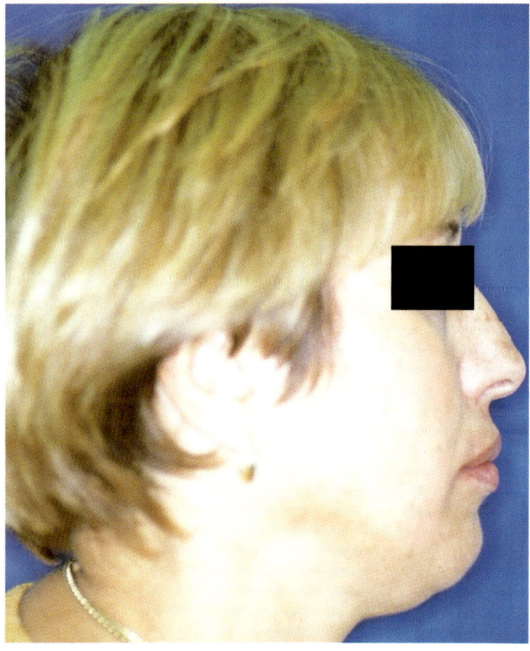

Figure 5.4

Face—side view.

- High lip line
- Temporomandibular joint was normal, mandibular motions were within normal limits
- Maximum opening of 50 mm
- Incompetent lips—habitually apart

INTRA-ORAL AND FULL-MOUTH PERIAPICAL RADIOGRAPH EXAMINATION

Maxilla (Figure 5.5):

- Parabolic arch
- High palate
- Spacing between the anterior teeth
- Missing third molar teeth
- Porcelain fused to metal crowns on the right premolar teeth
- Amalgam restorations on the right molars and left first premolar and second molar

Mandible (Figure 5.6):

- Parabolic arch
- Missing left third molar tooth
- Amalgam restorations on the molar teeth

Occlusal examination (Figures 5.7 and 5.8) revealed that the patient was Angle class I. The interocclusal rest space was 2–3 mm, overjet was 7 mm and overbite was 4 mm (Figure 5.9). There was a 1.0 mm discrepancy between centric relation and centric occlusion with both anterior and vertical components. There was a midline discrepancy. The maxillary right central incisor was extruded (see Figure 5.1). There was spacing between the maxillary incisor teeth and they were also slightly rotated (see Figure 5.1). Lateral jaw movements were guided by the canine and premolar teeth

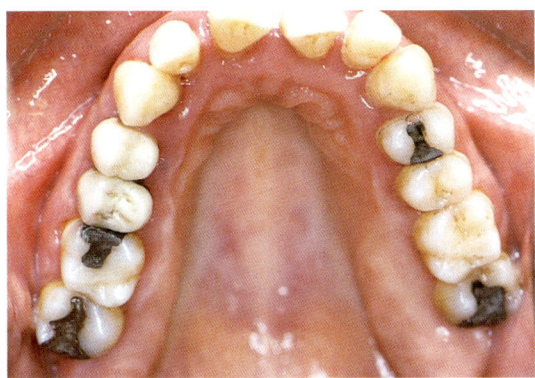

Figure 5.5

Maxillary arch—palatal view.

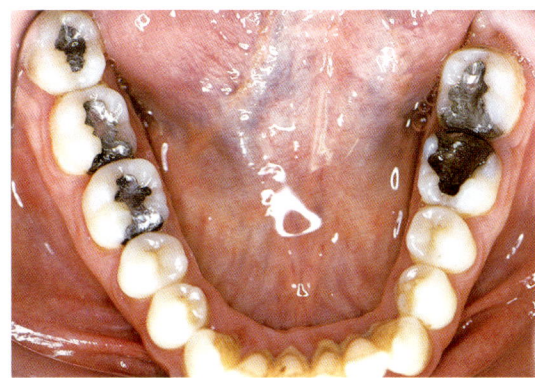

Figure 5.6

Mandibular arch—lingual view.

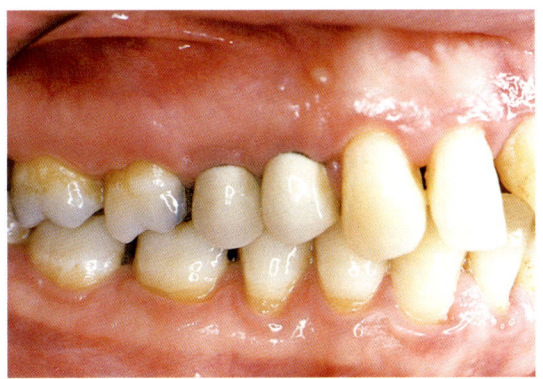

Figure 5.7

Occlusion—right side.

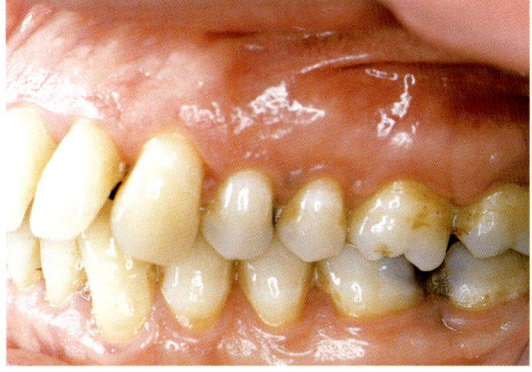

Figure 5.8

Occlusion—left side.

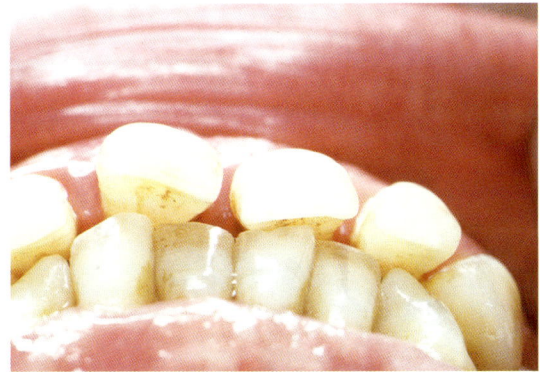

Figure 5.9

Occlusion—anterior view of overbite and overjet.

on the left side, and by group function followed by the canine teeth with incisal contacts on the right side. Protrusive movements were guided by the canines and incisors. No non-working side interferences were noted.

Fremitus:

- Maxillary right central incisor—grade II–III both in centric occlusion and protrusive jaw movements
- Maxillary left central incisor, left lateral incisor, and right lateral incisor—grade I

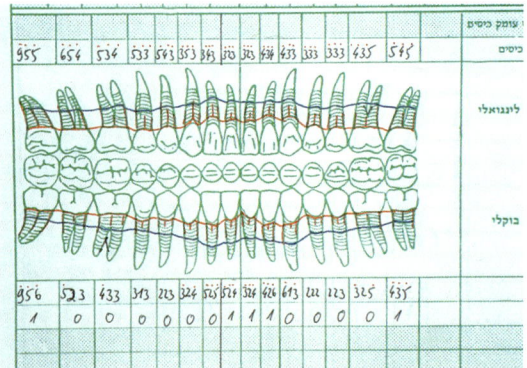

Figure 5.10

Periodontal chart—pre-treatment, maxilla.

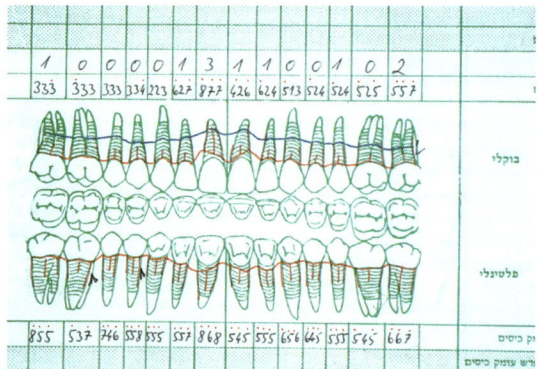

Figure 5.11

Periodontal chart—pre-treatment, mandible.

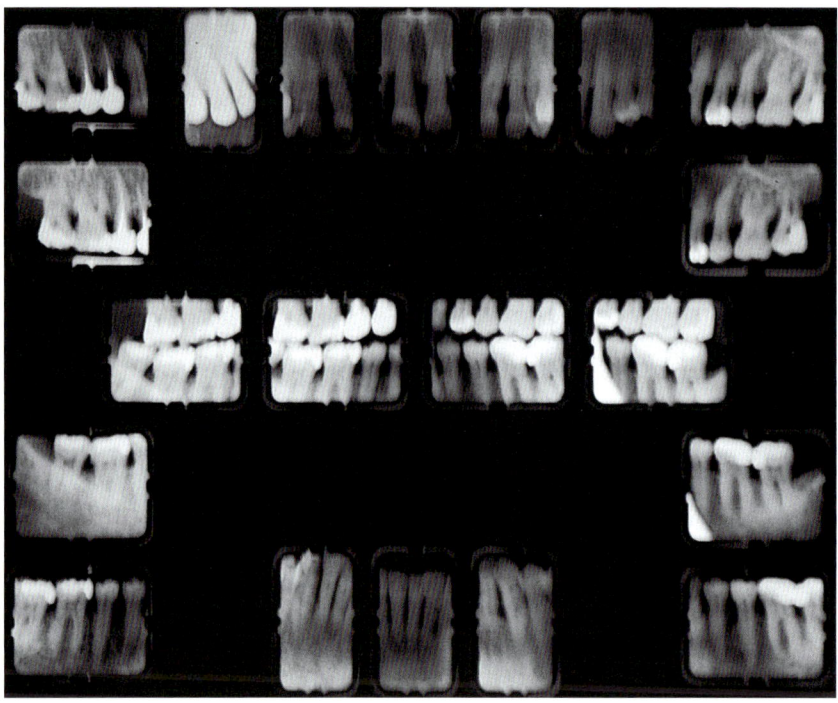

Figure 5.12

Radiographs of maxilla and mandible—pre-treatment.

both in centric (occlusion) and protrusive jaw movements

Periodontal examination (Figures 5.10 and 5.11) revealed calculus and plaque, probing depths of up to 8.0 mm on the maxillary teeth and up to 9.0 mm on the mandibular teeth with bleeding on probing on almost all of the teeth. There was slight gingival recession around most of the teeth. The maxillary left first premolar and left first molar had class I furcation involvement on the mesial.

FULL-MOUTH PERIAPICAL
SURVEY (Figure 5.12)

- Endodontic treatment—maxillary right premolars slightly short of apex
- Horizontal and vertical bone loss around most (of the) molar teeth

INDIVIDUAL TOOTH PROGNOSIS

- Hopeless:

$$\frac{1}{}\bigg|$$

- Poor:

$$\frac{7\ 6\ 5\ 4\ \big|\ 1\ 2\ 6\ 7}{7\ 8\ \big|}$$

- Fair:

$$\frac{2\ \big|\ 4\ 5}{2\ 1\ \big|\ 1\ 2\ 6}$$

- Good: the remaining teeth

SUMMARY OF FINDINGS

The 47-year-old patient, who suffered from pulmonary valve regurgitation, came to the clinic complaining of recent spacing between her front teeth, a foul odor in her mouth, and pain when chewing on the left side of her mouth. She presented with poor oral hygiene, plaque and calculus, and severe inflammation accompanied by deep probing depths, furcation involvements, and bleeding upon probing. The teeth were mobile and had fremitus in closing and jaw movements. The maxillary right central incisor was extruded and had a suppurating periodontal abscess.

DIAGNOSIS

- Advanced adult periodontitis
- Secondary occlusal trauma with primary origin of occlusal trauma from chewing on nuts
- Loss of posterior support, reduced occlusal support
- Deep bite
- Decreased vertical dimension of occlusion
- Acute dentoalveolar periodontal abscess—maxillary right central incisor tooth
- Faulty esthetics

ABOUT THE PATIENT

The patient was highly motivated for dental treatment due to the poor esthetic condition of her teeth. However, the poor oral hygiene she presented with, just 2 years following periodontal treatment and surgery, attested to the fact that she was unaware of the importance of good dental hygiene, and the direct relationship that it had to the success or failure of her dental treatment.

TREATMENT PLAN

PHASE 1: INITIAL PREPARATION

- Initial periodontal therapy including:
    oral hygiene instruction
    scaling and root planing
    caries excavation
- Occlusal adjustment of the (maxillary right central incisor) by selective grinding to reduce occlusal trauma

The first re-evaluation led to the second phase of the treatment plan.

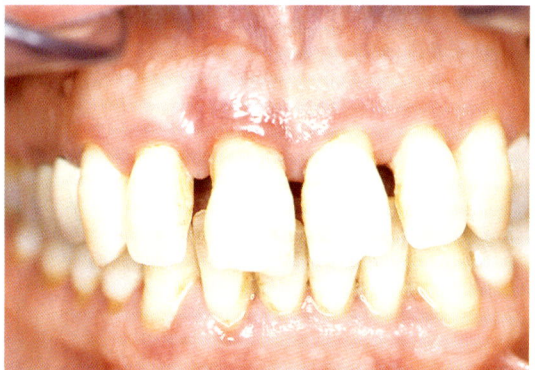

Figure 5.13

Anterior teeth after initial preparation, labial view.

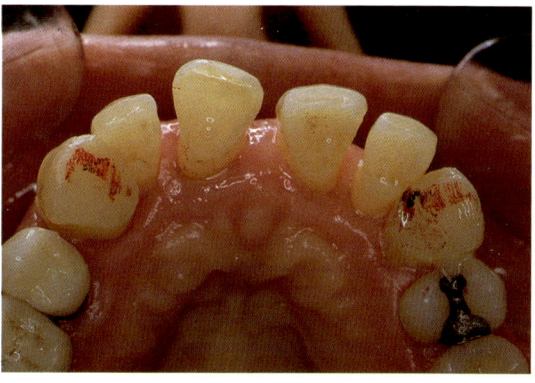

Figure 5.15

Anterior teeth, lingual view, canine platform.

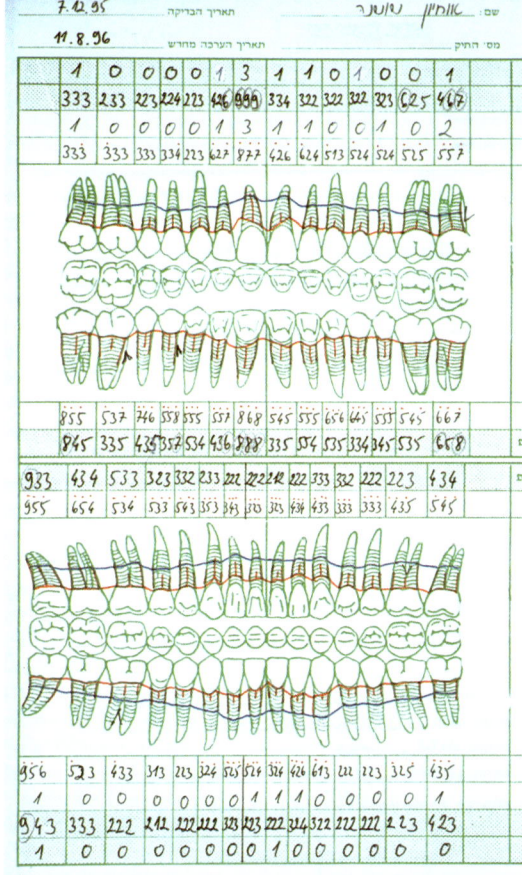

Figure 5.14

Periodontal chart—first re-evaluation.

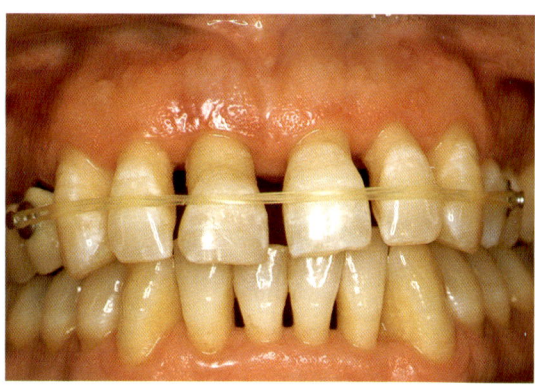

Figure 5.16

Anterior teeth, orthodontic treatment to close spaces and retract teeth.

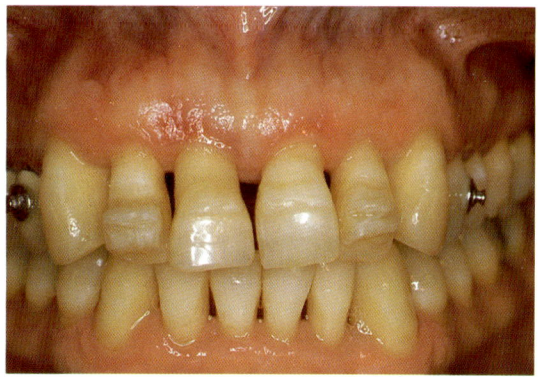

Figure 5.17

Anterior teeth, orthodontic treatment completed.

PHASE 2

- Eruption of the posterior teeth
- Retraction of the maxillary anterior teeth
- Temporary fixed maxillary prosthesis
- Re-establishment of an acceptable vertical dimension of occlusion, and a physiologic occlusal plane

TREATMENT

Initial treatment consisted of scaling, root planing, curettage, oral hygiene instruction, and extraction of the mandibular right third molar. At re-evaluation, after initial preparation, bleeding on probing had diminished to a great extent. However, the probing depths remained deep and showed almost no improvement (Figures 5.13 and 5.14).

In order to increase vertical dimension to enable posterior tooth eruption along with their supporting bone and provide space for maxillary anterior tooth retraction, a canine platform was constructed on the maxillary cuspid teeth (Figure 5.15). As eruption of posterior teeth took place, orthodontic treatment was then started to retract the maxillary anterior teeth and close the spaces (Figure 5.16). Lingual buttons were placed on the first premolars and elastics were then used to close the spacing between the teeth (Figure 5.17). To prevent drifting of the elastics gingivally, composite stops were placed on the labial surfaces of the anterior teeth. This treatment was accompanied by constant scaling, root planing, and curettage. Since the patient had a pulmonary valve regurgitation problem, this necessitated the use of prophylactic antibiotics (ERIC: coated erythromycin 1 g an hour before treatment, and 500 mg 6 hours after treatment) for each visit.

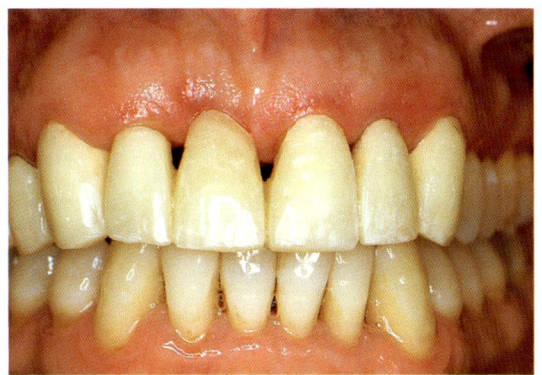

Figure 5.18

Maxillary teeth showing provisional restoration.

When the orthodontic treatment was completed and the anterior spacing eliminated, the maxillary teeth from the second right premolar to the left cuspid were prepared for full coverage, and a provisional fixed restoration was inserted. At the same time, the hopeless maxillary right central incisor was extracted (Figure 5.18).

At the second re-evaluation, the recorded probing depths were greater than 5 mm and the decision was made to undertake periodontal surgery (Figure 5.19). The goal of the periodontal surgery was to achieve an open clean-up and pocket elimination. During the periodontal surgery, the decision was made to resect the disto-buccal roots of both second molars in order to eliminate the trifurcation involvements of these teeth and improve their prognosis (Figures 5.20 and 5.21). Selective grinding and reshaping of the buccal cusps of the maxillary molar and premolar teeth was performed to diminish the strong lateral forces upon them.

At the following re-evaluation, it was noted that the maxillary right first premolar still showed unacceptable probing depths. Orthodontic treatment was then started to

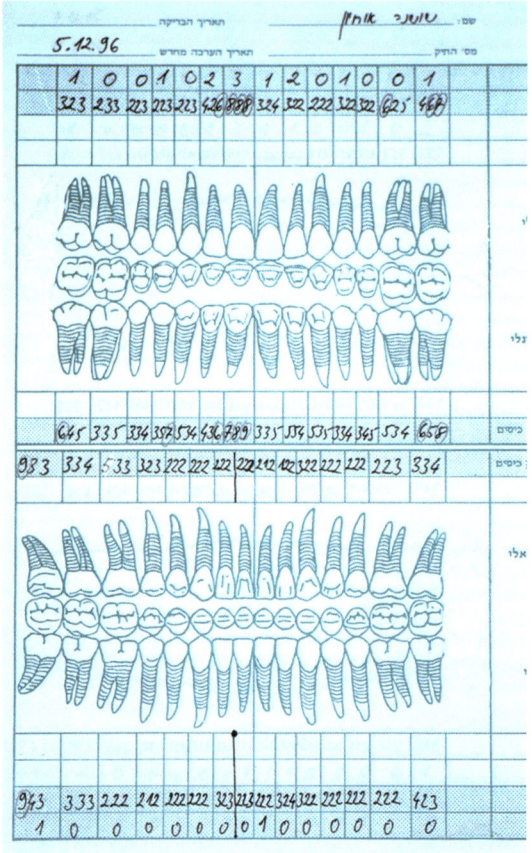

Figure 5.19

Periodontal chart: maxilla and mandible, re-evaluation.

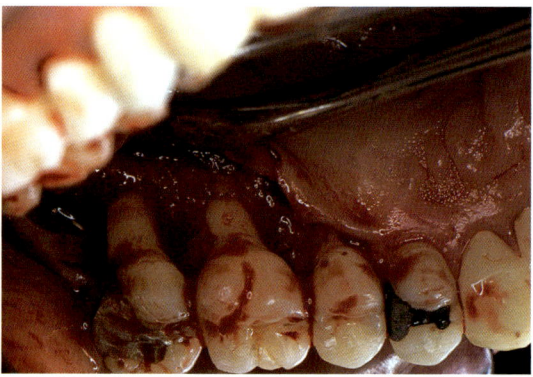

Figure 5.20

Periodontal surgery, maxillary left posterior quadrant.

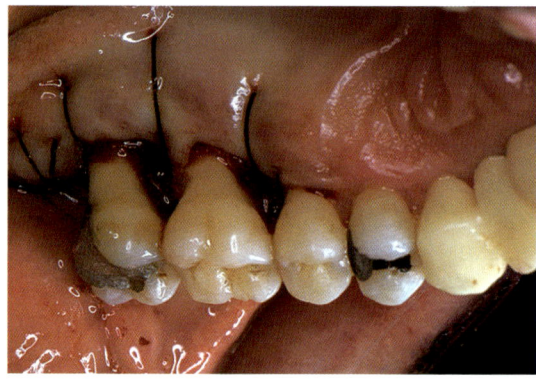

Figure 5.21

Periodontal surgery—maxillary left posterior quadrant, suturing.

extrude the tooth and, it was hoped, the supporting bone with it as a future implant site development (Figure 5.22). After the orthodontic treatment, charting revealed that the probing depths were still unchanged and it was then decided to extract the tooth. Upon extraction, a crack in the buccal root was seen along the palatal side, which explained why the tooth did not respond to all the treatment.

Periodontal surgery (soft tissue augmentation) was then carried out in the maxillary central incisor area to reshape the area,

taking tissue from the palate ('pouch technique') (Figure 5.23).

Since the vertical dimension had been increased during treatment, a minimal occlusal adjustment was made to return the patient to her original vertical dimension of occlusion.

At the final re-evaluation, it was determined that probing depths and mobility had been greatly diminished, and the final treatment was carried out. This included finalizing the teeth preparations. Copper band elastomeric impressions were made

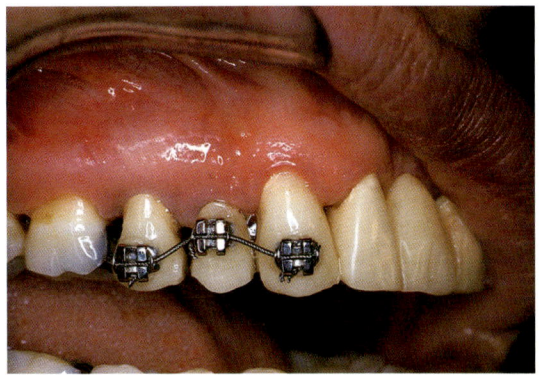

Figure 5.22

Orthodontic treatment to extrude maxillary first premolar.

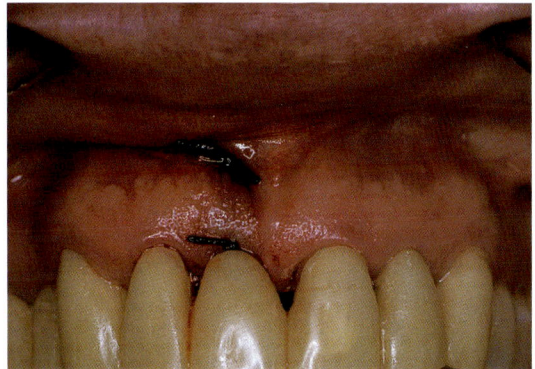

Figure 5.23

Maxillary right central incisor area—soft tissue graft, suturing.

of the prepared teeth, and stone dies and pattern resin copings produced. These copings were fitted in the mouth and used to record centric occlusion, and a polyether impression was taken for the working model. A master model was cast from this impression with the stone dies in place. This model was articulated to the model of the mandibular teeth made with an alginate impression. Metal copings were then cast and fitted on the individual prepared teeth with the pontics attached to the adjacent tooth. These were connected with pattern resin and soldered, and the soldered prosthesis fitted in the mouth. A centric record in Duralay at the vertical dimension of occlusion was made in the mouth and another polyether full arch impression done for the tissue details. This impression was cast and mounted to the lower model and the articulator by means of a facebow transfer and the Duralay centric record. The shade was chosen and the porcelain baked. The bridge was then fitted and final adjustments were done in the mouth in the biscque bake stage. The prosthesis was then glazed and temporarily

cemented in the mouth with Temp-Bond for a period of 2 weeks. The prosthesis was then cemented permanently with zinc oxyphosphate cement (Figures 5.24–5.27).

SUMMARY

The patient presented with what she thought was a simple problem of a loose front tooth and the start of spacing in her maxillary anterior teeth. Even though she had periodontal surgery 2 years previously, she was not aware of the importance of good oral hygiene and her periodontal condition had thus deteriorated. The initial treatment consisted of oral hygiene instruction and scaling and curettage. When the probing depths did not improve, orthodontic treatment was initiated as well as periodontal surgery in order to eliminate the deep pockets around the teeth. Even after this treatment, the maxillary first premolar did not respond and had to be extracted. Only then, it was discovered that the root was cracked and thus had been untreatable.

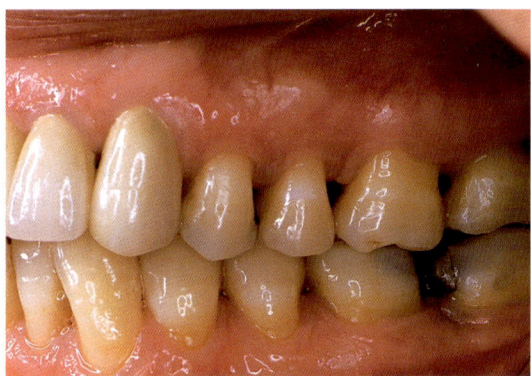

Figure 5.24

Treatment completed—permanent restorations, left side.

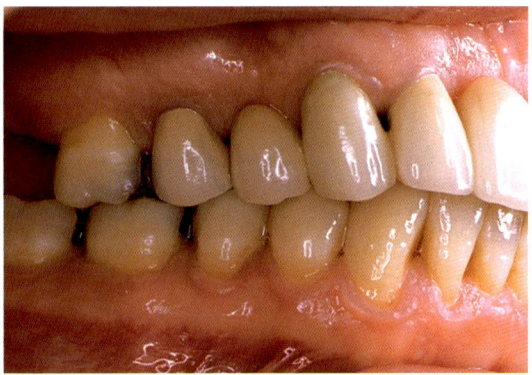

Figure 5.25

Treatment completed—permanent restorations, right side.

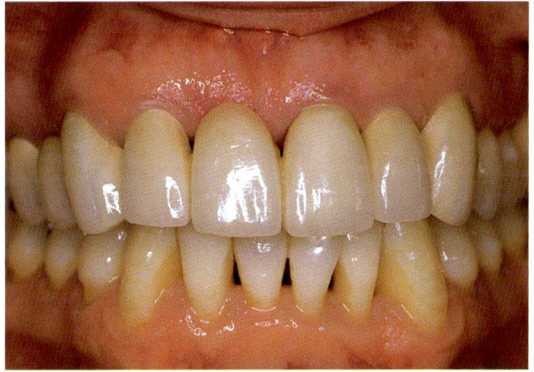

Figure 5.26

Treatment completed—permanent restorations, anterior view.

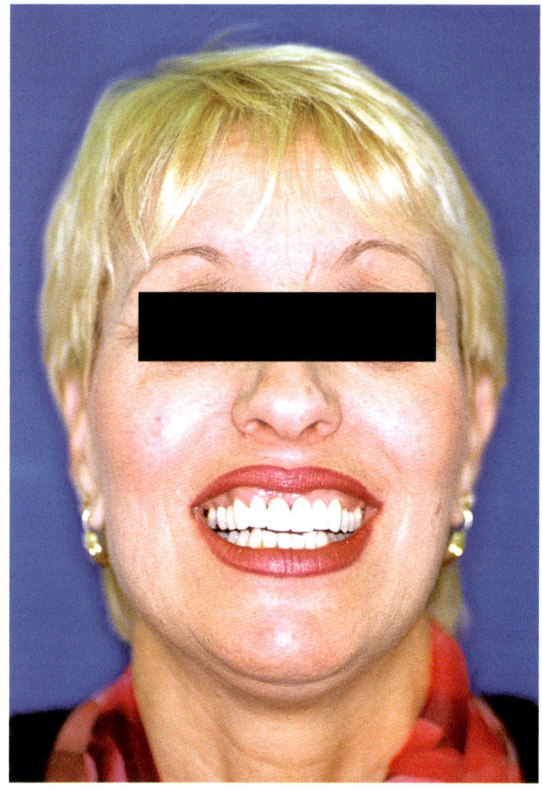

Figure 5.27

Treatment completed—face, frontal view.

What appeared to be a relatively easy treatment turned out to be rather involved, with orthodontic therapy and periodontal surgery needed in order to achieve an esthetic and functional result.

CASE DISCUSSION
AVINOAM YAFFE

This case presentation describes a rather bizarre situation of a 47-year-old woman with a 'tiny' chief complaint that led to a comprehensive treatment plan in order to restore esthetics and regain long-lasting physiologic occlusion. In order to achieve the goal of physiologic and esthetic occlusion with the periodontal condition that the patient presented with, we utilized the potential of tooth eruption both to reduce periodontal defects and minimize the damage of increasing the crown-to-root ratio. In order to compensate for the reduced posterior support both by periodontal involvement and missing teeth, the anterior teeth were incorporated into support by retracting them lingually, thus improving their position over the alveolar ridge and redirecting the occlusal forces in a more favorable position. By improving the overall periodontal condition, improving oral hygiene habits, and compensating for reduced posterior support by including the anterior group of teeth in vertical support, we have accomplished an esthetic long lasting physiologic occlusion.

CASE DISCUSSION
HAROLD PREISKEL

Patients requiring antibiotic prophylaxis pose particular problems due to the need to reduce the number of courses of antibiotic therapy to a minimum. While the patient was understandably concerned about her appearance, she appeared to have no idea of the severity of the problems in her mouth, or of what would be required to correct them. This is another example of what skilled operators can achieve with patient motivation, and with success on that front everything else falls into place. The combination of periodontal therapy and orthodontic treatment with skilled prosthodontics has produced not only a happy patient but also an esthetic and functioning dentition. Long may it last!

PATIENT 6   COMPLICATED ADVANCED ADULT PERIODONTITIS

Treatment by Miriam Oppenheimer

THE PATIENT

The patient, a male 49-year-old clerk, presented for dental treatment. His main complaints were the following:

'I have difficulty eating.'
'My front tooth is loose and hurts when I chew.'
'The spaces between my teeth appear to be getting bigger.' (Figures 6.1 and 6.2)
'Due to the spaces between my front teeth, I have problems speaking clearly.'

PAST MEDICAL HISTORY

The patient had mitral valve prolapse with mitral valve regurgitation requiring antibiotic prophylaxsis before any dental procedures.

HABITS

The patient clenches his teeth.

DIET

The patient drinks about five mugs of coffee and tea per day, with three teaspoons of sugar.

PAST DENTAL HISTORY

The patient was referred to the Graduate Prosthodontics Dental Clinic by a private dentist who felt that the case was too difficult for him to treat. The patient had recently lost two molar teeth and thought that most of his teeth had been extracted due to caries.

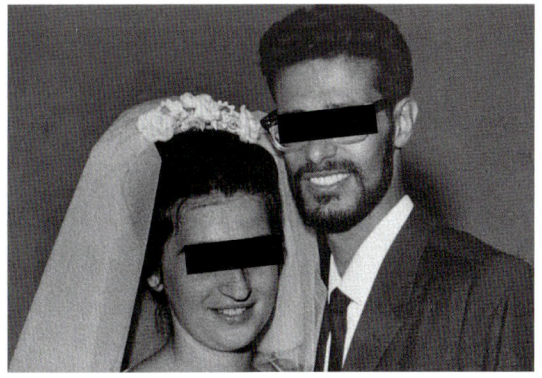

Figure 6.1

Frontal facial view of patient (on right) 20 years previously.

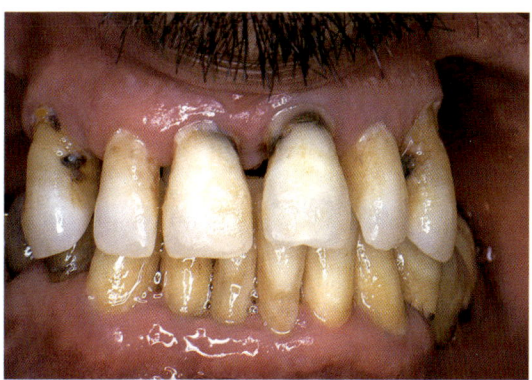

Figure 6.2

Anterior teeth showing spacing.

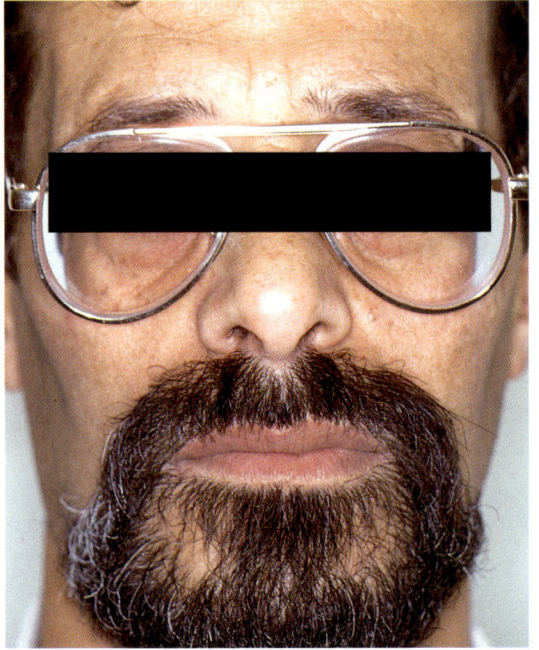

Figure 6.3

Frontal facial view.

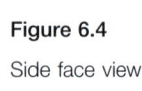

Figure 6.4

Side face view.

EXTRA-ORAL EXAMINATION
(Figures 6.3 and 6.4)

- Slight facial asymmetry
- Normally functioning muscles of mastication
- Temporomandibular joints were normal with freedom of eccentric movements
- Maximum opening between the incisors was 56.0 mm

INTRA-ORAL AND FULL-MOUTH PERIAPICAL RADIOGRAPH EXAMINATION

Maxilla (Figure 6.5):

- Missing teeth:

$$\underline{8\ 7\ 6\ 5\ 4\ \Big|\ 4\ 5\ 6\ 7\ 8}$$

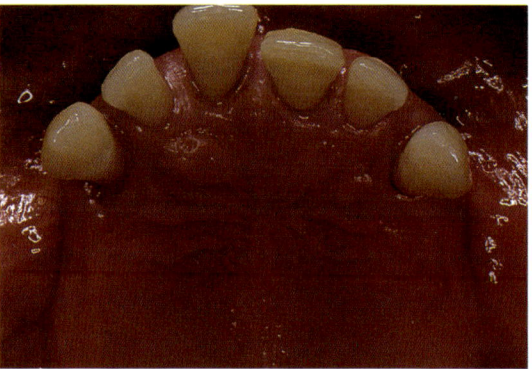

Figure 6.5

Maxillary arch.

- Flaring of the anterior teeth
- Palatal surfaces show wear facets
- Crown and root caries
- Resorbed alveolar ridges especially on the left side (Figure 6.6)
- Flat hard palate

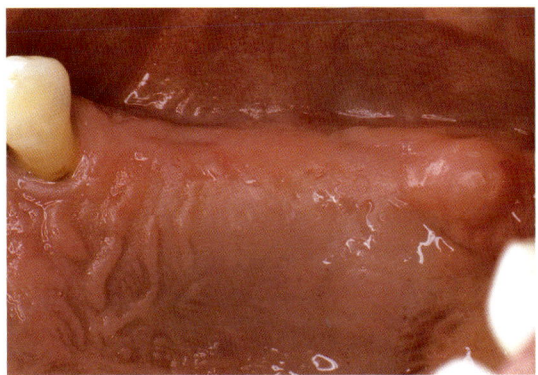

Figure 6.6

Maxillary arch—left posterior quadrant.

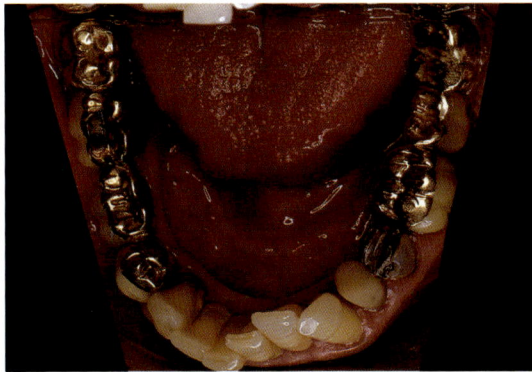

Figure 6.7

Mandibular arch.

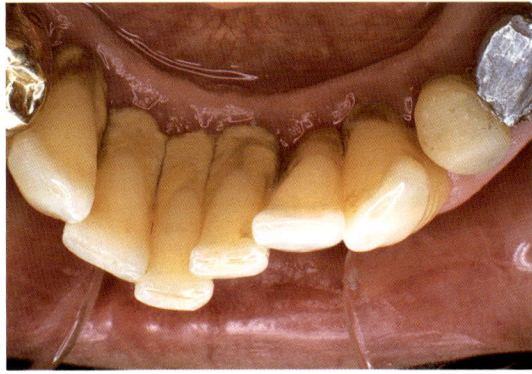

Figure 6.8

Mandibular arch—anterior teeth.

Mandible (Figures 6.7–6.8):

- Missing teeth:

$$\frac{\quad\quad|\quad\quad}{7\mid 5\,6}$$

- Crowding of the anterior teeth
- Anterior teeth were loose and rotated
- Extrusion
- Tipping
- Rotation
- Extensive caries
- Clenching
- Faulty restorations:

$$\frac{\quad\quad\quad|\quad\quad\quad}{8\,X\,6\,5\,4\mid 4\,X\,7\,8}$$

FULL MOUTH PERIAPICAL SURVEY
(Figure 6.9)

- Failing endodontic therapy accompanied by periapical lesions
- Ridge resorption in the edentulous areas

Occlusal examination revealed that the patient was Angle class II division I, with an overbite of 9.0 mm and an overjet of 4.0 mm The interocclusal rest space was 3.0 mm and, as noted, the maximum opening between the incisors was 56.0 mm, which if added to the 9.0 mm overbite would mean that the maximum opening movement was actually 65.0 mm. There was no discrepancy between centric occlusion (IC) and centric relation (CR). Fremitus and mobility were evident on the anterior maxillary teeth. There were two planes of occlusion in the mandible and a marked step in the occlusal plane distal to the cuspid teeth. There was loss of posterior occlusal support.

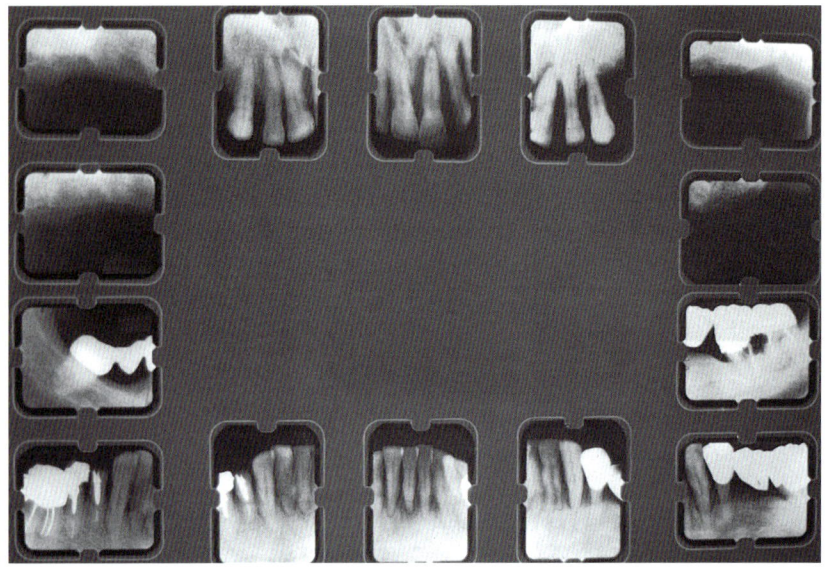

Figure 6.9

Radiographs of maxilla and mandible—pre-treatment.

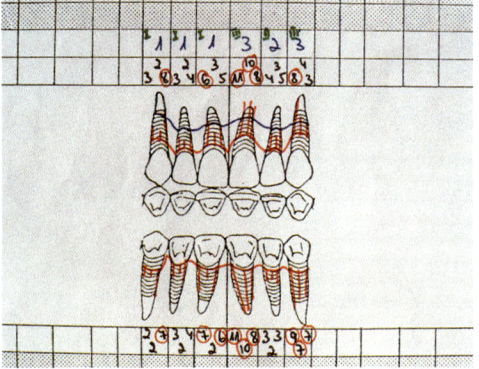

Figure 6.10

Maxillary periodontal chart.

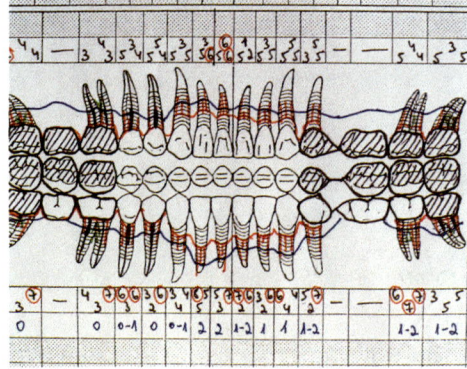

Figure 6.11

Mandibular periodontal chart.

Periodontal examination (Figures 6.10 and 6.11) revealed poor oral hygiene accompanied by large amounts of plaque and calculus. Probing depths of up to 11.0 mm were noted on the maxillary teeth and up to 7.0 mm on the mandibular teeth, with bleeding on probing on most of the teeth. There was 60% bone loss around some teeth. The condition was more severe in the maxilla than the mandible. There was reduced periodontal support due to infraboney pockets, furcation involvement and gingival recession.

INDIVIDUAL TOOTH PROGNOSES

The prognoses for the remaining teeth were the following:

- Very poor:

$$\frac{1 \mid 1\ 2\ 3}{\mid 8}$$

- Fair:

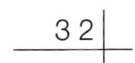

- Good: the remaining teeth

DIAGNOSIS

- Advanced adult periodontitis
- Missing teeth accompanied by edentulous ridge resorption
- Loss of posterior support
- Loss of vertical dimension
- Secondary occlusal trauma with primary origins
- Faulty restorations
- Irregular occlusal plane
- Caries
- Periapical lesions

ABOUT THE PATIENT

The patient was of a philosophical nature; he was interested in his dental treatment, followed instructions, but not always, and was generally cooperative. He wanted to keep as many of his remaining teeth as possible, and specifically requested not to have a complete maxillary denture. He was not interested in implants because his finances were limited. He also had never worn a removable prosthesis and was concerned as to how he would adjust to one.

POTENTIAL TREATMENT PROBLEMS

The patient had never worn a removable prosthesis, had limited finances for dental treatment, had poor eating habits, and clenched his teeth. He also was completely unaware of the severity of his problem. He suffered from advanced adult periodontitis with infraboney pockets, mobility, and fremitus. There were many missing teeth and the remaining residual ridges were resorbed, he had extensive caries and faulty restorations, all of which contributed to the difficulty of the treatment.

TREATMENT PLAN ALTERNATIVES

Maxilla:

- Fixed and removable prostheses if there was a marked improvement in the periodontal condition and the transitional restorations were maintainable
- A complete maxillary overdenture
- An implant supported fixed or removable prosthesis—rejected by the patient due to cost

Mandible:

- Fixed prosthesis supported by implants and natural teeth—rejected by patient due to cost
- Crowns on

8 654|

copings on |48

and a removable partial denture.
- Telescopic removable denture—rejected due to the cost
- Complete overdenture supported by copings

FINAL TREATMENT PLAN

A final treatment plan was chosen which consisted, in the first phase, of oral hygiene instruction, changing dietary habits, and fluoride rinses. This was followed by scaling and curettage, root planing, extraction of the left maxillary incisor tooth and immediate replacement with an orthodontic appliance, removal of caries, and provisional restorations. This would be followed by re-evaluation. The second phase of treatment would depend upon improvement in the patient's periodontal condition and his determination to change his dietary habits and oral hygiene. To improve the periodontal condition and change the force direction of the maxillary anterior teeth, to be parallel to the long axis of the tooth, the maxillary anterior teeth would be orthodontically moved in a palatal direction. Then, after making a transitional fixed anterior prosthesis with an incisal platform, provisional partial removable dentures would be constructed for both the maxilla and mandible to restore lost occlusal support. Another re-evaluation would then be made to determine whether periodontal surgery would be necessary. The prognosis of the mandibular anterior teeth and the mandibular left third molar would be assessed together with the condition of the maxillary remaining teeth to support a permanent fixed and removable prosthesis.

TREATMENT

The initial phase of treatment was completed with oral hygiene instruction, the introduction of new dietary habits, fluoride rinses, scaling and curettage, root planing, extraction of the left maxillary incisor tooth and immediate replacement with an orthodontic appliance (Figures 6.12 and 6.13). Caries was removed and provisional restorations were then fabricated for both jaws (Figures 6.14 and 6.15). The patient exhibited increased dental hygiene awareness and the soft tissues showed great

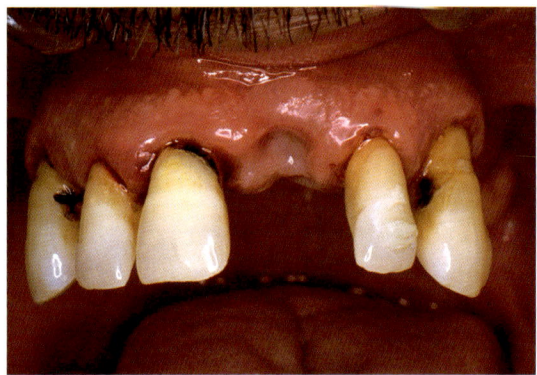

Figure 6.12

Maxillary anterior teeth after extraction of left central incisor.

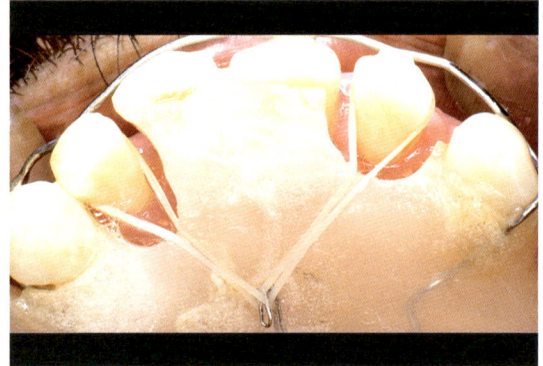

Figure 6.13

Clinical view of Hawley appliance—pre-treatment.

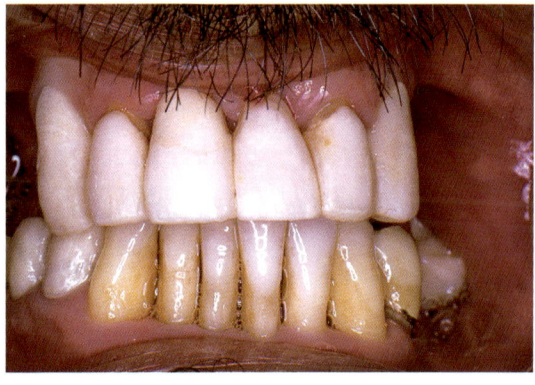

Figure 6.14

Maxillary anterior teeth after orthodontic treatment with provisional crowns.

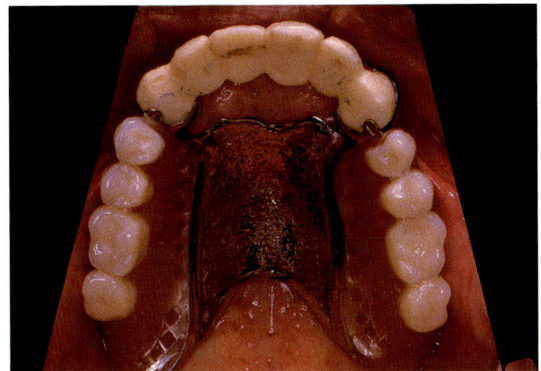

Figure 6.15

Maxilla with transitional crowns and removable partial denture.

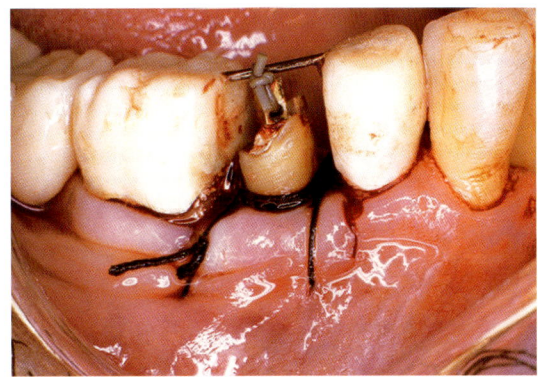

Figure 6.16

Periodontal surgery–crown lengthening procedure and orthodontic extrusion of right mandibular second premolar.

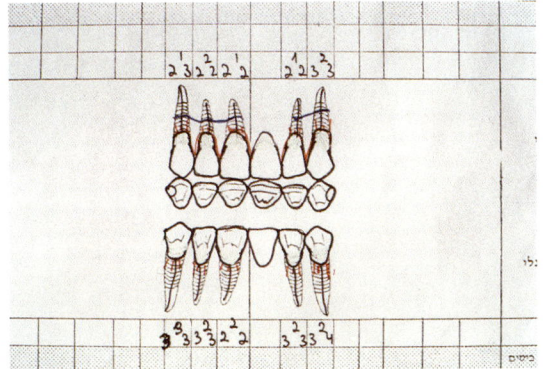

Figure 6.17

Periodontal chart at re-evaluation—maxilla.

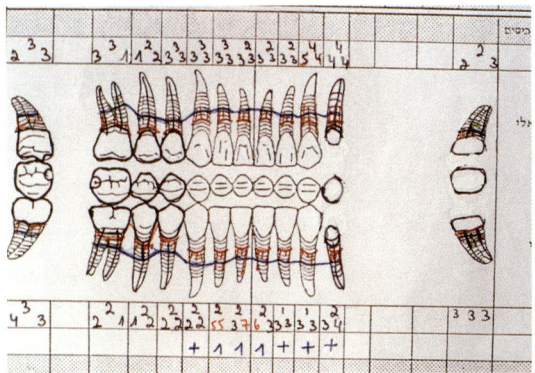

Figure 6.18

Periodontal chart at re-evaluation—mandible.

improvement. At this stage, periodontal surgery was performed on the maxillary anterior teeth and on the mandibular molars, for pocket elimination. The right second premolar was then treated with periodontal surgery–crown lengthening procedure (CLP) and with orthodontics to extrude the root in order to have the margins of the permanent restoration on sound tooth structure (Figure 6.16). At periodontal re-evaluation after healing, the probing depth was found to be less than 3.0 mm on the remaining teeth and the final phase of treatment was initiated (Figures 6.17 and 6.18). The prosthodontic

phase consisted of a mandibular complete overdenture over copings on the remaining teeth, and a fixed partial maxillary prosthesis supporting a posterior removable prosthesis. The remaining mandibular incisors were then extracted and added to the mandibular partial denture (Figure 6.19). The remaining maxillary and mandibular teeth were reprepared and copper band elastomeric impressions made. Stone dies were cast and Duralay transfer copings made. A centric relation record was made using these copings at the vertical dimension of occlusion, as determined by the provisional

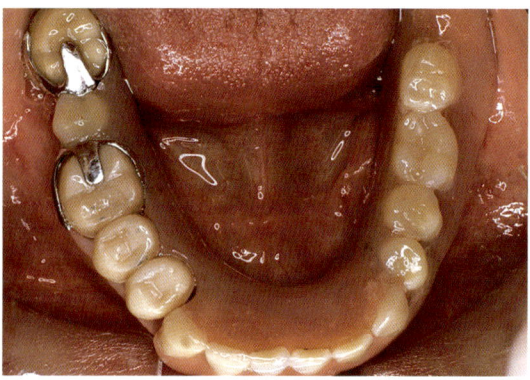

Figure 6.19

Provisional removable partial mandibular denture.

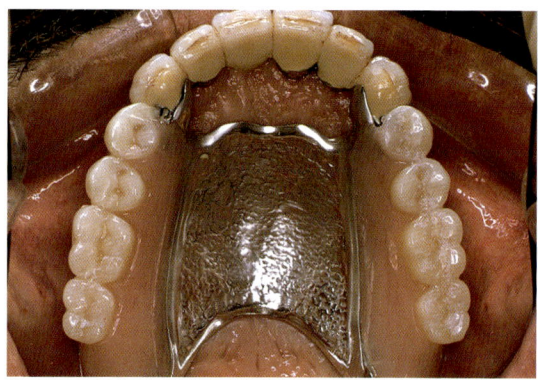

Figure 6.20

Treatment completed—maxilla.

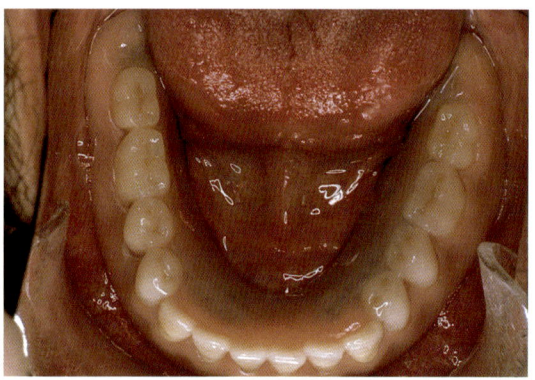

Figure 6.21

Treatment completed—mandible.

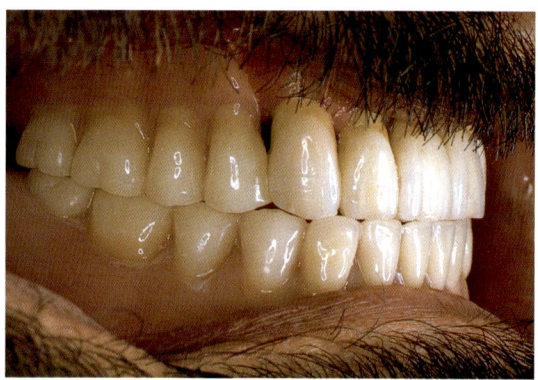

Figure 6.22

Treatment completed—right side.

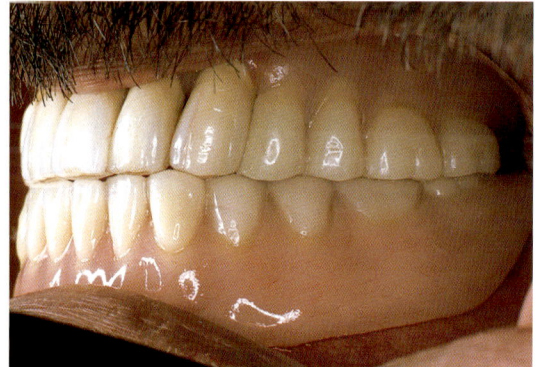

Figure 6.23

Treatment completed—left side.

restorations. The metal copings were fitted in the mouth, connected with Duralay, soldered and rechecked in the mouth after soldering. Elastomeric master impressions were then made of each jaw in order to fabricate the removable frameworks for the prostheses. The frameworks were fitted, and a facebow index together with a centric relation record at the vertical dimension of occlusion was made. The models were mounted on a Hanau articulator. The denture teeth were set up on the acrylic resin denture bases and checked clinically

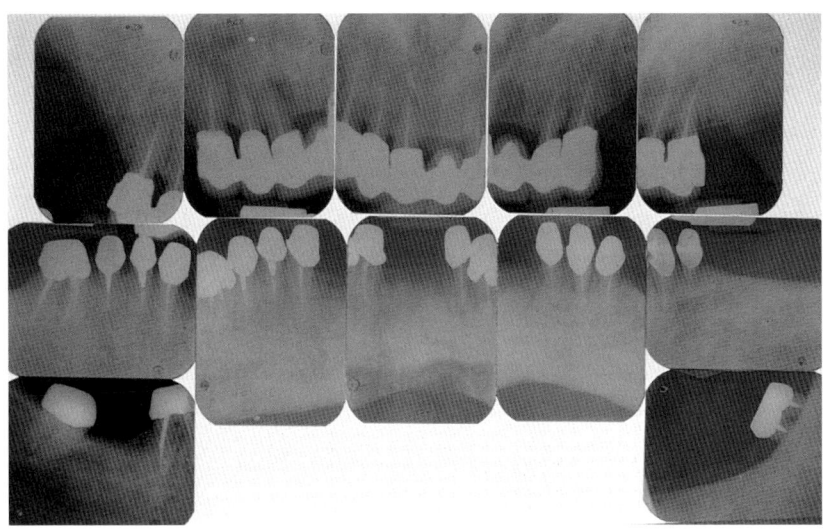

Figure 6.24

Radiographs of patient—post-treatment.

for function and esthetics. The removable maxillary partial denture and mandibular complete overdenture were processed. The restorations were then inserted and have been followed up since then with no deterioration (Figures 6.20–6.24).

SUMMARY

The patient presented with a severe case of advanced adult periodontitis, many missing teeth, crowding, mobility and fremitus of teeth, faulty restorations, and poor dietary habits. He was a clencher. He had difficulty in eating and was in pain. A compromise solution had to be found in this case because of the limited financial means available to the patient for his dental treatment. He also wanted to retain as many of his remaining teeth as possible. The solution consisted of eliminating the infection, orthodontic treatment to improve tooth position, changing his dietary pattern, and construction of a partial maxillary removable denture supported by a fixed anterior bridge and a complete mandibular overdenture on gold copings on the remaining teeth.

CASE DISCUSSION
AVINOAM YAFFE

This was a challenging patient, being effected both by caries and advanced periodontal disease complicated by loss of posterior support, aggravated by drifting and flaring of teeth. This case was treated by stretching the biological response of the patient to its maximum, allowing it to benefit from mechanical improvement by redirection of the forces to improve the crown-to-root ratio and creating a flat occlusion to minimize lateral forces. The continued success of this treatment will be dependent on the cooperation of the patient, by controlling his oral hygiene as well as his diet. Thus the overall prognosis of this case is guarded.

CASE DISCUSSION
HAROLD PREISKEL

Patients who seek professional help only when their dentition is in a terminal state pose particular difficulties. These problems are accentuated if the patient is unaware of the severity of the dental problem, eats a cariogenic diet, and has medical complications. In this instance, the need for antibiotic prophylaxsis dictated that as much work as possible be undertaken during each period of antibiotic cover to avoid unnecessary administration of the agent.

Very sensibly, disease control procedures were undertaken to begin with. Additional measures included changing dietary habits and fluoride rinses followed by a re-evaluation. Once the patient exhibited increased dental awareness, demonstrated cooperation, and the soft tissue showed a corresponding improvement, the stage could be set for planning the definitive treatment. This therapy included periodontal surgery, and the extrusion of a maxillary root to provide more tooth substance for the permanent restoration. The definitive treatment plan also included construction of an upper partial denture and a mandibular overdenture covering precious metal copings.

A mandibular overdenture opposing natural teeth could be vulnerable to the destabilizing influences of an irregular occlusal plane. Indeed, the planning and orientation of the occlusal plane is an important part of the therapy and this seems to have been undertaken. The planning of the treatment appears to have been thought out in depth and well executed. It is the long term that gives rise for concern, although the overdenture approach provides considerable versatility of treatment options should the patient's home care become less enthusiastic. The patient, like many who present with a dentition in a terminal state, would not usually have been in such a situation if their home care had been meticulous and they had always sought regular professional help. The prospect of losing all the teeth certainly concentrates the mind, but once the danger has passed the danger of old habits reverting is never far away. The overdenture, by its very nature, covers root surfaces and gingivae as well as the mucosa, so that plaque control is essential for long-term success. I was therefore happy to read of the outcome of this therapy, particularly the follow-ups that were taken.

PATIENT 7   ADVANCED PERIODONTITIS IN THE RELATIVELY YOUNG

Treatment by Rodica Greenberg

THE PATIENT

The patient, a 36-year-old computer engineer, presented himself for examination, consultation, and treatment with the following complaints (Figures 7.1 and 7.2)

'My mouth is uncomfortable.'
'My gums bleed all the time.'
'The spaces between my teeth are getting bigger.'
'My teeth are loose.'
'Flies fly into my mouth and I can't do anything about it because I can't close my lips together.'

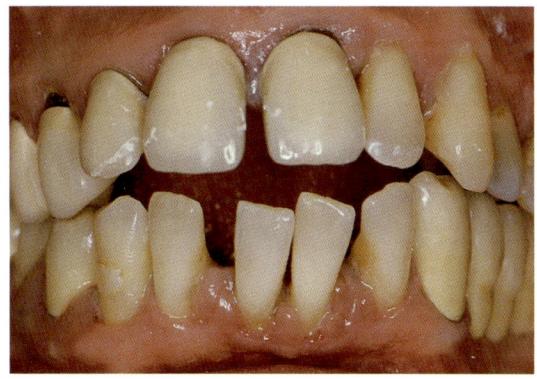

Figure 7.1

Anterior teeth—labial view.

PAST MEDICAL HISTORY

Neurofibromatosis, type 2 (bilateral acoustic neuromas), originally treated with phenytoin, but about 2 weeks after starting treatment, the medication was changed to Valporal (valproic acid) due to the gingival overgrowth caused by the phenytoin. Due to the neurofibromatosis there was paresthesia of the left facial nerve, which made it impossible for the patient to close his mouth and his left eye, and also caused problems for him in controlling his tongue.

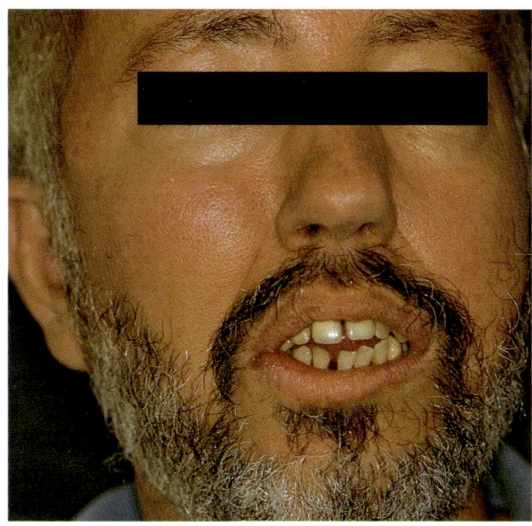

Figure 7.2

Face—frontal view.

Past dental history

The existing prostheses were completed about 7 years previously, but the patient could not remember the exact dates.

EXTRA-ORAL EXAMINATION
(Figure 7.2)

- Facial asymmetry
- Slightly convex profile
- Normally functioning muscles of mastication
- Normal temporomandibular joints
- Maximum opening 48 mm
- Incompetent lips

INTRA-ORAL AND FULL-MOUTH PERIAPICAL RADIOGRAPH EXAMINATION (Figures 7.1, 7.3–7.5)

- Angle class I
- Open bite minus 4.0 mm (Figure 7.1)
- Overjet minus 4.0 mm
- Interocclusal rest space 3.0 mm
- Maximum opening between the incisors 48 mm
- Mobility class 1–2 on the maxillary anterior teeth
- Class 2 mobility of the mandibular anterior teeth
- Discrepancy between centric occlusion (IC) and centric relation (CR) 0.5 mm

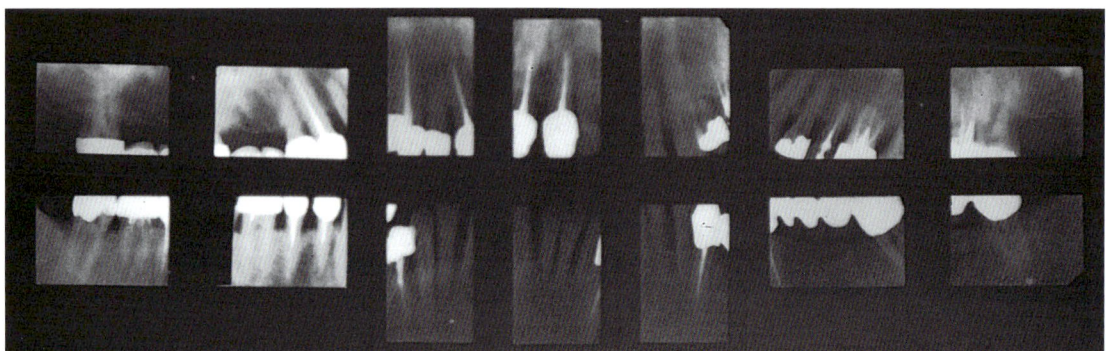

Figure 7.3

Radiographs of maxilla and mandible—pre-treatment.

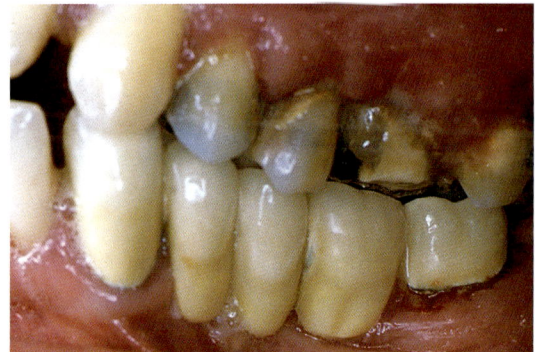

Figure 7.4

Left side—pre-treatment.

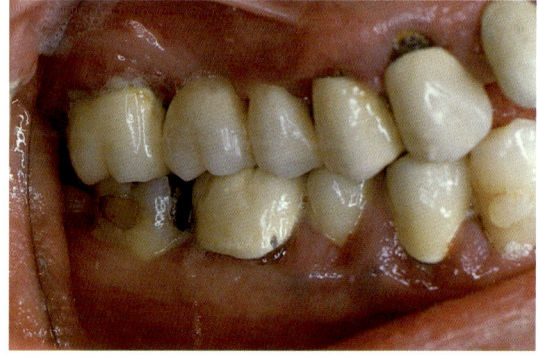

Figure 7.5

Right side—pre-treatment.

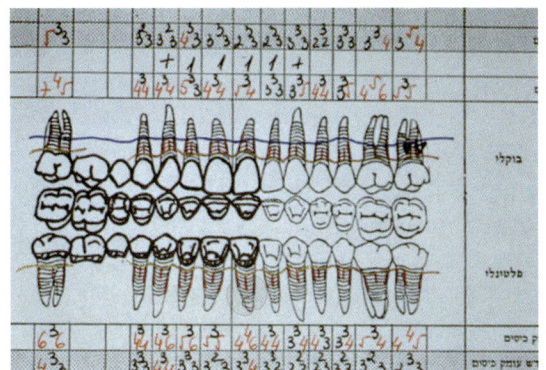

Figure 7.6

Periodontal chart—maxilla.

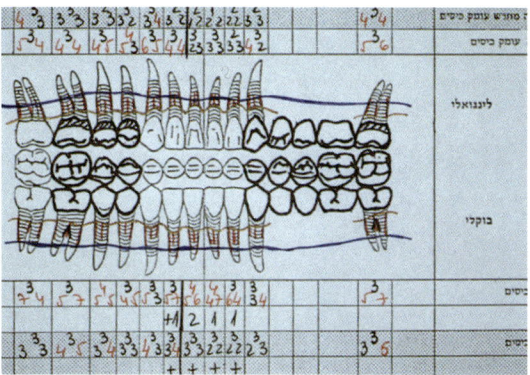

Figure 7.7

Periodontal chart—mandible.

Periodontal examination (Figures 7.6 and 7.7) revealed probing depths of up to 7.0 mm on most of the remaining teeth, with bleeding of the gingiva on probing on most of the teeth, with the condition being more severe in the maxilla than the mandible:

- Missing teeth:

$$\begin{array}{c|c} 8\,6\,5 & 8 \\ \hline 8 & 4\,5\,6\,7 \end{array}$$

- Caries
- Low maxillary sinuses
- 60% bone loss around some teeth
- Anterior spacing

INDIVIDUAL TOOTH PROGNOSIS

- Hopeless: none
- Poor:

$$\begin{array}{c|c} 7\,5\,3\,2\,1 & 1\,2\,3 \\ \hline 1 & 1 \end{array}$$

- Fair: the remaining teeth
- Good: none

DIAGNOSIS

- Advanced adult type periodontitis
- Missing teeth

- Reduced posterior occlusal support
- Flaring of anterior teeth
- Caries
- Faulty restorations
- Poor esthetics
- Open bite
- Neurofibromatosis type 2

ABOUT THE PATIENT

The patient understood the severity of his dental condition but was highly motivated as he thought that the dental treatment would enable him to be able to close his mouth. However, he absolutely refused to consider a removable prosthesis.

POTENTIAL TREATMENT PROBLEMS

- Advanced periodontitis and poor oral hygiene, accompanied by many missing teeth
- Existing restorations were faulty
- Open anterior bite
- Due to facial nerve damage, the patient could not close his lips or eyelids. During swallowing, his tongue moved anteriorly to close the space, putting pressure on

the anterior teeth and causing the food bolus to go down into the esophagus before it had been triturated completely. Consequently, the patient was constantly dripping liquids from the sides of his mouth

- His difficulty in hearing (left side) and seeing (right side) made it more difficult to teach him proper oral hygiene

TREATMENT ALTERNATIVES

Maxilla:

- Fixed anterior partial prosthesis and a removable posterior partial prosthesis, supported by implants
- Fixed anterior partial prosthesis and a removable posterior partial prosthesis, supported by the anterior fixed prosthesis with either clasps and rests, or attachments
- Fixed maxillary restoration as a shortened arch with only a premolar occlusion on the left side
- Fixed maxillary restoration with a weak terminal abutment on the right side

Mandible:

- Fixed anterior partial prosthesis with removable tooth supported posterior partial prosthesis
- Fixed tooth and implant supported partial prosthesis
- Fixed partial prosthesis with the cuspid as the terminal abutment on the left side
- Fixed mandibular restoration with a weak terminal abutment on the left side

TREATMENT PLAN

Following initial preparation, including oral hygiene instruction, scaling and root planing, and a periodontal re-evaluation, a final treatment plan was then chosen which consisted of selective grinding and orthodontic treatment to improve the occlusal relationship and close the existing spaces between the anterior teeth. This would improve the anterior tooth position and enable these teeth to participate in vertical dimension support. Following the orthodontic treatment a provisional full arch fixed maxillary and mandibular prostheses would be done and carefully followed over a period of at least 6 months to ascertain the ability of the abutment teeth to support the fixed prostheses. If this phase was successful, complete arch maxillary and mandibular fixed prostheses would be constructed.

TREATMENT

Initial preparation included scaling, curettage, root planing, and oral hygiene instruction. At the end of this stage, an obvious improvement in the soft tissue could be discerned. At this time a periodontal re-evaluation was done and it was observed that the pockets depths had greatly diminished and that the bleeding on probing had disappeared.

The orthodontic phase of treatment was then started using elastics to retract the mandibular and maxillary anterior teeth (Figure 7.8) and close the spaces. This was done in order to achieve better esthetics and move the teeth into a better position in the alveolar bone for occlusal support and with the intent to prepare the site for future development should implants be needed.

When the orthodontic stage was successfully completed (Figure 7.9), the supporting teeth were prepared and temporary restorations were placed (Figure 7.10). Periodontal evaluation was again

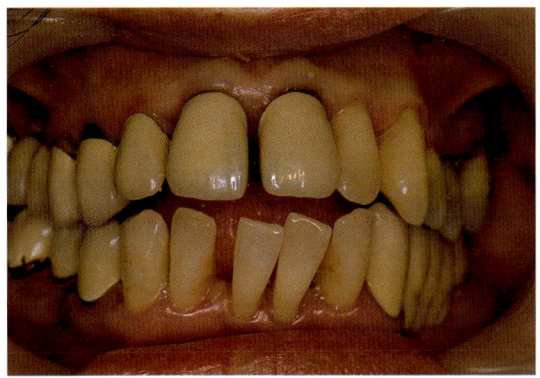

Figure 7.8

Teeth before orthodontic treatment.

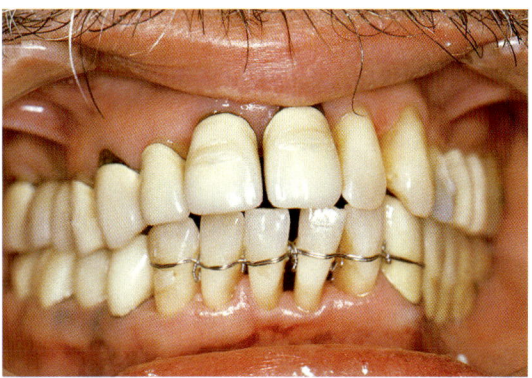

Figure 7.9

Teeth after orthodontic treatment.

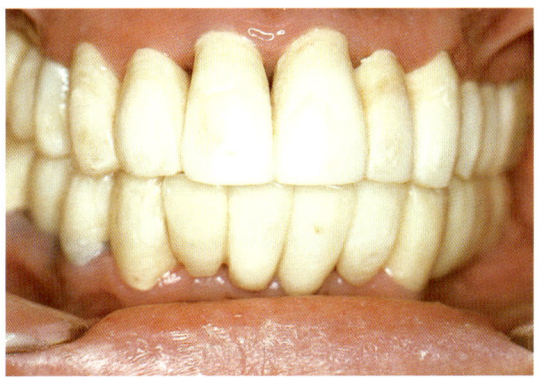

Figure 7.10

Transitional crowns.

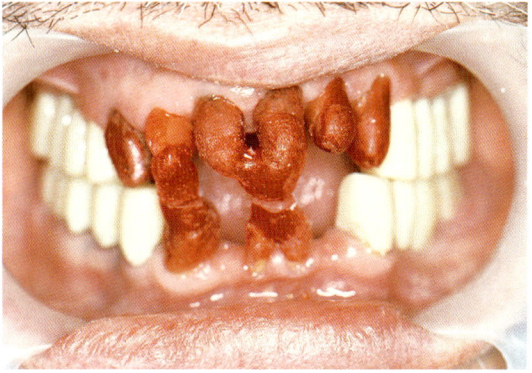

Figure 7.11

Fitting of Duralay copings.

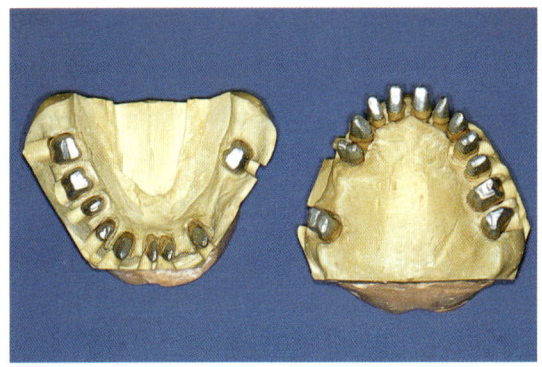

Figure 7.12

Working models.

performed and disclosed that the probing depths were less than 3.0 mm in all areas.

Copper band elastomeric impressions were then taken of all the prepared teeth and Duralay copings were made. These copings were used to record centric relation at the vertical dimension of the temporary restorations (Figure 7.11), and for the final impression for the working die model (Figure 7.12). These models were mounted on a semi-adjustable articulator (Hanau) utilizing a facebow registration, and centric records were taken at the vertical dimension

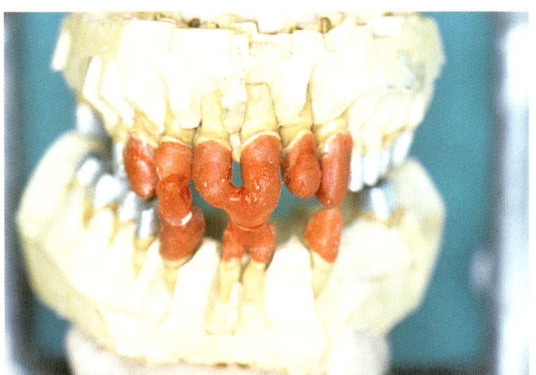

Figure 7.13

Working models mounted on Hanau articulator.

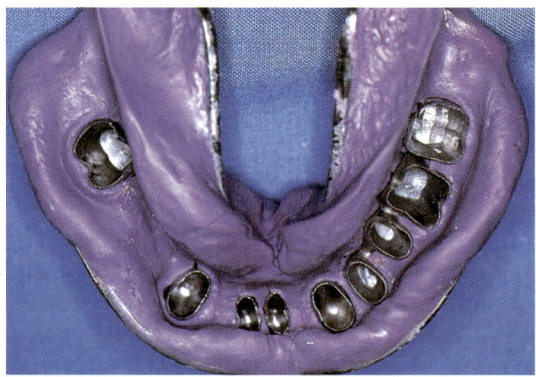

Figure 7.14

Impression of soldered castings for tissue detail—mandible.

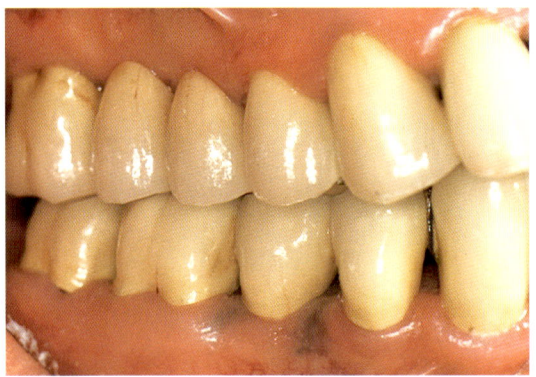

Figure 7.15

Treatment completed—right side.

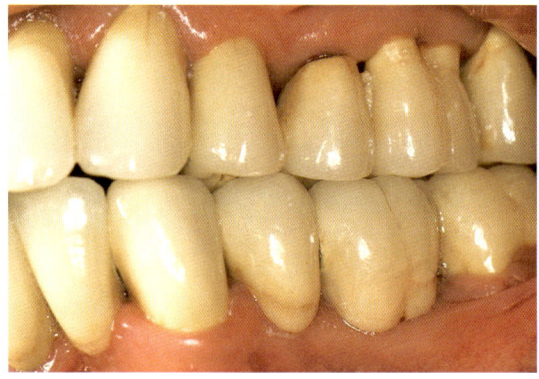

Figure 7.16

Treatment completed—left side.

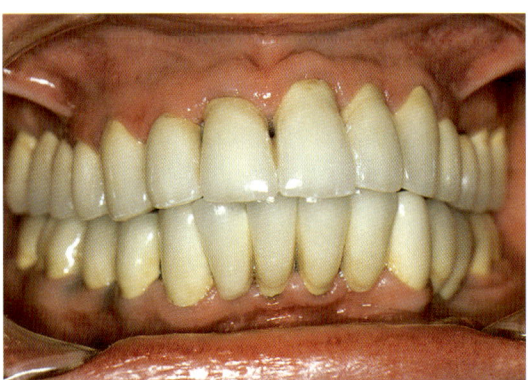

Figure 7.17

Treatment completed—anterior view.

of occlusion utilizing Duralay with a Neylon technique (Figure 7.13). The metal copings were then fitted and soldered and, after try-in of the soldered metal framework and centric records had been made, another elastomeric impression was done for the final tissue detail model (Figure 7.14). The porcelain was baked and the occlusion checked at the biscuit bake stage in the mouth and all adjustments needed were then made. The porcelain was then glazed and the crowns and bridges were cemented with Temp-Bond. The crowns and bridges were then cemented with zinc oxyphosphate cement for permanent cementation in 1995 (Figures 7.15–7.17).

The patient has been returning for follow-up and maintenance twice a year since then.

SUMMARY

The patient, a 36-year-old computer engineer, came to the Graduate Prosthodontics Clinic of the Hebrew University Dental School of Medicine for treatment. He presented with a severe problem of advanced adult periodontitis. He had many missing teeth, much alveolar bone loss around the remaining teeth, and faulty restorations in both jaws. There was considerable bone resorption and probing of up to 7.0 mm His fixed restorations were inadequate. There was mobility and fremitus in the maxillary anterior teeth and mobility of the mandibular anterior teeth. His dental condition was further complicated by his medical condition (neurofibromatosis type 2), which rendered him unable to close his mouth properly, and caused trauma to the anterior teeth during swallowing. With orthodontic and periodontal treatment accompanied by occlusal therapy, the patient received fixed partial prostheses that provided him with a physiological occlusion at the optimum vertical dimension of occlusion for his periodontal condition.

CASE DISCUSSION
AVINOAM YAFFE

The patient presented himself for treatment suffering from advanced periodontitis aggravated by the loss of many teeth and complicated by an anterior open bite. The treatment goals were to restore esthetic function and give the patient a long-lasting physiologic occlusion. By meticulous oral hygiene, scaling and root planing, his periodontal condition was greatly improved. Then by means of orthodontic treatment that moved the teeth lingually, and selective grinding to reduce the open bite, the esthetic and functional goals were achieved. In reducing the vertical dimension, the crown-to-root ratio of the posterior teeth (which were periodontally involved) was improved. Reasonable overjet and overbite were also achieved, gaining mutual protection of the anterior teeth during jaw movements. These procedures enabled us to achieve an esthetic and physiological occlusal scheme that will last for many years.

CASE DISCUSSION
HAROLD PREISKEL

Relatively young patients with advanced periodontal disease present challenging problems. Very sensibly, the initial treatment was not side tracked from attention to disease control procedures until a satisfactory outcome of this aspect of the treatment had been assured. Whether or not an active tongue thrust was contributing to the initial breakdown of the arcade is not mentioned, but it appears that there were no speech difficulties when the teeth were retracted into a more ideal relationship. I assume that the rebuilt occlusion provided the patient with a competent lip seal, which was lacking when he first attended for therapy. Providing some anterior guidance was an added bonus. However, the maintenance of the restorations, particularly the lower anterior fixed prosthesis, will require particular care on the part of the patient. An excellent result appears to have been obtained.

PATIENT 8   ADVANCED ADULT PERIODONTITIS

Treatment by Eyal Tarazi

THE PATIENT

The patient, a 64-year-old radiologist and a recent immigrant, came to the Graduate Prosthodontics Clinic for dental treatment (Figure 8.1). His chief complaints were:

'I am extremely sensitive to hot and cold foods on the lower left side.'
'Due to my missing teeth, I have difficulty eating on the right side.'
'Usually I only eat soft food.'
'Food packs underneath my bridge.'

PAST MEDICAL HISTORY

The patient was healthy, and did not take any medication. He had no known sensitivity or allergy to food or medications. About 40 years ago, he suffered from hepatitis A.

PAST DENTAL HISTORY

His last dental treatment was 7 years previously. His upper anterior teeth were restored 15 years previously. The mandible was treated about 18 years previously. As for his esthetic appearance, he stated, 'It's hard to explain, but because it's been like this for a long time, I feel that it's natural.'

EXTRA-ORAL EXAMINATION
(Figure 8.2)

- Asymmetrical face, with lower third being greater than the middle third

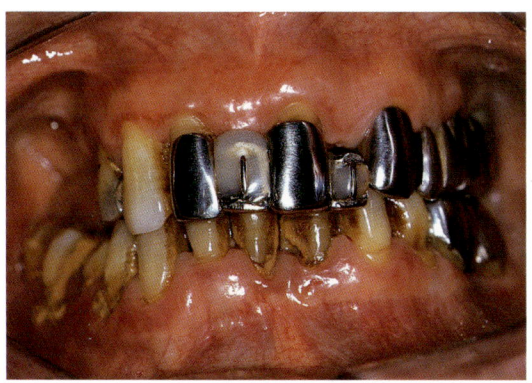

Figure 8.1

Anterior teeth—labial view.

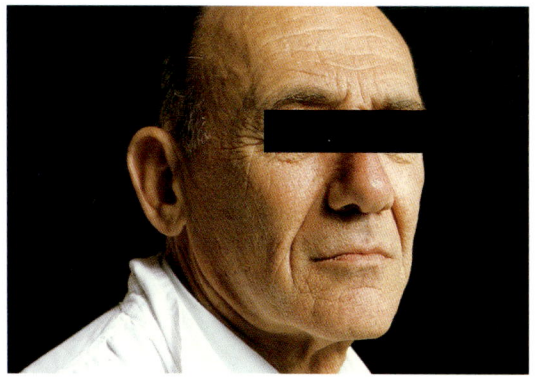

Figure 8.2

Face—frontal view.

- Long chin and prominent nose, in profile
- He 'smiled' with his lips closed
- Tenderness of the left masseter muscle during palpation
- Maximum opening of 52 mm, with deviation to the left on opening
- Mandibular motions within normal limits

INTRA-ORAL AND FULL-MOUTH PERIAPICAL RADIOGRAPH EXAMINATION

Maxilla (Figures 8.3, 8.5 and 8.6):

- Wide parabolic arch
- Deviation of the mid-palatal suture to the right side
- Narrowed space for the right central incisor
- Left first premolar pontic restored by two units
- Right first premolar tilted mesially and in close proximity to the canine
- Flat palate and residual ridges
- Restorations: fixed all metal partial prosthesis:

$$\frac{2\text{-}X \mid 1\text{-}X\text{-}3\text{-}X\text{-}X\text{-}5\text{-}X\text{-}X\text{-}8}{}$$

Mandible (Figures 8.4–8.6):

- Wide parabolic arch
- Crowding on the left side
- Spacing in the right side because of missing teeth
- Distal tilting of the right canine and lateral
- Rotations, overlapping and tooth abrasion
- High floor of the mouth
- Retained deciduous root instead of right second premolar
- Caries:

$$\frac{}{\mid 8}$$

- Restorations: fixed all metal (gold) partial prosthesis:

$$\frac{}{\mid 5\text{-}X\text{-}7}$$

Occlusal examination revealed that the patient was Angle classification class II occlusion on the right side and class I occlusion on the left side. The interocclusal rest space was 3–4 mm. Overjet was 3–5 mm and overbite was 4–6 mm. There was a 1.0 mm hit and slide from centric relation to centric occlusion anteriorly and vertically. The mandibular anterior segment showed overeruption.

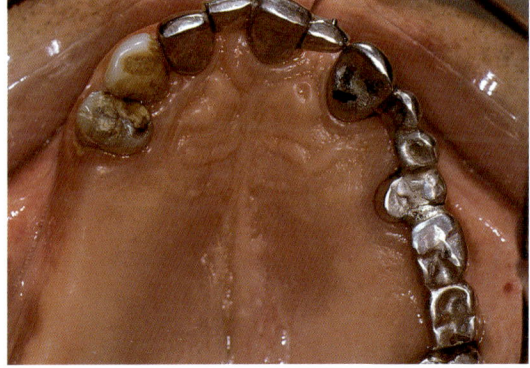

Figure 8.3

Maxillary arch—palatal view.

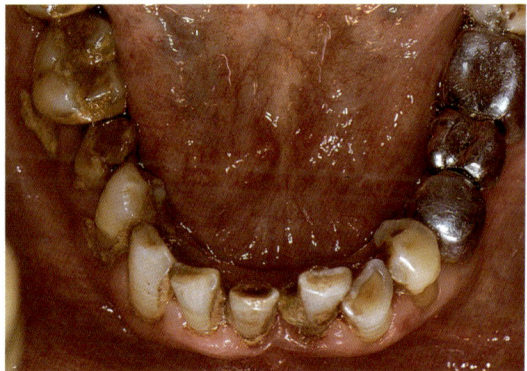

Figure 8.4

Mandibular arch—lingual view.

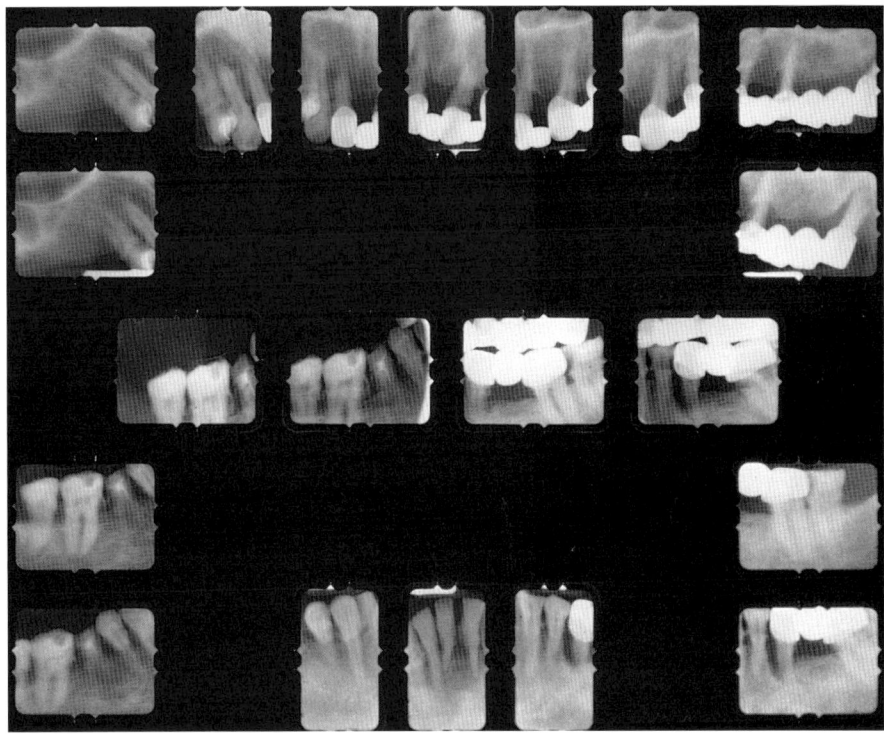

Figure 8.5

Radiographs of maxilla and mandible, pre-treatment.

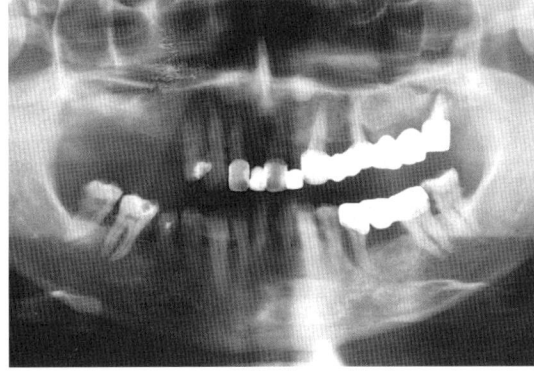

Figure 8.6

Panoramic radiograph—pre-treatment.

Lateral jaw movements were guided by the canine and premolar on the left side, and by the canine with incisal contacts on the right side. Protrusive movements were guided by the canines and the incisors. No non-working side interference was noted.

Fremitus:

- Maxillary cuspids—grade II
- Maxillary left central incisor—grade III
- Left second premolar—grade III
- Left third molar—grade III

Periodontal examination (Figures 8.7–8.12) revealed large amounts of calculus and plaque, probing depths of up to 10.0 mm on the maxillary teeth and up to 8.0 mm on the mandibular teeth, with bleeding of the gingival tissues on probing on most of the teeth. There was gingival recession around almost all of the teeth.

The maxillary left third molar had class 2 furcation on the mesial and distal. The mandibular left second and third molars, and the right first molar all had class 1 furcation involvements.

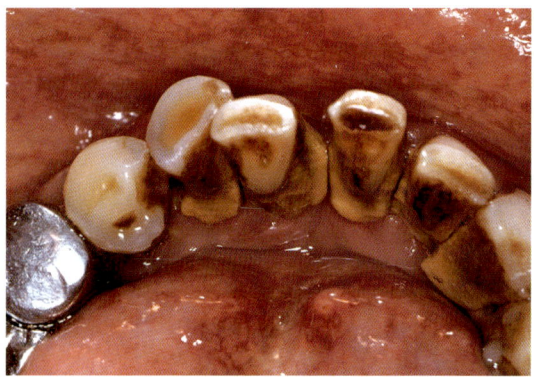

Figure 8.7

Mandibular anterior teeth—lingual view, showing calculus accumulation.

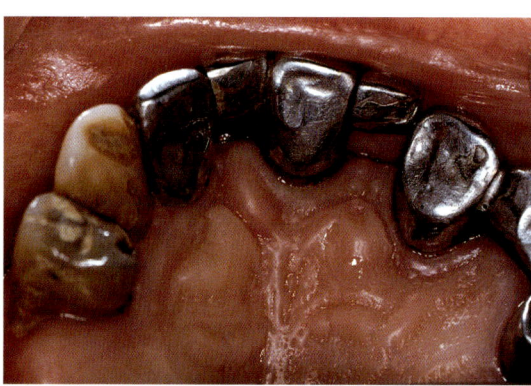

Figure 8.8

Maxillary anterior teeth showing periodontal inflammation.

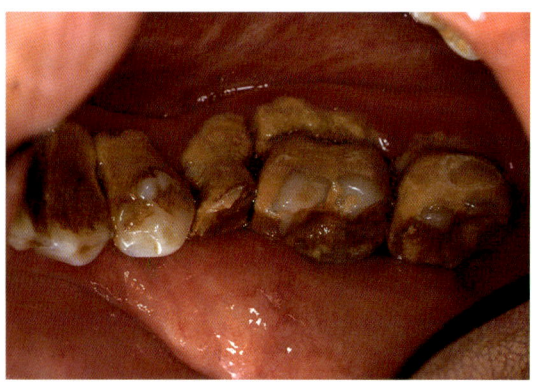

Figure 8.9

Mandibular right posterior teeth showing calculus accumulation.

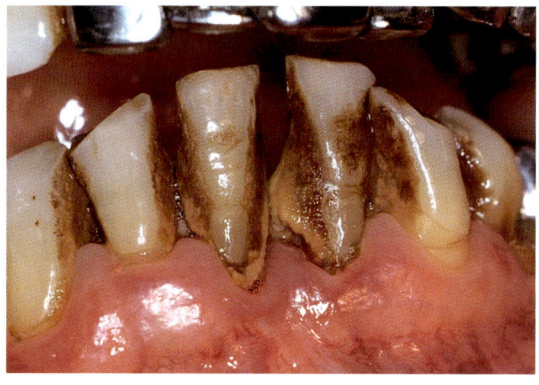

Figure 8.10

Mandibular anterior teeth—labial view, showing calculus accumulation.

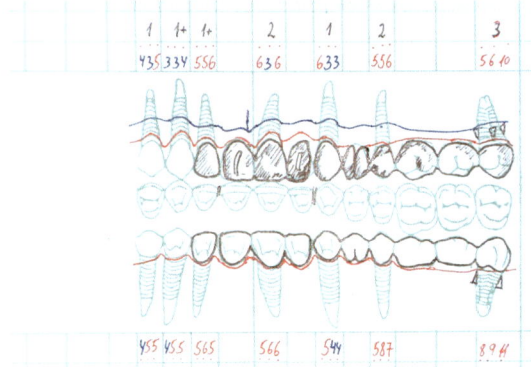

Figure 8.11

Periodontal chart—maxilla, re-evaluation.

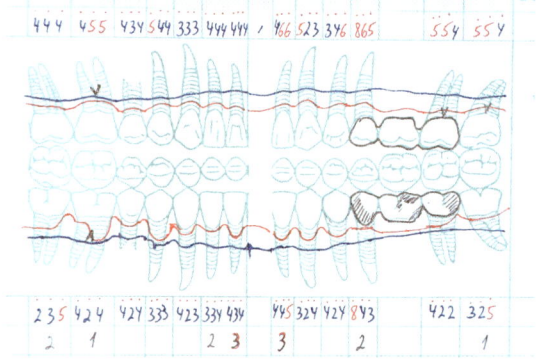

Figure 8.12

Periodontal chart—mandible, re-evaluation.

DIAGNOSIS

- Advanced adult type periodontitis
- Multiple defective restorations
- Carious lesions and secondary caries
- Abrasion and abfraction
- Missing teeth—partially edentulous arches
- Deep bite
- Compromised posterior occlusion
- Decreased vertical dimension of occlusion
- Poor occlusal plane
- Secondary occlusal trauma
- Acute pulpitis—lower left third molar
- Chronic apical periodontitis—upper left molar
- Esthetic impairment (although it did not appear to effect the patient)

ABOUT THE PATIENT

He was a highly motivated immigrant who wanted to improve his oral condition, and was highly disciplined and very patient. His expectations were to improve his oral condition by all means, and despite his poor financial condition, he insisted on a fixed oral rehabilitation. He had a very sensitive gag reflex. Initial language problems were later surmounted.

EMERGENCY TREATMENT PLAN

- Control of acute conditions
- Endodontic therapy—lower third molar
- Extraction of the upper left third molar

TREATMENT PLAN

PHASE 1: INITIAL PREPARATION

- Initial periodontal therapy
- Oral hygiene instruction

- Scaling and root planing
- Caries excavation
- Occlusal adjustment by selective grinding to reduce occlusal trauma

RE-EVALUATION I

PHASE 2: TREATMENT PLAN

- Replacement of inadequate restorations by provisional restorations
- Further elimination of occlusal trauma by splinting and stabilization with provisional restorations
- Re-establishment of an acceptable vertical dimension of occlusion, and a physiologic occlusal plane
- Creation of anterior contacts by the use of a lingual platform

RE-EVALUATION II

PHASE 3: TREATMENT PLAN

- Adjunctive orthodontics—forced eruption of the upper right premolar, to eliminate the deep osseous deformity
- Insertion of two implants on each side of the maxilla

PHASE 4: TREATMENT PLAN

Provisional restorations.

PHASE 5: TREATMENT PLAN

Prosthetic phase.

PHASE 6: TREATMENT PLAN

Recall and maintenance.

TREATMENT

Initial treatment consisted of scaling, curettage, oral hygiene instruction, and extraction of the third left maxillary molar. This phase of treatment took almost 6 months due to communication problems, until the patient was able to improve his oral hygiene to the extent that the treatment could continue (Figure 8.13). The left second mandibular premolar was also extracted. Root canal therapy was carried out on the second and third left mandibular molars, and the right

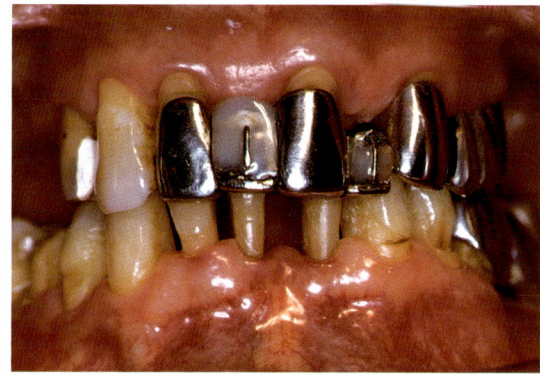

Figure 8.13

Anterior teeth after transitional restorations.

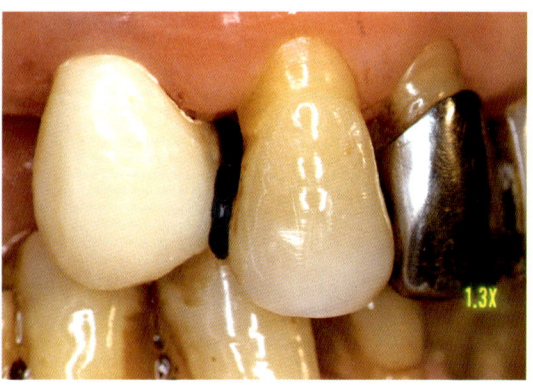

Figure 8.14

Maxillary canine and first premolar after minor orthodontic tooth movement.

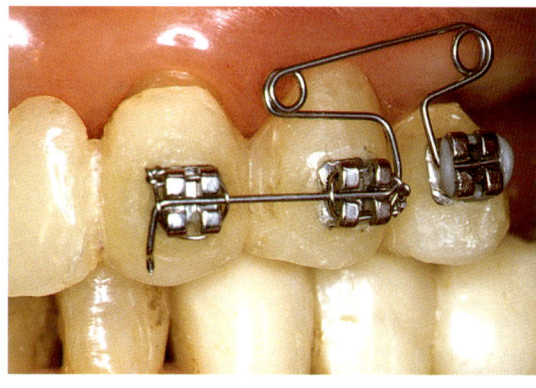

Figure 8.15

Orthodontic treatment to extrude maxillary left second premolar.

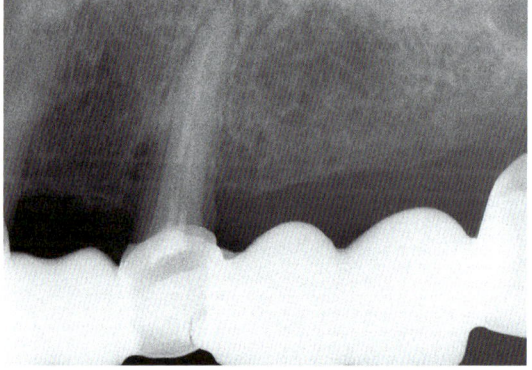

Figure 8.16

Radiograph before extrusion of maxillary left second premolar.

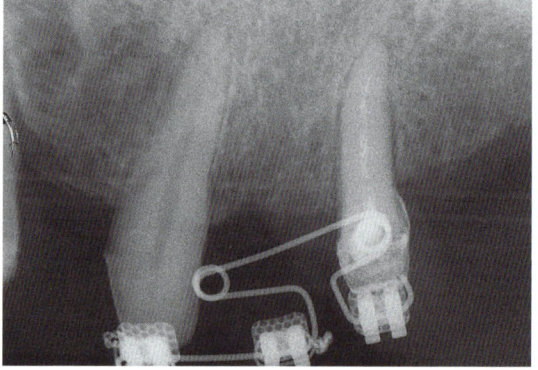

Figure 8.17

Radiograph after extrusion of maxillary left second premolar, showing accompanying bone.

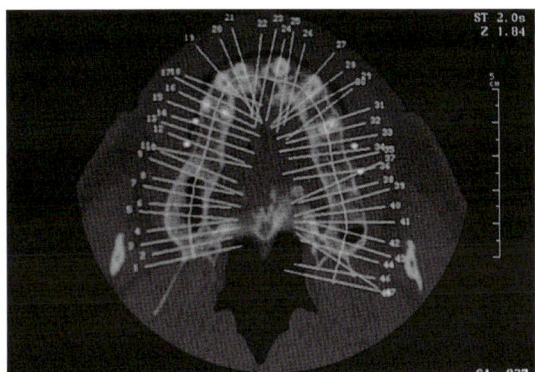

Figure 8.18

CT radiograph of maxilla for implant placement.

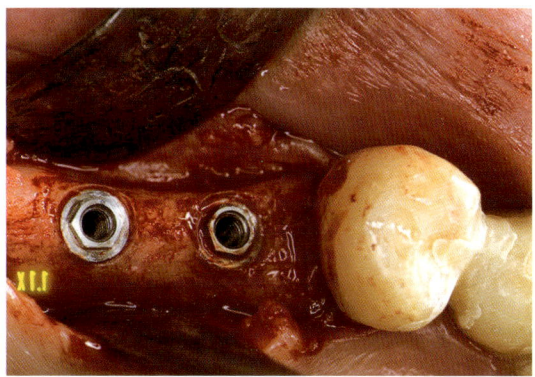

Figure 8.19

Implants—mandible left posterior region.

first maxillary premolar. When that stage was completed, minor orthodontic treatment was undertaken to open up root proximity between the right first maxillary premolar and the right canine (Figure 8.14). At that stage all the remaining maxillary teeth and the mandibular teeth from the left third molar to the right cuspid were prepared for provisional restorations. On the left side, the second maxillary premolar was forced to erupt. This was achieved by first separating the first and second premolars (Figure 8.15), and then by use of a coil spring. The second premolar was extruded along with the accompanying bone into position. This procedure eliminated the deep infrabony pocket around the second premolar (Figures 8.16 and 8.17).

Due to the severe gag reflex, and in spite of great effort on his part, the patient could not adapt to the provisional maxillary partial removable prosthesis that was made for him, and it was discarded. At that point it was decided that a maxillary removable prosthesis was not viable, and the treatment plan of fixed maxillary posterior prostheses on implants was chosen.

Computerized tomographic (CT) radiographs were made of the maxilla utilizing an acrylic stent with gutta percha points in the areas that required implants (Figure 8.18). The CT radiographs indicated that the bone type was class IV, and on the left side, the width of the bone was inadequate for implant placement. An autogenous bone graft from the chin was placed on the left side 6 months before the implant insertion. Two Brånmark implants (Nobel Biocare USA, Inc: Yorba Linda, CA) were then placed on each side in the maxilla in the premolar and molar areas (Figure 8.19). In the right side, self-tapping 15 and 13 mm long, 3.75 mm diameter implants were used, and on the left side self-tapping 12 mm long and 5.0 mm diameter implants were inserted.

New provisional transitional prostheses were then constructed after the uncovering of the implants. At that point, copper band elastomeric impressions were taken of all the prepared teeth and Duralay copings were made. These copings were used to record centric relation at the vertical dimension of the temporary restorations, together with the teeth position in the arch for the final impression for the working model. A polyether complete arch impression in a custom tray was made to pick up the Duralay and implant impression copings. The metal copings were then cast, fitted and soldered. After try-in of the soldered metal framework, another polyether impression was made for tissue detail for the final master model. These models were mounted on a semi-adjustable articulator (Hanau) utilizing a facebow registration and centric records were taken at the vertical dimension of occlusion utilizing Duralay with a Neylon technique. The porcelain was baked and the occlusion checked at the biscuit bake stage in the mouth and all adjustments needed were then made. The porcelain was then glazed and the crowns and bridges were cemented with Temp-Bond on the prepared teeth for a period of 3 weeks. The implant-supported bridges were screwed in to the implants and were not attached to the natural teeth supported bridges. The crowns and bridges were then permanently cemented with zinc oxyphosphate cement for permanent cementation (Figures 8.20–8.29).

SUMMARY

The patient presented with various problems. Due to a language problem, communication was very difficult. Even though at the beginning the patient was very satisfied with his appearance, as the treatment continued, he became more and more involved in his treatment. The treatment was long and extensive, encompassing a long initial treatment due to the language barrier. Once the patient understood the importance of good oral hygiene, he collaborated and became an important accessory to his care. The treatment extended over more than a 2-year period, but both the patient and the dentist thought that the result justified their efforts.

CASE DISCUSSION
AVINOAM YAFFE

This 64-year-old-patient presented for treatment in the Graduate Prosthodontics clinic. He had advanced adult periodontitis which was complicated by missing teeth, decreased vertical dimension aggravated by deep bite and faulty restorations with midline deviation. All these findings demanded comprehensive integrated treatment planning that included orthodontic treatment for both periodontal and teeth alignment problems,

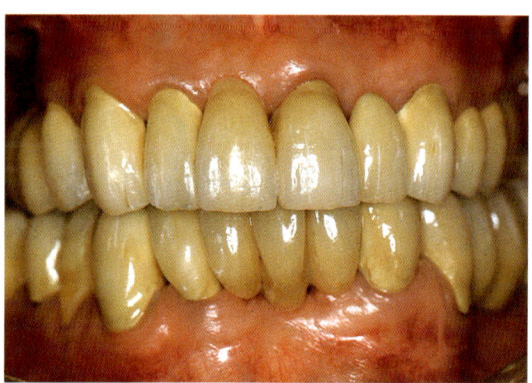

Figure 8.20

Treatment completed—permanent restorations, anterior view.

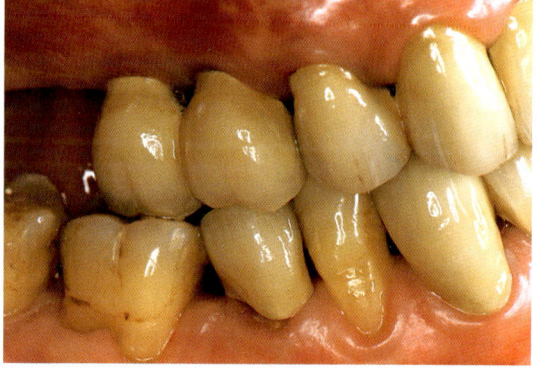

Figure 8.21

Treatment completed—permanent restorations, right side.

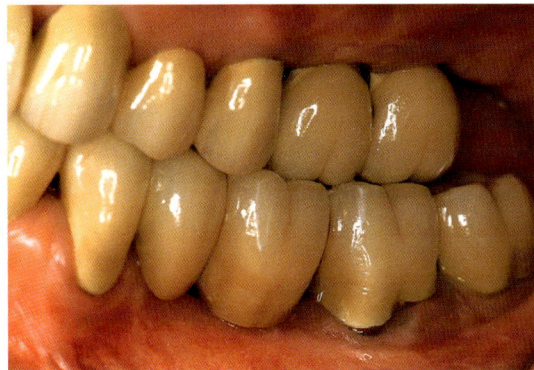

Figure 8.22

Treatment completed—permanent restorations, left side.

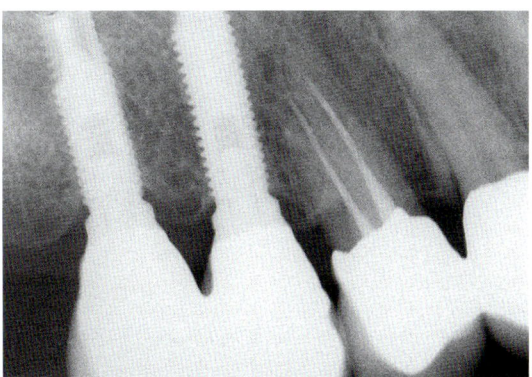

Figure 8.24

Post-treatment radiographs, maxillary right posterior area.

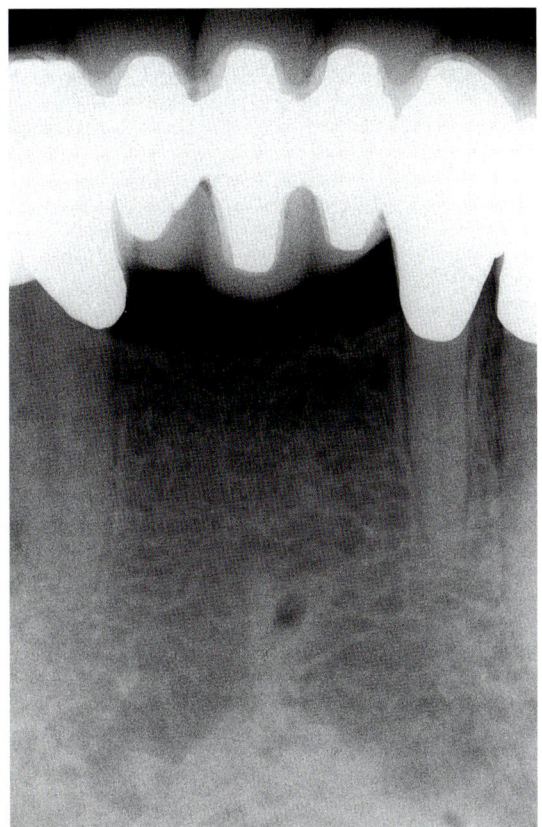

Figure 8.23

Post-treatment radiographs, anterior mandibular area.

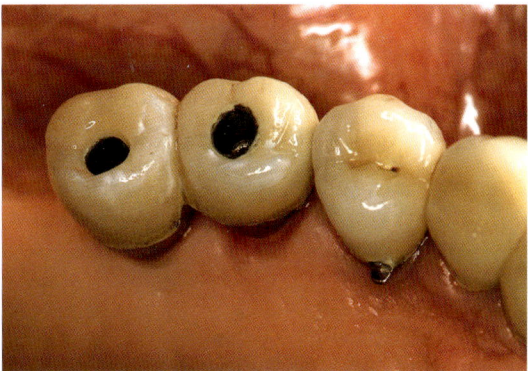

Figure 8.25

Maxillary right posterior area, clinical view.

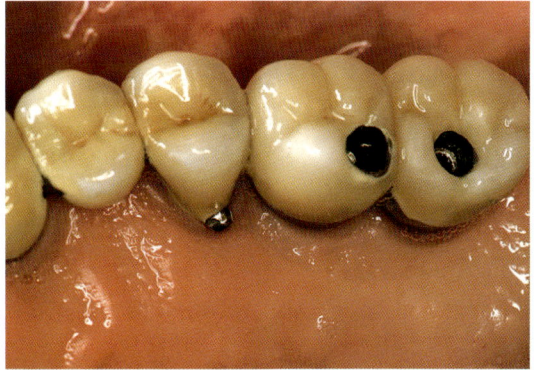

Figure 8.26

Maxillary left posterior area, clinical view.

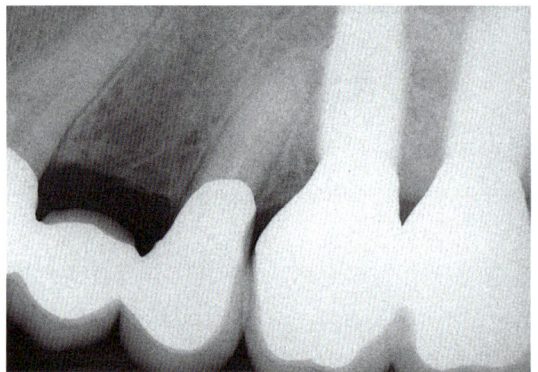

Figure 8.27

Post-treatment radiograph, maxillary left posterior area.

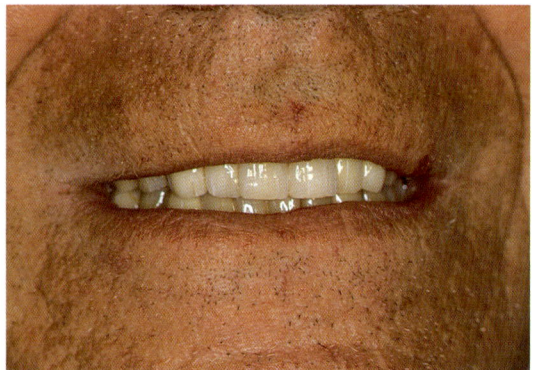

Figure 8.28

Patient's smile after treatment.

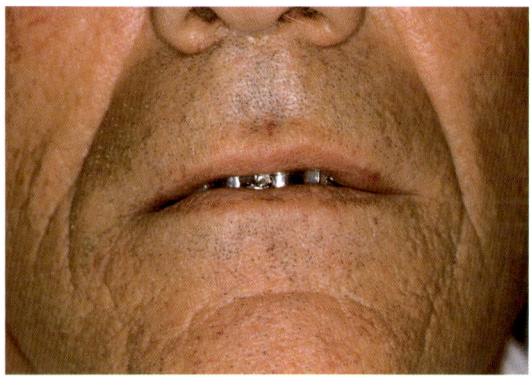

Figure 8.29

Patient's forced smile before treatment.

a new occlusal scheme to reduce lateral forces on remaining teeth, and reducing occlusal forces by including the anterior group of teeth in support. At the completion of treatment these objectives were met. The occlusal support was restored, a physiologic occlusal scheme was placed, and functional and esthetic demands were met, to both the patient's and the dentist's satisfaction.

CASE DISCUSSION
HAROLD PREISKEL

This highly educated patient received treatment involving a combination of skills and techniques that would stretch the capabilities of an experienced specialist, let alone a graduate working under supervision. A pronounced gag reflex and a language barrier that initially prevented direct communication were yet further obstacles to be overcome. The saga of this patient's therapy makes interesting reading, with the patient himself becoming ever increasingly involved in his own treatment and appreciating the impressive skills and care that he was receiving.

The gag reflex ruled out the use of a removable prosthesis that would have simplified the restoration of the maxillary arcade. Another, simpler, alternative might have been to have left a shortened arch in the new right posterior maxillary area. Instead I am sure that the patient benefited from the more complex but comprehensive restoration that was constructed and I trust that his ongoing maintenance will be continued with the same enthusiasm with which he participated in the initial treatment.

MODERATE TO ADVANCED ADULT PERIODONTITIS

Treatment by Eyal Tarazi

THE PATIENT

The patient, a 40-year-old woman employed as an administrator, presented herself for examination and consultation at the Hadassah Hebrew University School of Dental Medicine Graduate Prosthodontics Clinic with the following complaints:

'I have difficulty chewing.'
'I feel that my mouth is breaking down completely. I looked different when I was younger' (Figure 9.1).
'I also don't like the way I look' (Figure 9.2).

'I want a crown for the implant that I had done.'

PAST MEDICAL HISTORY

The patient's past medical history was non-contributory.

PAST DENTAL HISTORY

The patient had not seen a dentist for at least 7 years. A few months previously she had started periodontal treatment and had the mandibular right first molar extracted

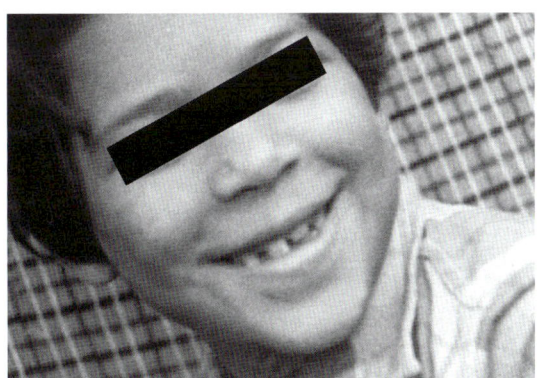

Figure 9.1

Picture of patient at age 10.

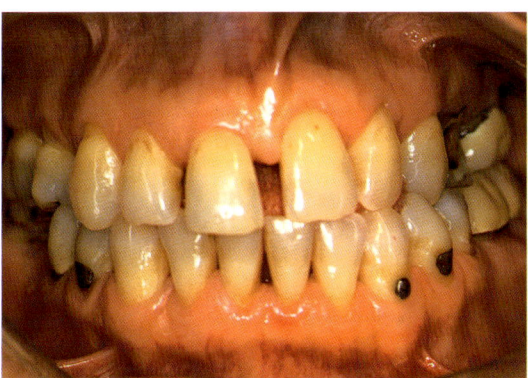

Figure 9.2

Frontal view of teeth, showing overbite.

and replaced by an implant. She was seeking a fixed restoration on the implant.

EXTRA-ORAL EXAMINATION
(Figure 9.3)

- Slight facial asymmetry
- Slightly convex profile
- Muscles and temporomandibular joints normal
- Maximum opening 46.0 mm with a 3.0 mm deviation to the left side on opening.

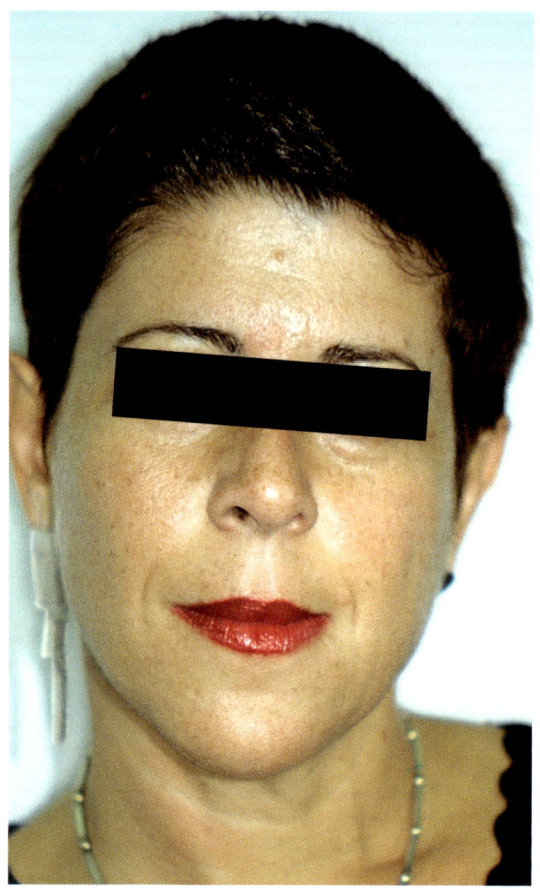

Figure 9.3

Frontal facial view.

- Smiling revealed spacing between the incisor teeth
- Due to slight drooping of the left upper lip, the patient exposed more of her teeth on the right side than the left side

INTRA-ORAL AND FULL-MOUTH PERIAPICAL RADIOGRAPH
EXAMINATION (Figures 9.4–9.8)

- Missing teeth (the maxillary missing premolars were congenitally missing):

$$\frac{8\ 7\ 5\ |\ 4\ 5\ 8}{8\ 6\ |\ 8}$$

- Caries
- 60% bone loss around the maxillary left first molar
- Spacing between the anterior teeth
- Maxillary right first premolar rotated 90°
- 8.0 mm implant in the first right mandibular area
- Mid-line discrepancy of the maxillary incisors

Occlusal examination revealed that the patient was Angle class 1, with an overbite of 2.0 mm and overjet of 3.0 mm. The interocclusal rest space was 3.0. Mobility class 1 and fremitus class I–II were found on the maxillary anterior teeth. A 0.5 mm discrepancy existed between centric occlusion (CO) and centric relation (CR). There was distal drifting of the maxillary canine teeth, with the left canine in the left first premolar position. In lateral movements there was cuspid protection and in protrusive movements there was anterior disclusion.

Periodontal examination (Figures 9.6 and 9.7) showed probing depths of up to 9.0 mm on the maxillary teeth and up to 4.0 mm on

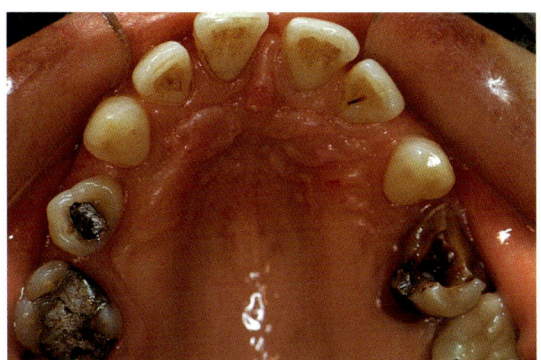

Figure 9.4

Maxillary arch.

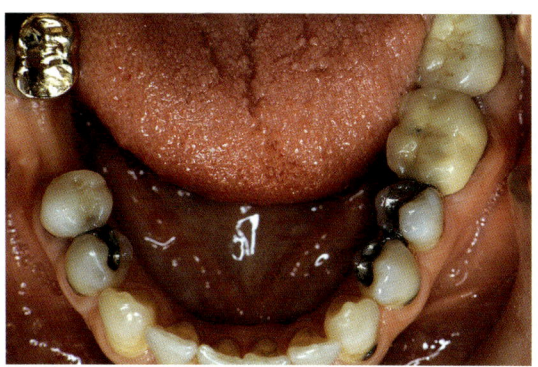

Figure 9.5

Mandibular arch.

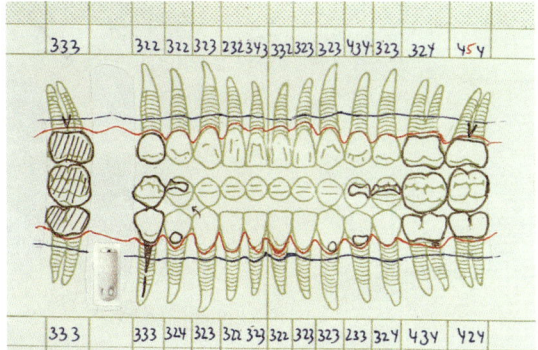

Figure 9.6

Periodontal chart—maxilla.

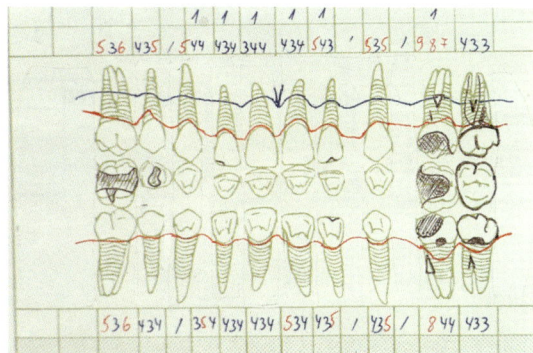

Figure 9.7

Periodontal chart—mandible.

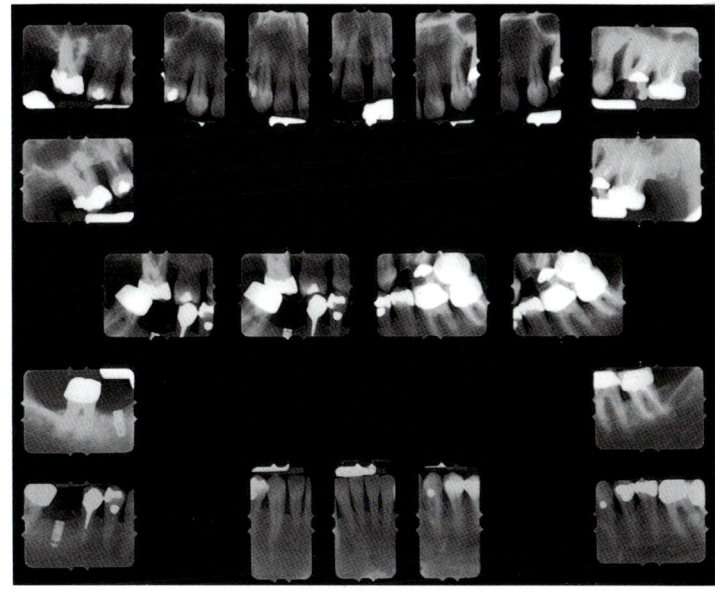

Figure 9.8

Radiographs of maxilla and mandible.

the mandibular teeth; bleeding on probing was more severe in the maxilla than in the mandible. The maxillary left first molar had class 2 furcation involvement on the buccal and mesial surfaces, and the left second molar had class 2 furcation involvement on the mesial and buccal surfaces.

INDIVIDUAL TOOTH PROGNOSIS

- Hopeless: none
- Poor: $\underline{\hspace{0.5cm}|6}$

- Fair: the rest of teeth

DIAGNOSIS

- Moderate with localized advanced adult periodontitis
- Congenital partial anodontia
- Missing teeth accompanied by loss of posterior occlusal support
- Faulty restorations
- Caries
- Reduced vertical dimension
- Flaring of maxillary anterior teeth
- Compromised esthetics
- Secondary occlusal trauma
- Perio-endo lesion on the maxillary first molar accompanied by probing depths of 9.0 mm

ABOUT THE PATIENT

The patient had come to the clinic complaining of difficulty in chewing and concern with her appearance. However, her main request was for a restoration of a single crown on the implant placed recently in her mandible. In order to address her complaints she was told that

a comprehensive treatment plan was necessary. After explanation and consultation, she accepted the suggested treatment plan. She was very cooperative in her dental treatment and was ready to do everything necessary in order to save her teeth.

POTENTIAL TREATMENT PROBLEMS

- Advanced periodontitis complicated by loss of teeth, aggravated by faulty restoration and flaring of anterior teeth
- There were large spaces between the maxillary anterior teeth due to the congenitally missing teeth and the subsequent drifting of her other teeth
- The existing restorations were inadequate
- The maxillary left first molar had a severe perio-endo lesion

TREATMENT GOALS

In order to attain a more favorable tooth position, orthodontic treatment would be required. Orthodontic treatment goals were:

- Close the anterior spaces
- Extrude teeth
- Level gingival margins
- Correct the misaligned center line of the maxillary teeth
- Open space posteriorly for fixed partial prostheses

A computerized digital picture was made, and different treatment options were then presented to the patient. The treatment plan chosen was to orthodontically close the anterior spaces, and leave the maxillary left cuspid in the premolar position. On the right side of the maxilla, it was decided to rotate the maxillary premolar in order to open space for an additional tooth to be placed.

TREATMENT ALTERNATIVES

Maxilla:

- Fixed posterior partial prostheses
- Fixed anterior partial prosthesis and a removable posterior partial prosthesis

Mandible:

- Fixed partial posterior prosthesis
- Fixed tooth and implant supported partial prosthesis

TREATMENT

Initial preparation included scaling, curettage, root planing and oral hygiene instruction. At the end of this stage, an obvious improvement in the soft tissue could be discerned. A periodontal re-evaluation was made and it was observed that the pocket depths had greatly diminished, while bleeding on probing had disappeared.

Endodontic therapy was undertaken on the palatal root of the maxillary left first molar; the mesial and disto-buccal tooth roots were resected. The maxillary second molar was also prepared and a transitional fixed acrylic resin restoration was made (Figure 9.9). In the mandible, the right second premolar and the right second molar were prepared for fixed restorations and a fixed transitional acrylic resin prosthesis was made (Figure 9.10). The implant in the right mandibular first molar area was left unexposed, in the bone.

Before the orthodontic phase of treatment started, a diagnostic set-up was made, and the anterior maxillary teeth were repositioned on a study model as a guide for the treatment goal (Figure 9.11).

Using fixed brackets and a labial arch wire, the maxillary incisor teeth were repositioned to their correct position (Figure 9.12) They were then retained in this position utilizing a modified Hawley appliance (Figures 9.13 and 9.14).

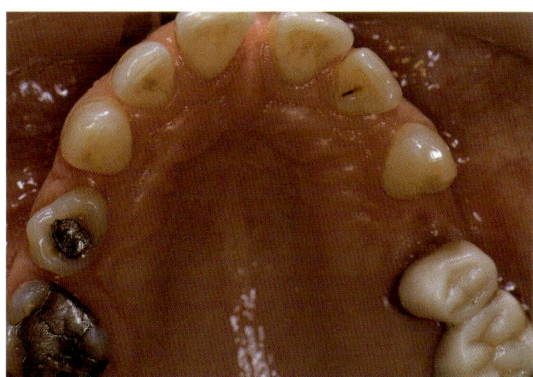

Figure 9.9

Maxilla showing transitional restorations.

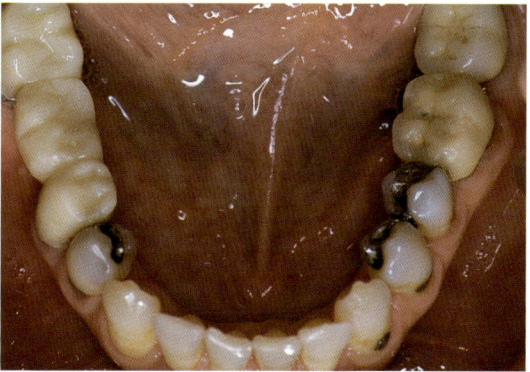

Figure 9.10

Mandible showing transitional restorations.

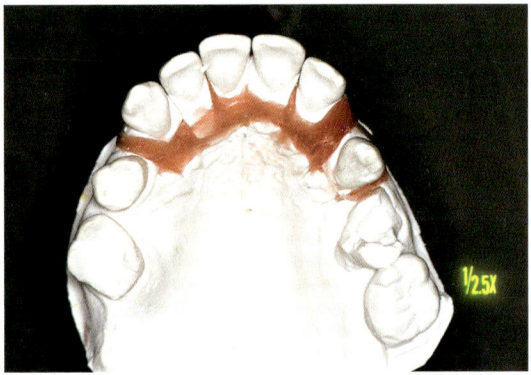

Figure 9.11

Palatal view of maxillary anterior teeth repositioned on model.

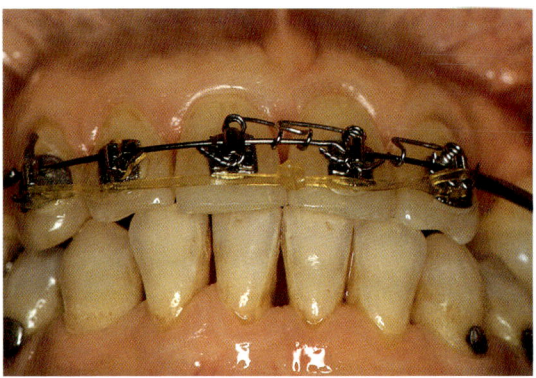

Figure 9.12

Orthodontic treatment—spaces closed.

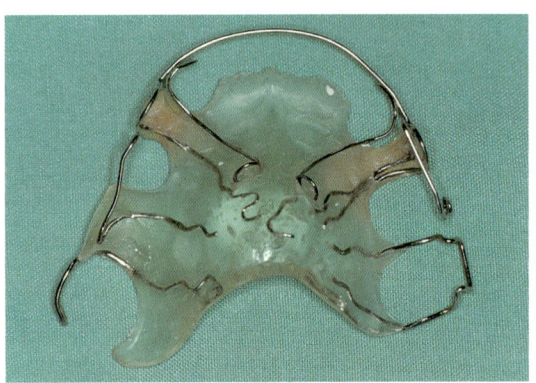

Figure 9.13

Modified Hawley appliance.

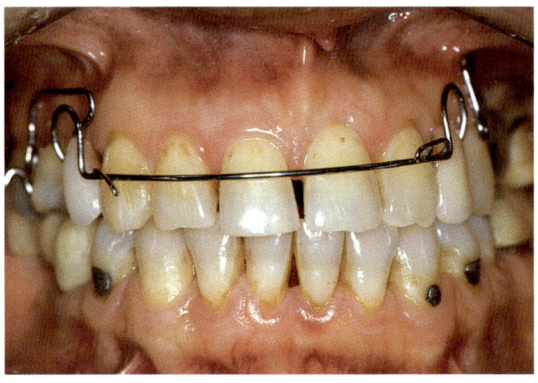

Figure 9.14

Modified Hawley appliance in mouth.

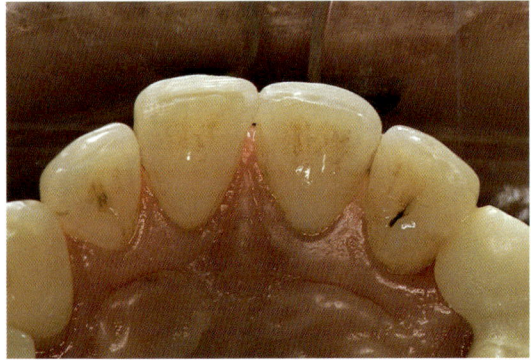

Figure 9.15

Maxilla—after closing of anterior spaces.

At completion of the orthodontic stage (Figure 9.15), two alternative treatment plans were considered. The first was to splint the anterior teeth with porcelain fused to metal crowns with precision attachments in the distal of the canines. This would enable the posterior splints to be fixed to the anterior splints. The second option was to use a lingual wire to splint the maxillary anterior teeth and have a free-standing posterior restoration.

The second option for retention of these teeth was chosen. The lingual surfaces of

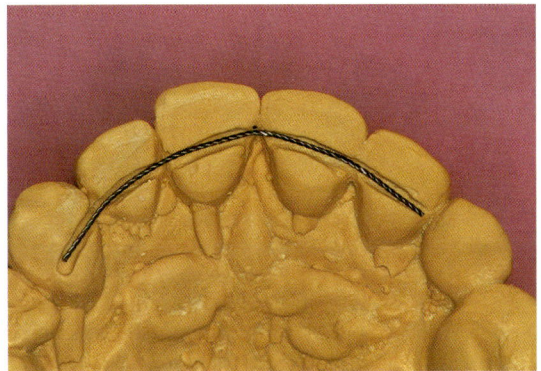

Figure 9.16

Wire splint for maxillary teeth retention (on model).

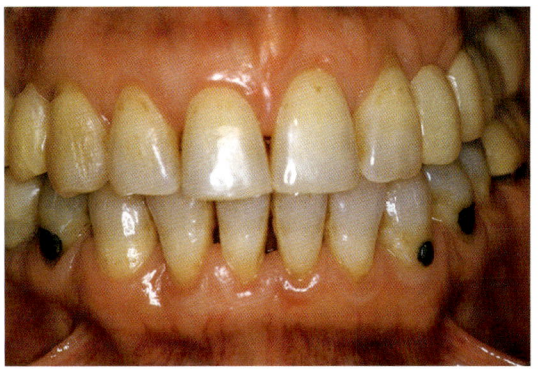

Figure 9.17

Transitional restorations—anterior view.

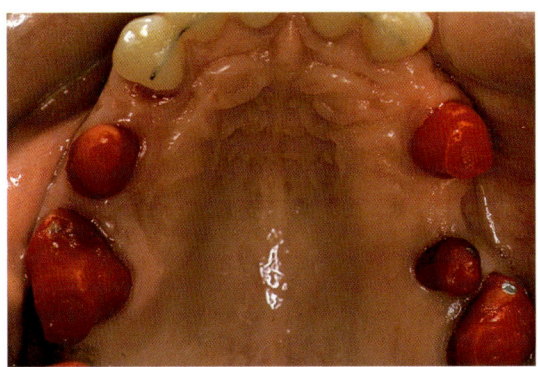

Figure 9.18

Duralay copings fitted in maxilla.

the anterior maxillary teeth were pumiced, etched, bonded, and built to occlusal contact with mandibular anterior teeth by adding microfil composite resin (Durafil vs). A groove was then made in the composite platform and a nitinol orthodontic wire was fitted and bonded in place (Figure 9.16).

The remaining maxillary teeth were prepared and a transitional acrylic resin restoration was prepared for fixed prostheses and transitional acrylic resin restorations were placed (Figure 9.17).

Copper band elastomeric impressions were then taken of all the prepared teeth and Duralay copings were made. These copings (Figure 9.18) were used to record the teeth position in the arch for the final impression for the working model and also centric relation at the vertical dimension of the temporary restorations. A polyether complete arch impression was made to pick up the copings and their relationship to the remaining teeth (Figures 9.19 and 9.20). The metal copings were then cast, fitted and soldered, and after try-in of the soldered metal framework another polyether impression was made for the final master model. These models were mounted on a semi-adjustable articulator (Hanau) utilizing a facebow registration. Centric records were made at the vertical dimension of occlusion utilizing Duralay with a Neylon technique. The porcelain was baked and the occlusion checked at the biscuit bake stage in the mouth and all adjustments needed were then made. The porcelain was then glazed and the crowns and bridges were cemented with Temp-Bond for a period of 3 weeks. The

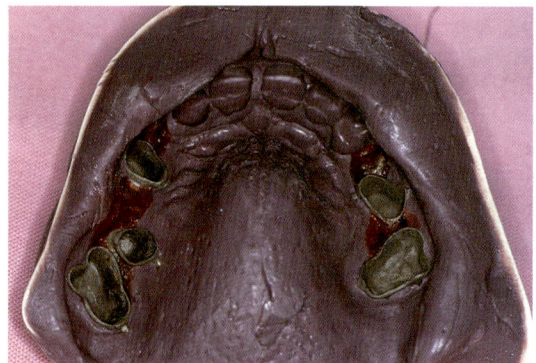

Figure 9.19

Polyether maxillary impression of metal copings.

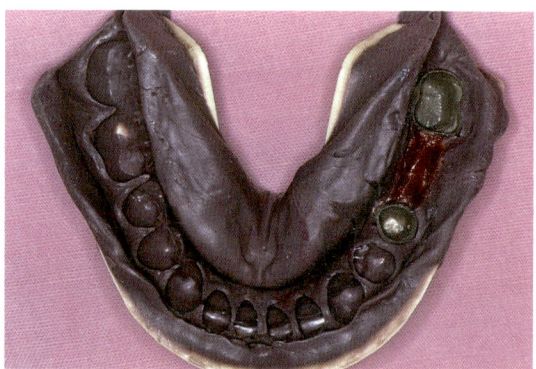

Figure 9.20

Polyether mandibular impression of metal copings.

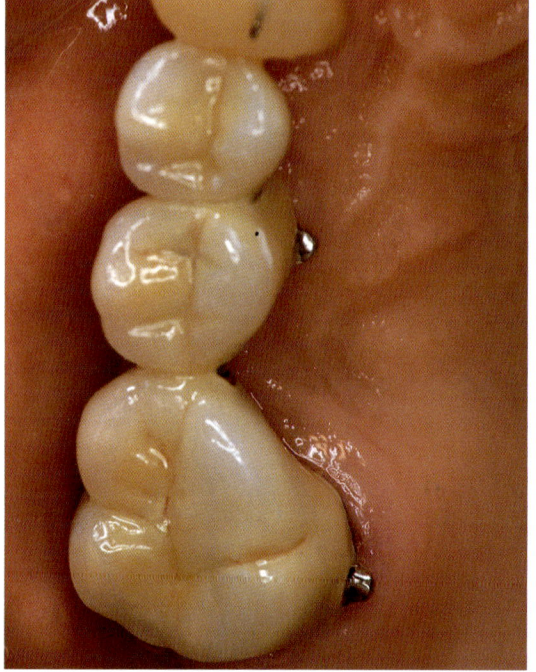

Figure 9.21

Maxillary restorations—right side.

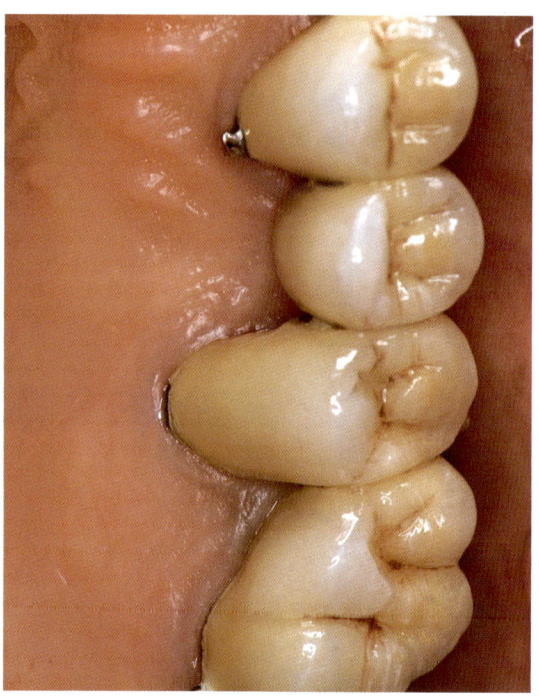

Figure 9.22

Maxillary restorations—left side.

crowns and bridges were then permanently cemented with zinc oxyphosphate cement for cementation (Figures 9.21–9.23).

The patient has been returning for follow-up and maintenance twice a year.

SUMMARY

The 40-year-old female patient came to the Graduate Prosthodontics Clinic of the Hebrew University Dental School of Medicine for a simple restoration of a

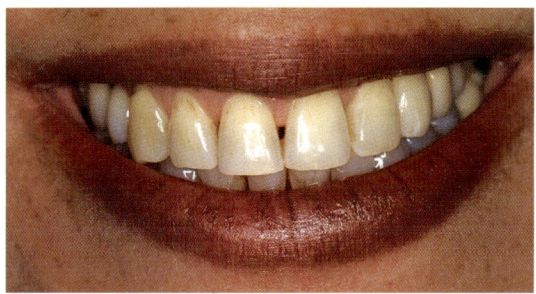

Figure 9.23

Frontal facial view of patient after treatment completion.

crown on a recently placed implant. The patient presented with moderate to advanced adult periodontitis. She had many missing teeth, advanced alveolar bone loss around some teeth, and faulty restorations in both jaws. There was mobility and fremitus in the maxillary anterior teeth.

After a complete examination, diagnosis, and consultation, the patient agreed to a comprehensive treatment plan, and not just a single crown for her implant.

With orthodontic and periodontal treatment accompanied by occlusal therapy, the patient received a physiologic occlusion at the optimum vertical dimension of occlusion.

CASE DISCUSSION
AVINOAM YAFFE

The patient presented herself to the Graduate Prosthodontics Program, seeking treatment for various complaints. She had been treated earlier by a periodontist who replaced a missing lower first right molar by an 8.0 mm implant, even though the adjacent teeth had been previously treated. The patient's advanced periodontal disease, accompanied by flaring of anterior teeth along with several missing teeth, was quite challenging. The orthodontic treatment addressed the patient's esthetic complaints and improved the periodontal condition. This facilitated participation of the anterior teeth in occlusal support in their new favorable position. The occlusal scheme was tailor made to address the periodontal situation. A functional physiologic occlusion was established.

CASE DISCUSSION
HAROLD PREISKEL

The treatment received by this patient underscores the importance of establishing a comprehensive program of therapy at the outset, together with achievable goals. The hazards of treating a patient on a quadrant or tooth-by-tooth basis is clearly evidenced by earlier attempts at treatment.

Computer simulation has been employed to augment the more standardized radiographic and diagnostic case investigation techniques. Modifying an existent diagnostic cast is a relatively straightforward and extremely effective way of assessing the results of therapy and was used to good effect. The patient's treatment has transformed her mouth from an unsightly, diseased and rapidly deteriorating situation into one of health, function, and good looks.

PATIENT 10   SEVERE ADVANCED ADULT PERIODONTITIS

Treatment by Erez Mann

THE PATIENT

The patient, a 58-year-old engineer, presented herself for examination and consultation at the Hadassah Hebrew University School of Dental Medicine Graduate Prosthodontics Clinic with the following complaint:

'My upper and lower front teeth are loose.'

She had been to several dentists, all of whom had told her that she would most probably need complete dentures or, at best, if some roots could be saved, complete overdentures.

PAST MEDICAL HISTORY

Past medical history was non-contributory.

EXTRA-ORAL EXAMINATION
(Figures 10.1 and 10.2)

- Normal facial symmetry
- Slightly convex profile

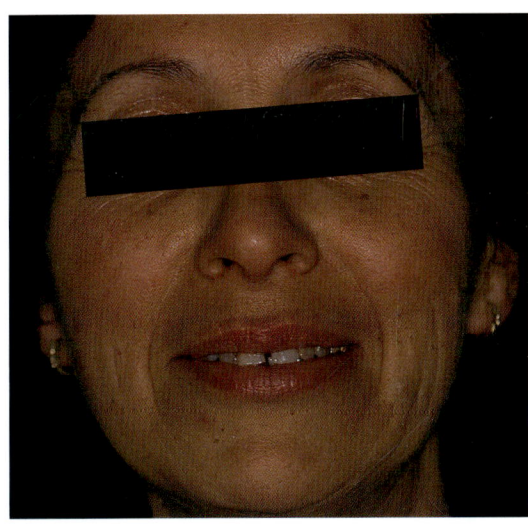

Figure 10.1

Frontal facial view.

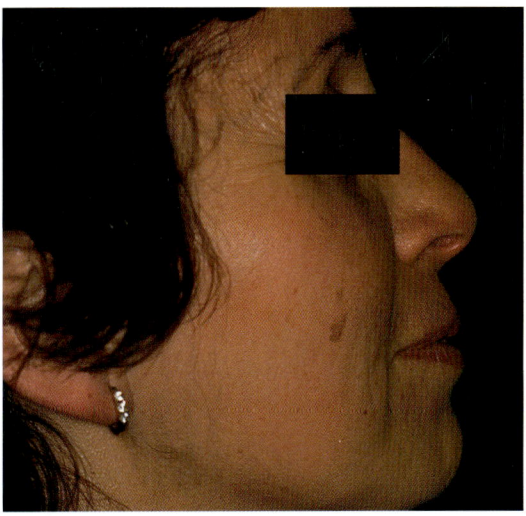

Figure 10.2

Side face view.

- Normally functioning muscles of mastication
- The temporomandibular joints were normal
- The maximum opening was 48 mm with a 2.0 mm deviation to the left side on opening and a 2.0 mm deviation to the right side in the closing movement

INTRA-ORAL AND FULL-MOUTH PERIAPICAL RADIOGRAPH EXAMINATION (Figures 10.3–10.11)

- Missing teeth:

$$\frac{7\ 6\ 4\ \ |\ 4\ 6\ 7\ 8}{7\ 6\ 5\ \ |\ 4\ 5\ 6\ 7\ 8}$$

- Caries
- Low maxillary sinuses
- 60% bone loss around some teeth
- Spacing between the anterior teeth

Occlusal examination revealed that the patient was Angle class 1, with an overbite of 2.0 mm and overjet of 3.0 mm (Figure 10.5). The interocclusal rest space was 3.0 mm and the maximum opening between the incisors was 48 mm. Fremitus class I–II was found on the maxillary anterior teeth and there was mobility of the mandibular anterior teeth. There was a 0.5 mm discrepancy between centric occlusion (IC) and centric relation (CR). The patient had a removable partial mandibular denture which was unsatisfactory and was not used (Figure 10.6).

Periodontal examination (Figures 10.7 and 10.8) revealed probing depths of up to 5.0 mm on the maxillary teeth and up to 5.0 mm on the mandibular teeth, with slight bleeding of the gingiva on probing (BOP) on some of the teeth, with the condition

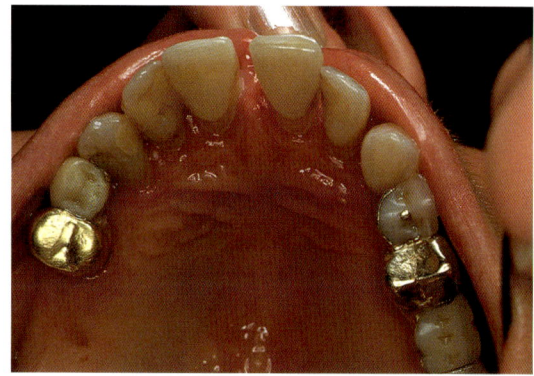

Figure 10.3

Maxillary arch.

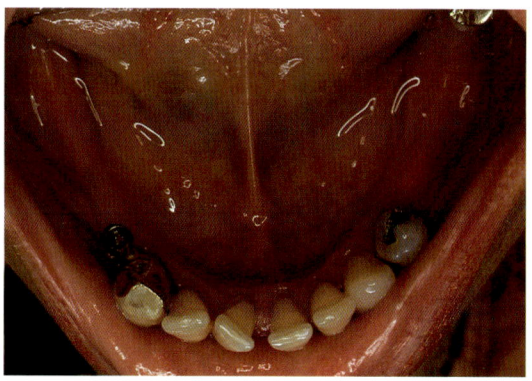

Figure 10.4

Mandibular arch.

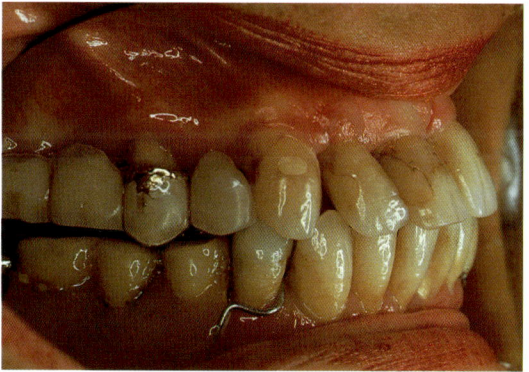

Figure 10.5

Anterior overjet and overbite.

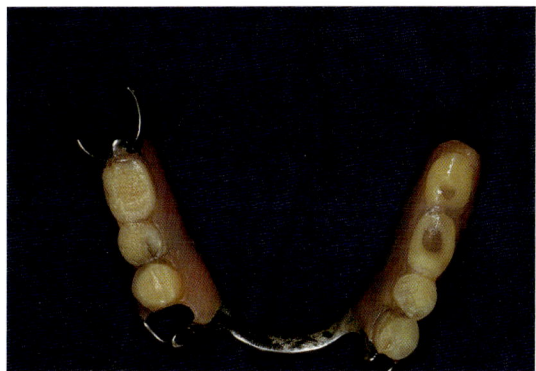

Figure 10.6

Patient's removable mandibular partial denture.

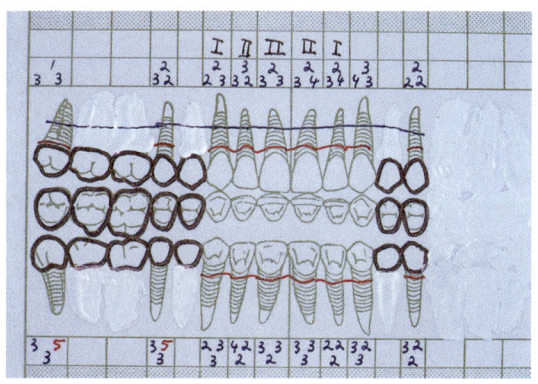

Figure 10.7

Maxillary periodontal chart.

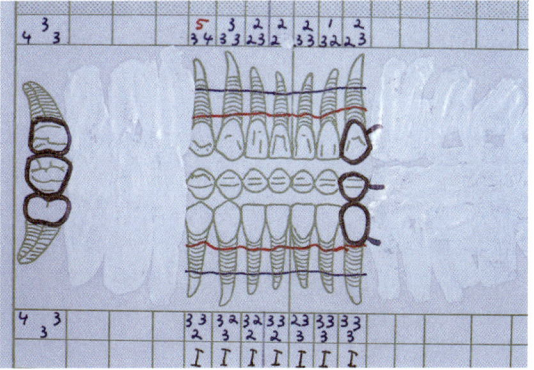

Figure 10.8

Mandibular periodontal chart.

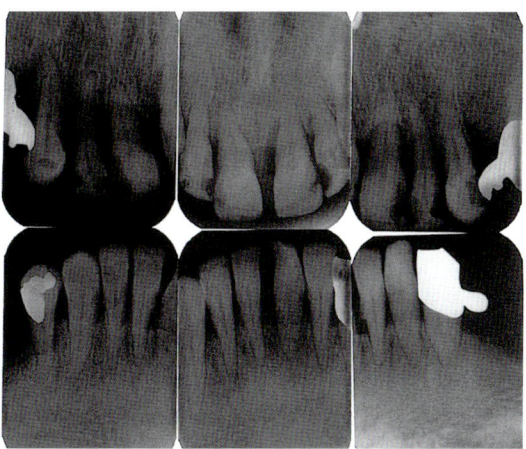

Figure 10.9

Radiographs of maxillary and mandibular anterior quadrant.

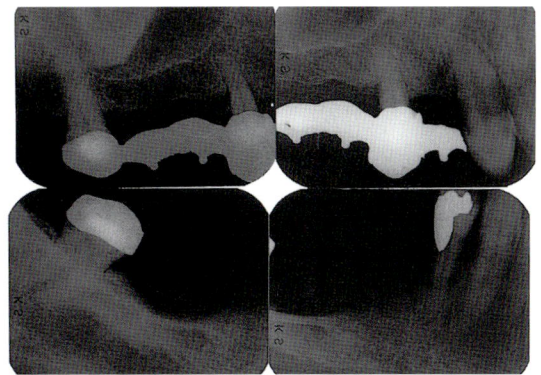

Figure 10.10

Radiographs of right posterior quadrant.

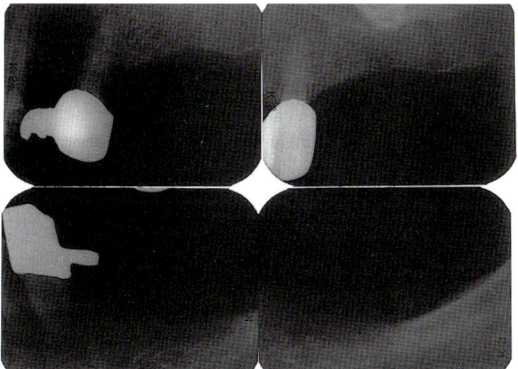

Figure 10.11

Radiographs of left posterior quadrant.

being more severe in the maxilla than the mandible.

INDIVIDUAL TOOTH PROGNOSIS

- Hopeless: none
- Poor:

$$\frac{8\,5\,3\,2\,1 \mid 1\,2\,3}{1 \mid 1}$$

- Fair: the rest of the teeth
- Good: none

DIAGNOSIS

- Advanced adult periodontitis
- Missing teeth accompanied by loss of posterior occlusal support, and flaring of maxillary anterior teeth
- Caries
- Faulty restorations
- Poor esthetics
- Reduced vertical dimension

ABOUT THE PATIENT

The patient understood the severity of her dental condition and came to the clinic hoping to avoid construction of complete maxillary and mandibular dentures, because that was what other dentists had told her was the only possible treatment. She was very cooperative in her dental treatment, and was prepared for any financial outlay necessary in order to save her remaining teeth.

POTENTIAL TREATMENT PROBLEMS

- The advanced periodontitis was accompanied by many missing teeth

- The existing restorations were inadequate
- The patient refused to wear a removable mandibular partial denture

TREATMENT POSSIBILITIES

Maxilla:

- Fixed anterior partial prosthesis and a removable posterior partial prosthesis supported by implants
- Fixed anterior partial prosthesis and a removable posterior partial prosthesis supported by the anterior fixed prosthesis with either clasps and rests, or attachments
- Fixed maxillary restoration as a shortened arch with only a premolar occlusion on the left side

Mandible:

- Fixed anterior partial prosthesis with removable tooth supported posterior partial prosthesis
- Fixed tooth and implant supported partial prosthesis
- Fixed partial prosthesis with the cuspid as the terminal abutment on the left side

TREATMENT PLAN

Following initial preparation including oral hygiene instruction, scaling and root planing, and periodontal re-evaluation a final treatment plan was then chosen which consisted of orthodontic treatment to improve the occlusal relationship and close the existing spaces between the anterior teeth. This would improve the anterior tooth position to facilitate participation in vertical dimension support and to reduce the root proximity between the mandibular right cuspid and the first premolar. Following the orthodontic treatment, a provisional fixed maxillary prosthesis terminating with a premolar occlusion on the left side would be done. The mandible would be treated with a provisional fixed prosthesis on the remaining teeth, which extended from the right third molar to the left cuspid. At the time the treatment plan was chosen the patient still refused to consider a removable mandibular prosthesis.

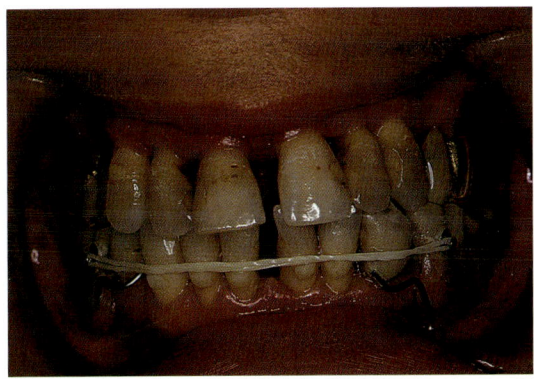

Figure 10.12

Elastic retraction of mandibular anterior teeth.

TREATMENT

Initial preparation included scaling, curettage, root planing and oral hygiene instruction. At the end of this stage, an obvious improvement in the soft tissue could be discerned. At this time a periodontal re-evaluation was done and it was observed that the pocket depth had greatly diminished and that the bleeding on probing had disappeared.

The orthodontic phase of treatment was then started using elastics to retract the mandibular anterior teeth (Figure 10.12). The maxillary incisor teeth were also treated orthodontically with a modified Hawley appliance (Figure 10.13). This retracted the maxillary anterior teeth and closed the spaces. This was done in order to achieve better esthetics and move the teeth into better position in the alveolar bone for occlusal support, and with the intent to prepare the site for future development should implants be needed (Figure 10.14).

When the orthodontic stage was successfully completed, (Figures 10.15 and 10.16) the supporting teeth were prepared and temporary restorations were placed (Figures 10.17–10.19). A coil spring was then inserted to separate the right mandibular cuspid from

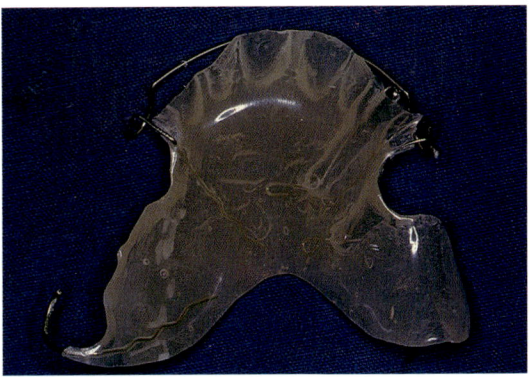

Figure 10.13

Hawley orthodontic appliance.

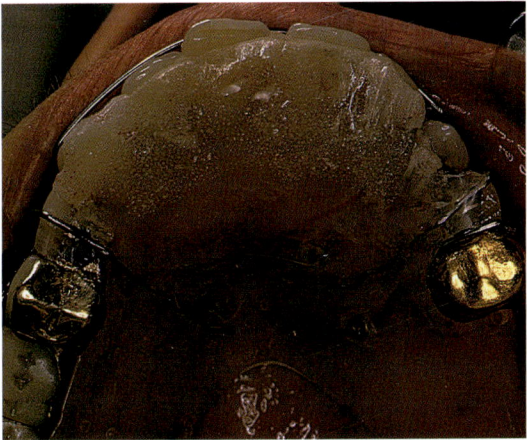

Figure 10.14

Clinical view of Hawley appliance—pre-treatment.

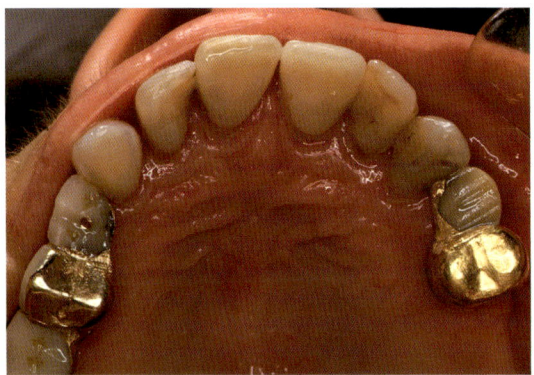

Figure 10.15

Maxillary anterior teeth after orthodontic treatment.

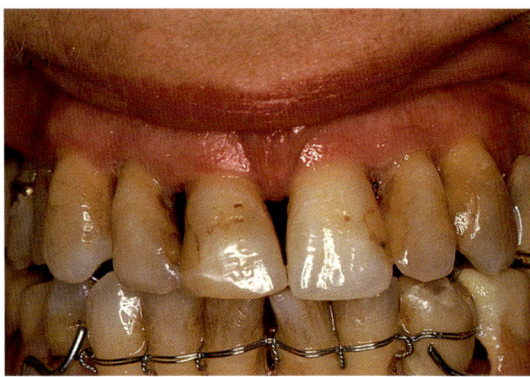

Figure 10.16

Anterior teeth after orthodontic treatment.

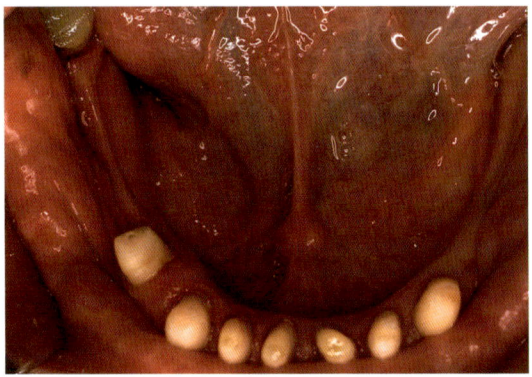

Figure 10.17

Final tooth preparation—mandible.

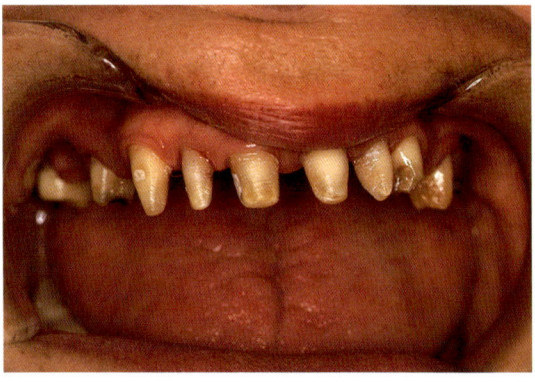

Figure 10.18

Final tooth preparation—maxilla.

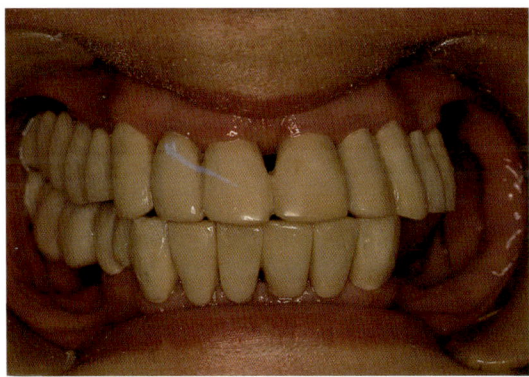

Figure 10.19

Transitional restorations—maxilla and mandible.

the right first premolar (Figure 10.20). Radiographs (Figure 10.21) and periodontal evaluation were again performed and disclosed that the probing depth were less than 3.0 mm in all areas. A transitional removable mandibular partial denture was also suggested to the patient, and again rejected.

Copper band elastomeric impressions were then taken of all the prepared teeth and Duralay copings were made. These copings (Figure 10.22) were used to record centric relation at the vertical dimension of the temporary restorations and for the final impression for the master model. The metal copings were

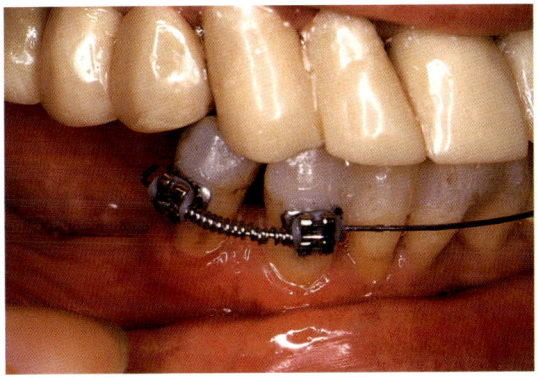

Figure 10.20

Coil spring to separate the right mandibular cuspid and premolar teeth.

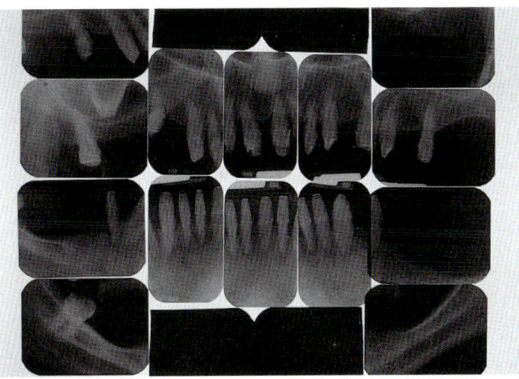

Figure 10.21

Completed teeth preparations—maxilla and mandible, radiographs.

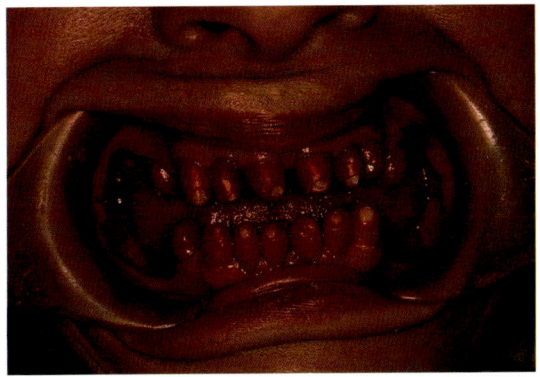

Figure 10.22

Duralay copings fitted—maxilla and mandible.

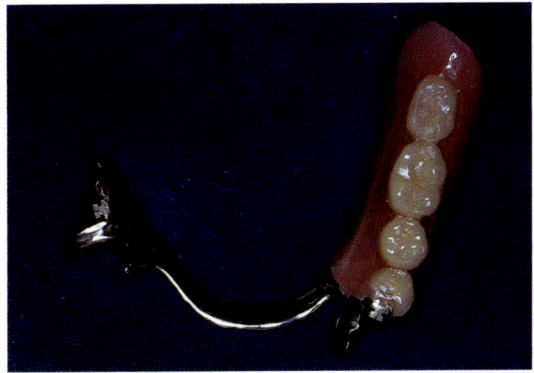

Figure 10.23

Removable partial mandibular denture.

then fitted and soldered and, after try-in of the soldered metal framework, another elastomeric impression was done for tissue detail and for the final master model. These models were mounted on a semi-adjustable articulator (Hanau) utilizing a facebow registration and centric records were taken at the vertical dimension of occlusion utilizing Duralay with a Neylon technique. At this point the patient was finally convinced of the importance of a partial removable mandibular denture and agreed to try and adjust to one. The porcelain was baked and the occlusion checked at the biscuit bake stage in the mouth and all adjustments needed were then made. Rest preparations were then milled into the fixed prosthesis in the lingual of the right molar area pontic as well as the distal surface of the left cuspid. The porcelain was then glazed and the final elastomeric impression for the removable mandibular partial denture was done. The framework for the partial denture was then cast and fitted and a bite tray constructed on it for centric registration record. This was done and the denture teeth were set up and checked in the mouth for esthetics and occlusion. The denture was then processed (Figure 10.23). The crowns and bridges were cemented with Temp-Bond and the partial removable mandibular denture inserted. The crowns and bridges were then cemented with zinc oxyphosphate cement for permanent cementation (Figures 10.24–10.29).

The patient has been returning for follow-up and maintenance twice a year since then and adjusted to her removable mandibular partial denture (Figures 10.30 and 10.31).

SUMMARY

The 58-year-old patient came to the Graduate Prosthodontics Clinic of the Hebrew University Dental School of Medicine as a last resort. She had been to three dentists who had all told her that it would be impossible to save any of her remaining teeth and that she would need complete dentures. She was told that there might be a chance to save some of her teeth to support an overdenture, but only if she went to the Dental Clinic at Hadassah. The patient presented with a severe problem of advanced adult periodontitis. She had many missing teeth, considerable alveolar bone loss around the remaining teeth, and faulty restorations in both jaws. There was much bone resorption but the

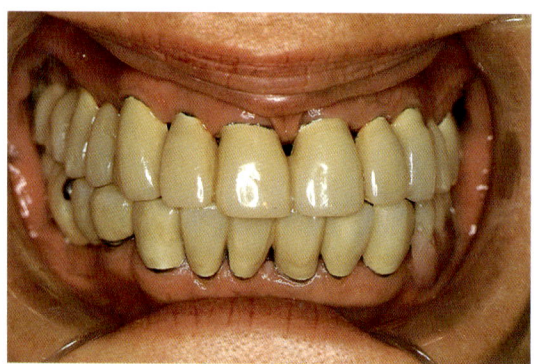

Figure 10.24

Case cemented—post-treatment, anterior view.

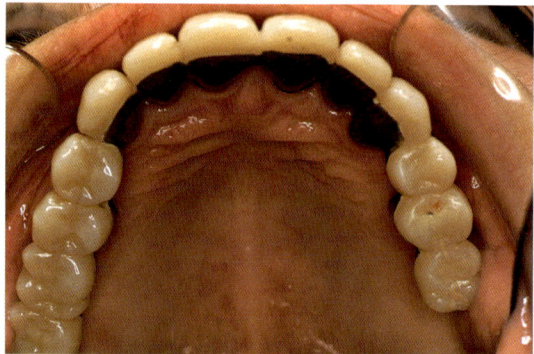

Figure 10.25

Case cemented—maxilla.

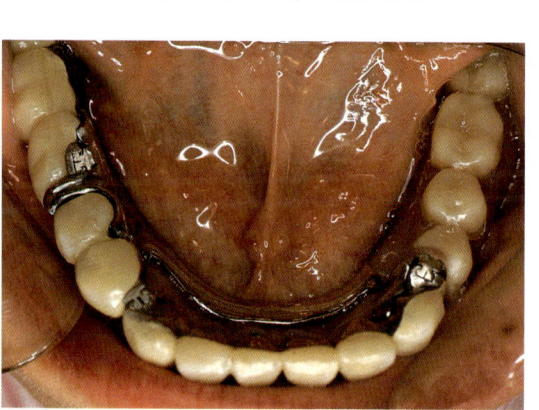

Figure 10.26

Case cemented—mandible.

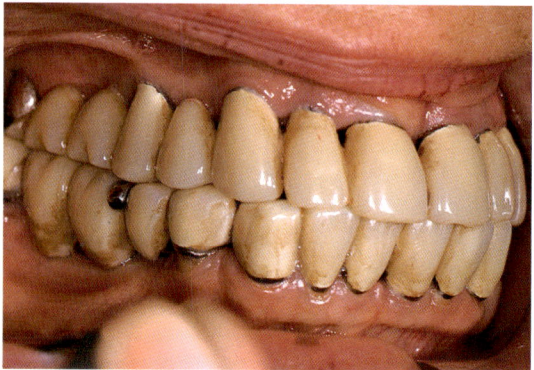

Figure 10.27

Case cemented—right side.

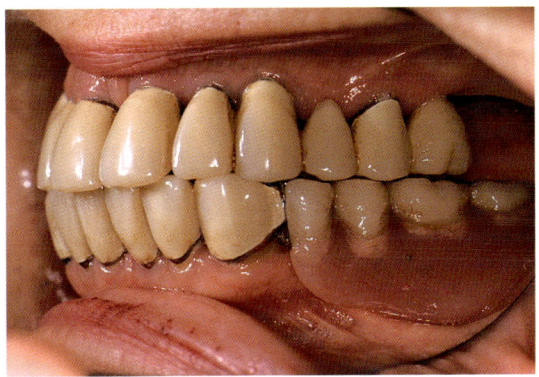

Figure 10.28

Case cemented—left side.

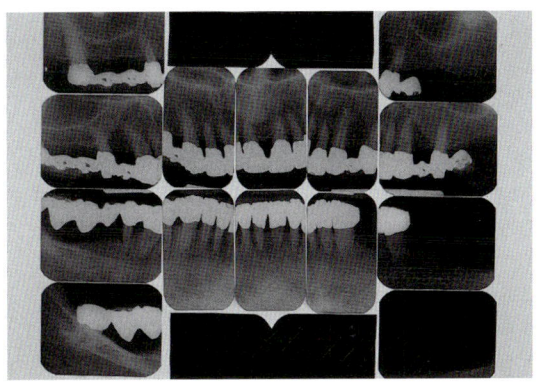

Figure 10.29

Radiographs of case—post-treatment.

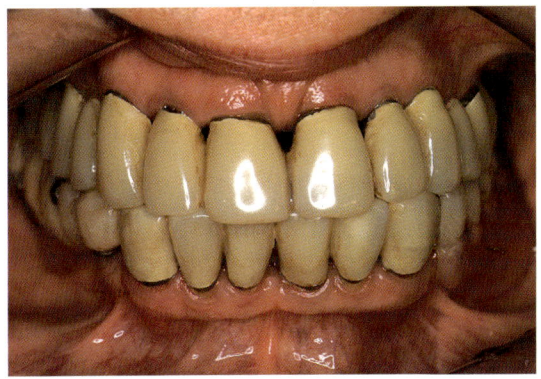

Figure 10.30

Patient clinically—five years post-cementation.

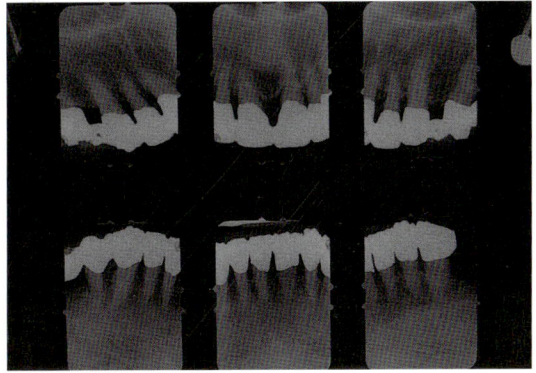

Figure 10.31

Patient radiographs—five years post-cementation.

probing depth around the remaining teeth was not excessive, mostly 4.0 mm or less, except for the right mandibular premolar and the right maxillary second premolar and third molar. Her fixed and removable restorations were inadequate and she hardly ever wore her removable partial mandibular denture. There was mobility and fremitus in the maxillary anterior teeth and mobility of the mandibular anterior teeth.

With orthodontic and periodontal treatment accompanied by occlusal therapy, the patient received a physiologic occlusion at the optimum vertical dimension of occlusion for this periodontal condition. The patient was adamant about not having a removable prosthesis and refused to use one during the course of treatment. Only when she was told that the case could not be completed ending in a cuspid occlusion on the left side, did she agree to try to use a removable partial mandibular denture. She successfully overcame her aversion to the removable denture and today, 10 years post-treatment, functions very well with her partial removable denture. As a compromise solution, the missing posterior mandibular teeth were replaced as pontics on a fixed prosthesis as opposed to the removable mandibular partial denture, as we felt that the patient might not wear the partial denture. If that did occur, at least she would have full occlusion on the right side.

CASE DISCUSSION
AVINOAM YAFFE

This patient represents a complicated case with advanced periodontal disease and missing teeth accompanied by drifting and flaring of anterior teeth with mobility and fremitus. The patient was treated with the intent to address both the occlusal and periodontal problem that affected her periodontal condition. Once the occlusion was stabilized and with successful oral hygiene instruction, scaling and curettage, the periodontal condition improved considerably—to such an extent that there was no need for any surgical periodontal procedures. The new position of the anterior teeth enabled them to participate in occlusal support, thus improving the prognosis of the treatment and serving the patient for the past 10 years with no signs of breakdown.

CASE DISCUSSION
HAROLD PREISKEL

Commenting on a treatment plan with the benefit of the successful 10-year follow-up is relatively simple as it is hard to argue with a good result. The treatment, however, was far from straightforward. In addition to the problems of advanced periodontitis, lack of posterior support, flaring of the maxillary teeth, and caries, the operators were faced with a patient who adamantly refused to wear a removable prosthesis. The fact that they were able to undertake a comprehensive plan of treatment and motivate the patient to the extent of wearing a removable prosthesis, is eloquent testimony to their communication skills as well as their clinical expertise. Bearing in mind that the patient was treated in the early 1990s, the use of orthodontics to improve a potential implant site must be considered well ahead of its time.

PATIENT 11   SEVERE ADVANCED ADULT PERIODONTITIS

Treatment by Zvi Gutmacher

THE PATIENT

The patient, a 46-year-old farmer, presented himself for examination and consultation at the Hadassah Hebrew University School of Dental Medicine Graduate Prosthodontic Clinic with the following complaints:

'I can't chew my food so I swallow it in large pieces.'
'I can't bite food with my front teeth, and I grind my teeth.'
'I hate the way I look due to my buck teeth.' (Figure 11.1)

PAST DENTAL HISTORY

The patient attended the dentist only when a tooth was painful or broken.

PAST MEDICAL HISTORY

Past medical history was non-contributory.

EXTRA-ORAL EXAMINATION

- Normal facial symmetry

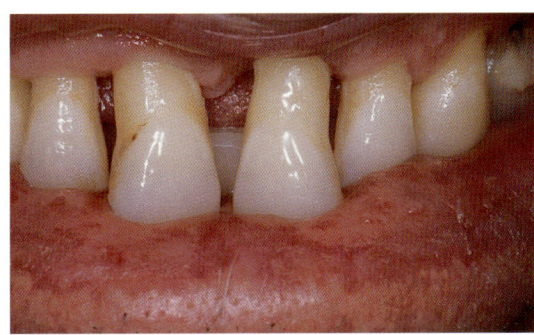

Figure 11.1

Anterior teeth showing spacing

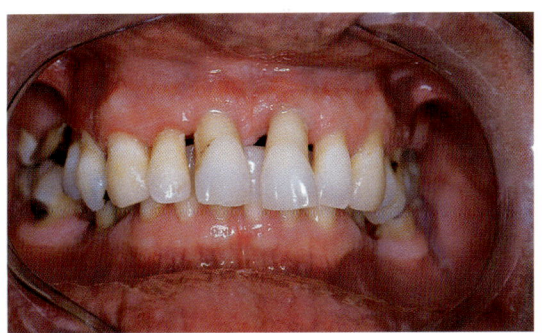

Figure 11.2

Anterior teeth

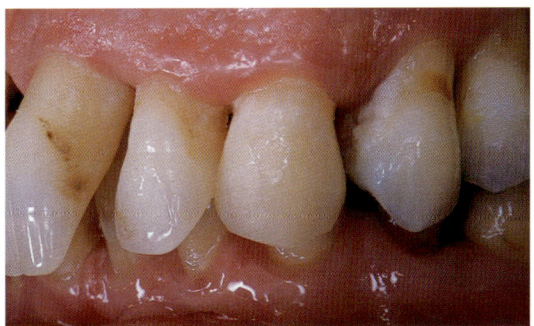

Figure 11.3

Scissor bite left side

- Straight profile with accentuated labio-mental fold, and trapped lower lip
- Normally functioning muscles of mastication
- Temporomandibular joints were normal
- The patient also exhibited solar keratosis in the lower lip

INTRA-ORAL AND FULL-MOUTH PERIAPICAL RADIOGRAPH EXAMINATION (Figures 11.1–11.9)

Clinical and radiographic examination revealed:

- Missing teeth:

$$\frac{6 \mid 6\,8}{6 \mid 6}$$

- Residual roots:

$$\frac{ \mid }{7 \mid 7}$$

- Extensive caries and loss of crown structure
- Low maxillary sinuses
- Widened periodontal ligament around the mandibular third molars
- 60% bone loss around some teeth
- Furcation involvement of the mandibular right second molar tooth
- Radio-opacity in the maxillary left sinus area

Occlusal examination revealed that the patient was Angle class II division I, with an overbite of 10.0 mm and overjet of 7.0 mm. The interocclusal rest space was 5.0 mm and the maximum opening was 52.0 mm.

Fremitus and mobility were found on the maxillary incisor teeth as well as the left maxillary first premolar. In the intercuspal position (IC) a 'scissors bite' existed in

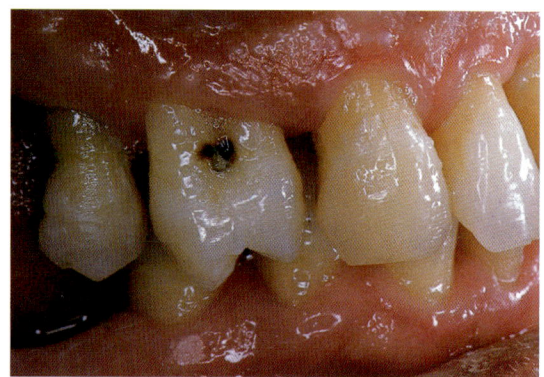

Figure 11.4

Scissor bite right side

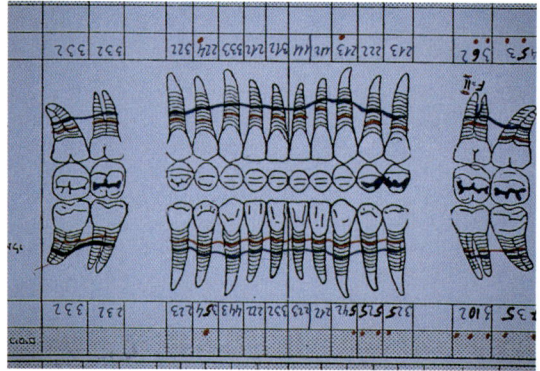

Figure 11.5

Mandibular periodontal chart

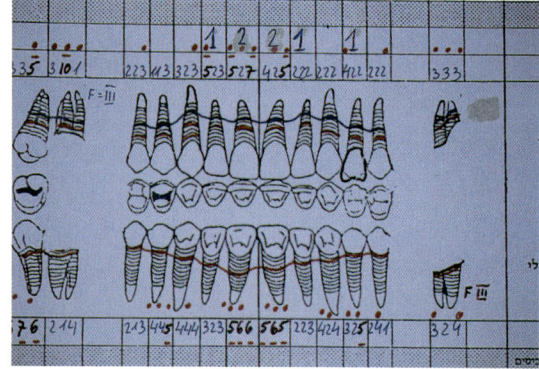

Figure 11.6

Maxillary periodontal chart

which the buccal outer line angle of the mandibular supporting cusp was lingual to the functional outer aspect (FOA) of the maxillary supporting cusp (Figures 11.3 and 11.4). There was no discrepancy between centric occlusion (IC) and centric relation (CR). Fremitus and mobility were found on several teeth.

The periodontal examination (Figures 11.5 and 11.6) revealed probing depths of up to 5.0 mm on the maxillary teeth and up to 10.0 mm on the mandibular teeth, with bleeding of the gingiva on probing (BOP) on most of teeth, with the condition being more severe in the mandible than the maxilla (Figures 11.7–11.9).

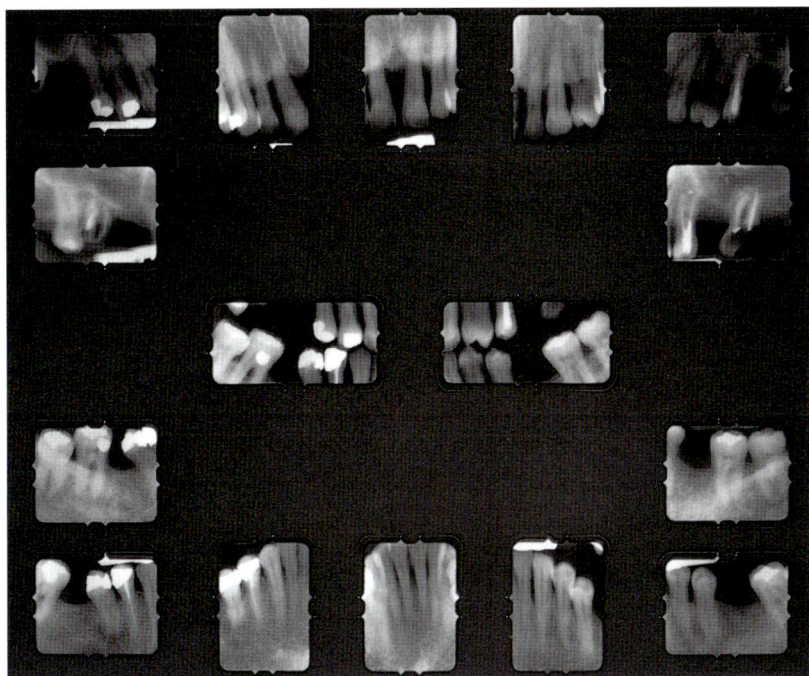

Figure 11.7

Radiographs of maxilla and mandible—pre-treatment

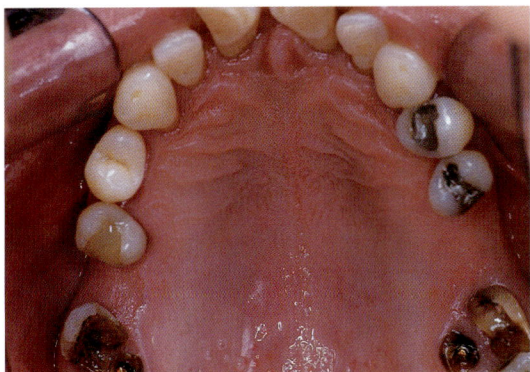

Figure 11.8

Maxillary arch

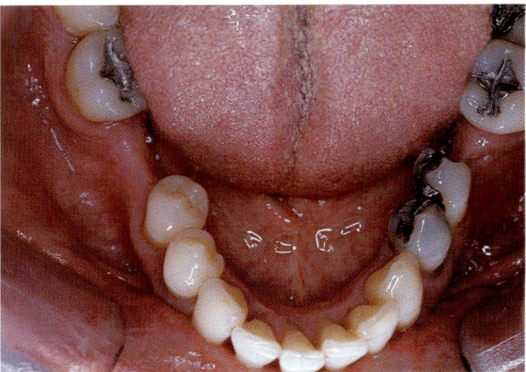

Figure 11.9

Mandibular arch

INDIVIDUAL TOOTH PROGNOSIS

- Hopeless:

$$\frac{7 \mid 1\ 1}{}$$

- Poor:

$$\frac{4\ 2 \mid 2\ 7}{}$$

- Good:

$$\frac{}{8 \mid 7\ 8}$$

- Fair: the remaining teeth

DIAGNOSIS

- Advanced adult periodontitis
- Missing teeth
- Loss of occlusal support
- Scissors bite – jaw size disparity
- Decreased vertical dimension
- Secondary occlusal trauma with primary origins
- Caries
- Faulty restorations
- Poor esthetics
- Periapical changes

ABOUT THE PATIENT

The patient was young and optimistic and understood the severity of his dental condition and came to the clinic hoping to avoid construction of complete maxillary and mandibular dentures because other dentists had told him that was the only possible treatment. His expectations regarding his treatment were functional and esthetic improvement to his mouth.

POTENTIAL TREATMENT PROBLEMS

- The advanced periodontitis was accompanied by missing teeth

- The disparity of jaw size caused the scissors bite and lack of occlusal support
- The deep overbite would cause biomechanical problems for the restorations and increasing the vertical dimension of occlusion would accentuate the unfavorable bucco-lingual relationship between the jaws and also worsen the crown–root ratio of the teeth, putting more stress on the periodontium
- Because of the primary and secondary occlusal trauma, a complete mouth rehabilitation would be difficult to do.

Note: from old radiographs we concluded that the existing radio-opacity in the maxillary left sinus area was due to a molar tooth that had endodontic therapy which was overfilled with cement entering the sinus. The tooth had subsequently been extracted.

TREATMENT ALTERNATIVES

Maxilla:

- Fixed anterior partial prosthesis and a fixed posterior partial prosthesis supported by implants
- Fixed anterior partial prosthesis and a removable posterior partial prosthesis supported by the anterior fixed prosthesis with either clasps and rests or attachments
- A fixed maxillary restoration as a shortened arch with only a premolar occlusion.

Mandible:

- Fixed partial prosthesis
- Removable tooth-supported partial prosthesis
- Fixed tooth and implant-supported partial prosthesis
- Fixed and removable partial prosthesis

TREATMENT PREREQUISITES

- In order to achieve a tooth-supported prosthesis, orthodontic treatment to change the bucco-lingual relationship of the maxillary and mandibular teeth was mandatory
- In order to do an implant-supported maxillary fixed prosthesis, maxillary sinus augmentation would be required

FINAL TREATMENT PLAN

A final treatment plan was then chosen which consisted of orthodontic treatment to improve the occlusal relationship, a fixed anterior maxillary prosthesis and a removable posterior maxillary prosthesis with semi-precision attachments, and a fixed partial prosthesis in the mandible.

The maxillary second molars that were considered hopeless would be restored with temporary restorations to augment posterior occlusal support during the orthodontic treatment.

TREATMENT

Initial preparation included scaling, curettage, root planing and oral hygiene instruction. At the end of this stage, an obvious improvement of the soft tissue could be discerned (Figure 11.10). At this time a periodontal recharting and evaluation was done and it was observed that the pockets depths had greatly diminished and that the bleeding on probing had disappeared (Figures 11.11 and 11.12).

The orthodontic phase of treatment was then started using a Hawley bite plane

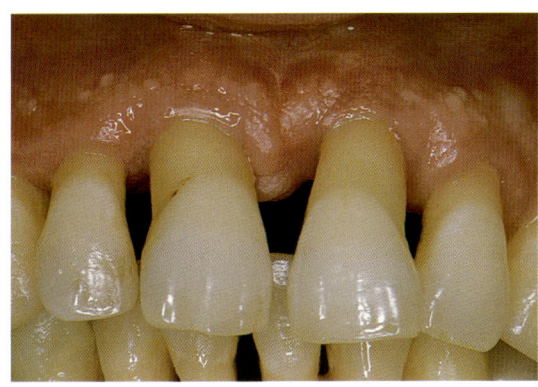

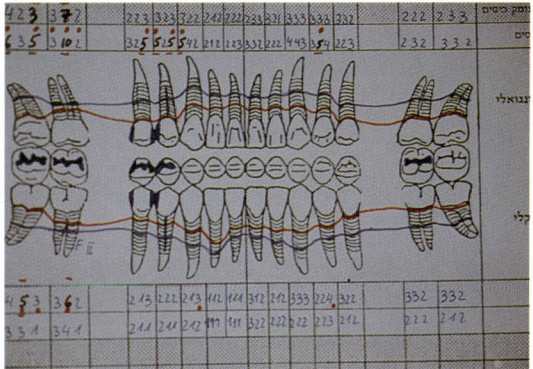

Figure 11.10

Maxillary anterior teeth after initial treatment

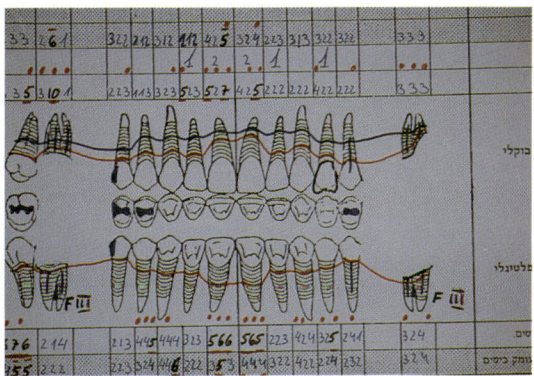

Figure 11.11

Periodontal chart at re-evaluation—maxilla

Figure 11.12

Periodontal chart at re-evaluation—mandible

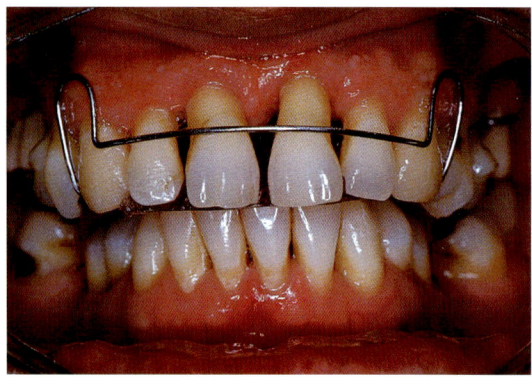

Figure 11.13

Clinical view of Hawley appliance—pre-treatment

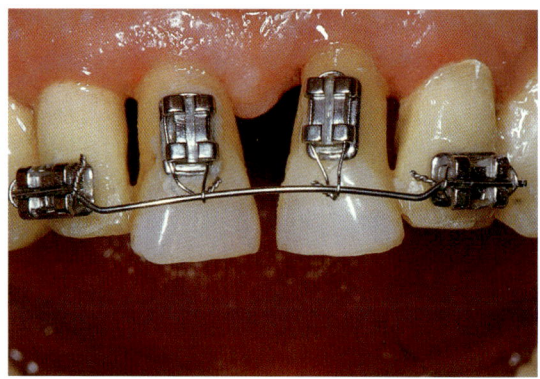

Figure 11.14

Maxillary teeth—orthodontic treatment, extrusion of central incisor teeth

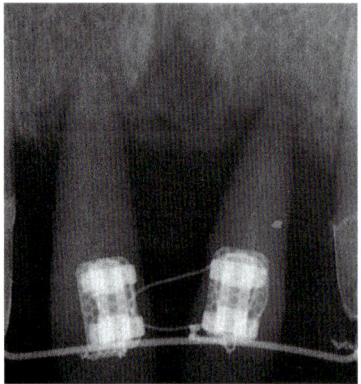

Figure 11.15

Maxillary teeth—radiograph, extrusion of central incisor teeth

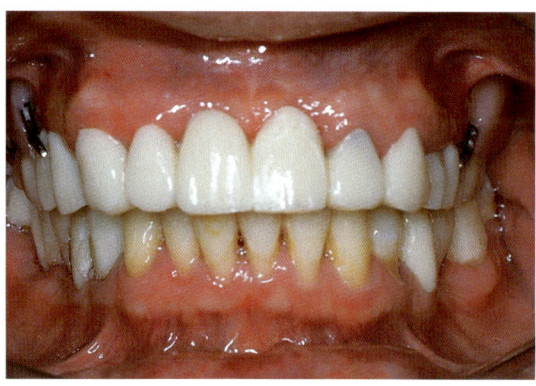

Figure 11.16

Transitional crowns and removable partial denture

retainer (Figure 11.13), the goals of which were to increase the vertical dimension of occlusion, add occlusal support, induce muscular relaxation, and make sure that retruded cuspal position (RC) and intercuspal position (IC) were co-incidental.

The maxillary incisor teeth, despite their hopeless prognosis, were also treated orthodontically to extrude them in order to achieve better esthetics and prepare the site for future development if implants were to be used in the future (Figures 11.14 and 11.15).

When the orthodontic stage was successfully completed, the supporting teeth were prepared and transitional (provisional) restorations were placed (Figure 11.16).

Radiographs and periodontal evaluation were again performed and disclosed that the probing depth were less than 3.0 mm in all areas except the mandibular second right molar. A transitional removable maxillary partial denture was also fabricated to get the patient acclimated to a removable prosthesis (Figure 11.17).

Periodontal surgery was performed on the mandibular right second molar for pocket elimination; it was decided that the tooth was hopeless and it was thus

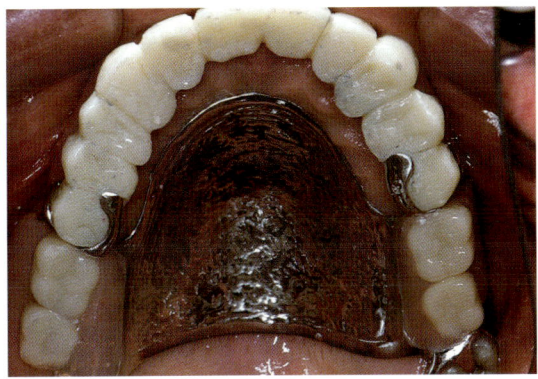

Figure 11.17

Transitional crowns and removable partial denture—maxilla

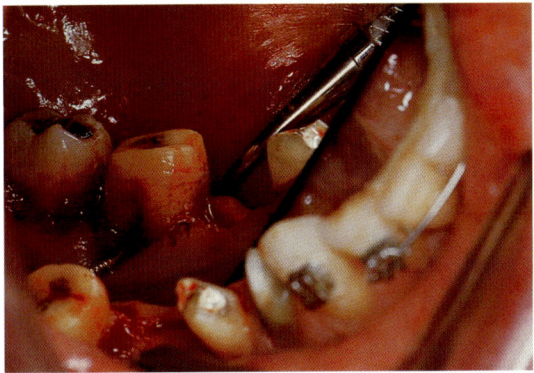

Figure 11.18

Periodontal surgery—right mandibular second molar

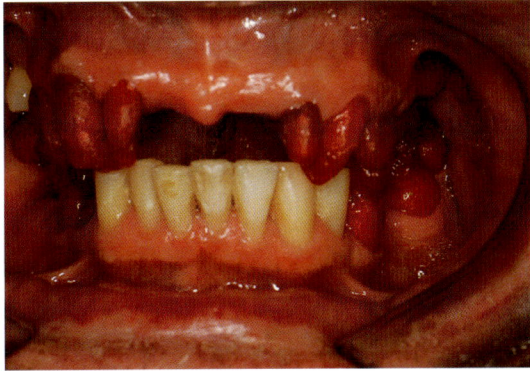

Figure 11.19

Duralay copings fitted—maxilla and mandible and centric relation record

extracted at the time of the periodontal surgery (Figure 11.18).

Following healing, the teeth were reprepared and copper band elastomeric impressions were then taken of all the prepared teeth and Duralay copings were made. These copings were used for the final impression for the master model. They were also used to record centric relation at the vertical dimension of the temporary restorations (Figure 11.19). The metal copings were then fitted and soldered and after try-in of the soldered metal framework (Figures 11.20 and 11.21), another elastomeric impression was done for tissue transfer for the final master model.

These models were mounted on a semi-adjustable articulator (Hanau) utilizing a facebow registration and centric records taken at the vertical dimension of occlusion utilizing Duralay with a Neylon technique (Figures 11.22 and 11.23).

The porcelain was baked and the occlusion checked at the biscuit bake stage in the mouth and all adjustments needed were then made. The porcelain was then glazed. An elastomeric impression in a close-fitting individual tray was made on the non-cemented fixed prosthesis and the edentulous areas, so that the removable maxillary partial denture framework could be fabricated on the crowns and bridges, as opposed to a stone model of them (Figure 11.24).

The framework for the partial denture was then cast and fitted and a bite tray constructed on it for centric record registration (Figure 11.25). This registration was done in Duralay using the Neylon technique (Figure 11.26) and the denture teeth were set up and checked in the mouth for esthetics and occlusion.

The denture was then processed and inserted into the mouth. The crowns and

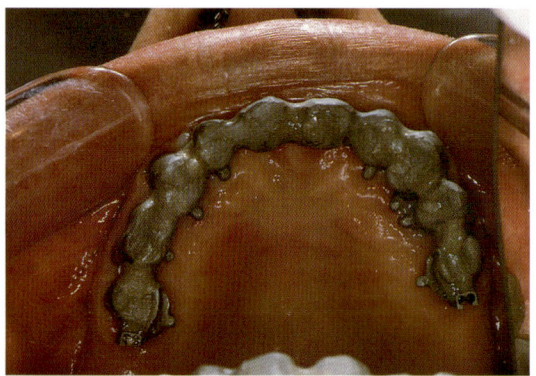

Figure 11.20

Metal copings try-in—maxilla

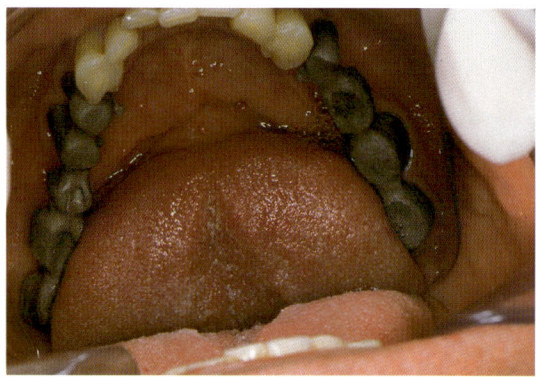

Figure 11.21

Metal copings try-in—mandible

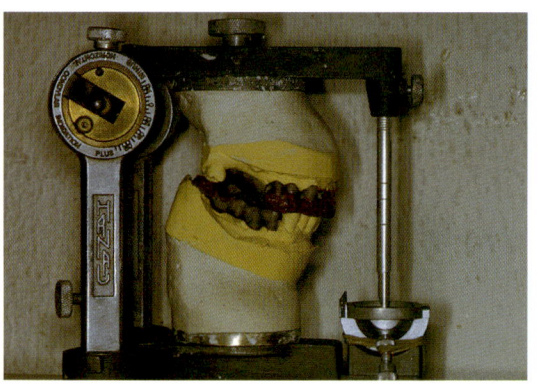

Figure 11.22

Centric relation record on Hanau articulator—right side

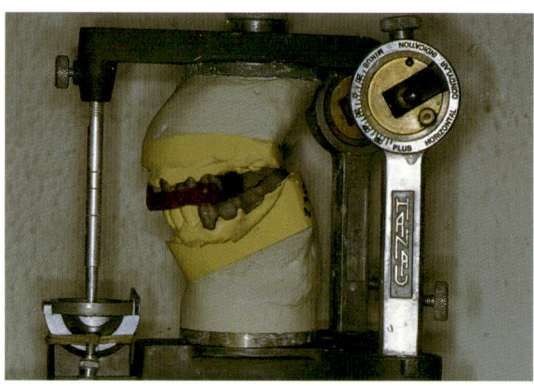

Figure 11.23

Centric relation record on Hanau articulator—left side

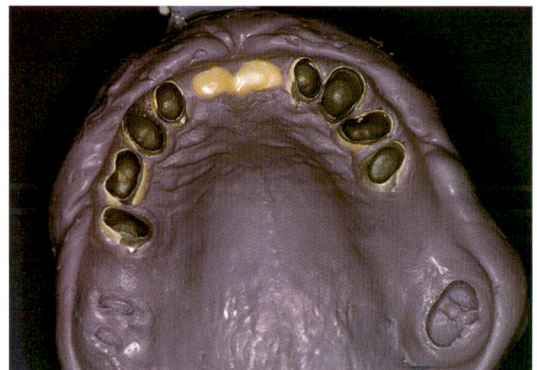

Figure 11.24

Elastomeric impression for maxillary removable partial denture framework

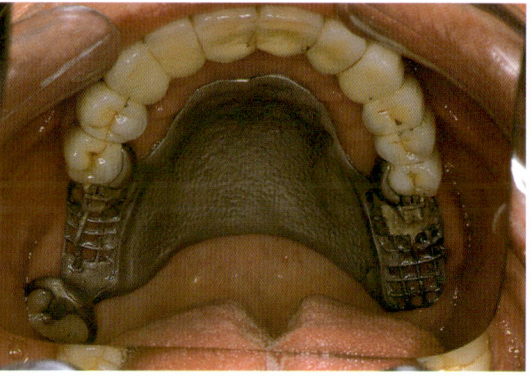

Figure 11.25

Fitting of maxillary removable partial denture framework

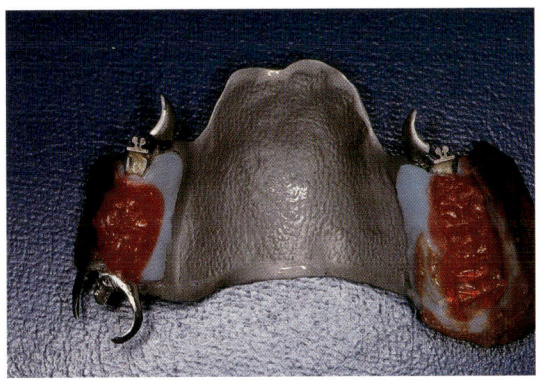

Figure 11.26

Centric relation record on occlusal tray on removable partial denture

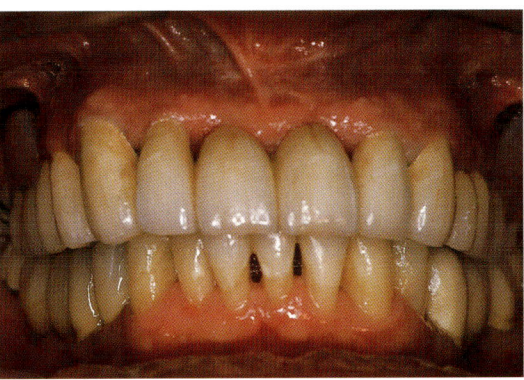

Figure 11.27

Case completed—anterior view

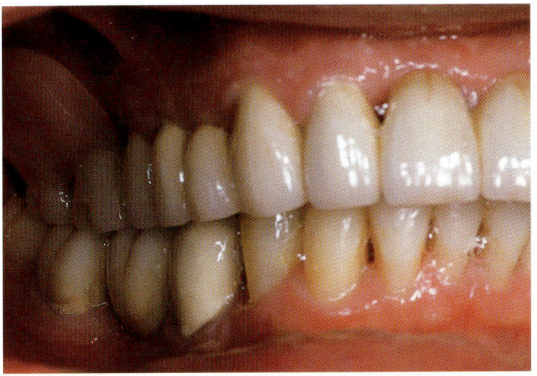

Figure 11.28

Case completed—left side

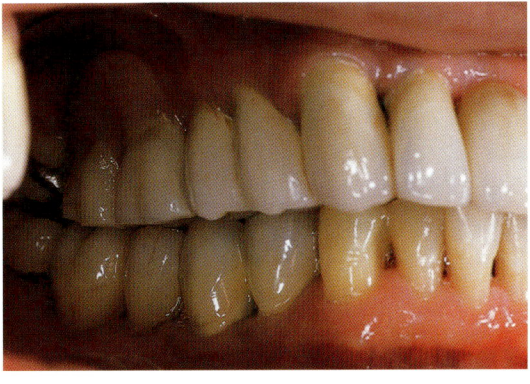

Figure 11.29

Case completed—right side

bridges were cemented with Temp-Bond and the partial removable maxillary denture inserted. The crowns and bridges were then cemented with zinc oxyphosphate cement for permanent cementation (Figures 11.27–11.30).

The patient has been returning for follow-up and maintenance twice a year.

SUMMARY

The patient presented with a severe problem of advanced adult periodontitis, missing teeth, scissors bite, and loss of posterior occlusal support. With orthodontic and periodontal treatment accompanied by occlusal therapy, the patient received a physiological occlusion at the optimum vertical dimension of occlusion.

CASE DISCUSSION
AVINOAM YAFFE

This patient was a relatively young individual, 46 years old, with a complicated dental situation due to many missing teeth, and

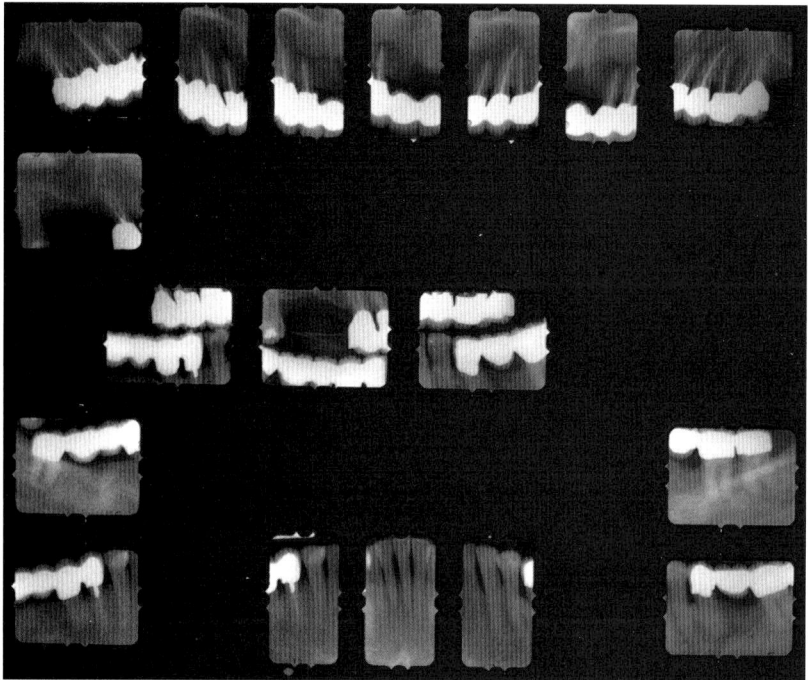

Figure 11.30

Post-treatment radiographs

loss of support, accompanied by a deep overbite and aggravated by a scissors bite that along with a severe periodontitis caused a total loss of vertical support.

There were several alternative methods of treatment possible for this patient:

- An overlay partial denture
- A removable partial denture after extraction of the maxillary anterior teeth
- Orthognathic surgery

The solution that was utilized in this case encompassed biomechanical considerations and the patient's well-being as well as satisfaction with the final result. The orthodontic treatment achieved support from the teeth in scissors bite as well as minimal bite opening (needed for the prosthetic treatment) and thus minimized the increased crown–root ratio caused by

the periodontal disease which would have been aggravated by the increased vertical dimension. The orthodontic treatment also included future site development before the extraction of the maxillary central incisor teeth. All this, along with the esthetic considerations, contributed to the successful treatment of the patient.

CASE DISCUSSION
HAROLD PREISKEL

The patient's treatment represents more than a complex plan of dental therapy. It marks the transition from a patient who had no motivation into one who was prepared to undertake multiple visits to a dental office involving an impressive amount of treatment over an extended period of time. The clinicians are to be congratulated on the patient motivation achieved and upon the successful outcome. It is always important to have a fallback position in case the patient's interest wanes and a simpler plan can be substituted. The step-by-step approach employed has considerable advantage in this respect.

Another laudable aspect of the therapy was an appreciation of the three-dimensional problems associated with a marked discrepancy of arch size. At an early stage it was important to establish how much of the deranged occlusion was as a result of loss of posterior occlusal support and how much as a result of the decrease of vertical dimension of occlusion. Of course the two are inter-related, with a decrease of vertical dimension accentuating the effect of a forward mandibular posture. The use of transitional restorations to determine maxillo–mandibular relationships is an important aspect of the treatment. Forward thinking has also been demonstrated with the extrusion of anterior teeth to be subsequently extracted to encourage bone growth for possible implant placement at a later date.

Alternative avenues of approach were discussed at the very outset. Having selected root-supported fixed prosthodontics as the primary support, a difficult decision involves the missing maxillary molars. Is it necessary to replace them or could a shortened arch be accepted? The shortened arch would be far simpler from the prosthodontic point of view, for no-one should underestimate the complications of producing a removable prosthesis. The maxillo–mandibular relations of this patient helped make the decision to replace the missing maxillary molars, leaving open the possibility of employing a distal cantilever pontic on each side to produce some molar support without the need for a denture. However, it can be seen that the upper left second pre-molar is root filled and we know from the work of Glantz and others that the prognosis of a restoration with a distal cantilever pontic is not good when the distal abutment is root filled. The clinicians therefore elected to construct a partial denture with all the difficulties involved, to say nothing of the maintenance requirements. They ensured that the patient understood the rationale of the treatment from the outset.

Individual techniques are simply tools of our trade; it is the planning and results that matter. This patient's treatment represents both a success in patient education and in clinical dentistry. I hope that the patient returns for routine maintenance.

III   EXTENSIVE LOSS OF TEETH

PATIENT 12 REFUSAL OF ORTHOGNATHIC SURGERY

Treatment by Miriam Calev

THE PATIENT

The patient, a 26-year-old housewife, came to the clinic for consultation. Her complaints were as follows:

'Everything related to my mouth bothers me.' (Figure 12.1)
'I am missing lots of teeth.'
'My front teeth stick out.'
'My palate hurts.'
'Due to my fear of dentists, I have neglected my teeth for many years.'

MEDICAL HISTORY

The medical history was non-contributory.

PAST DENTAL HISTORY

Past dental history was non-contributory.

EXTRA-ORAL EXAMINATION
(Figures 12.2 and 12.3)

- Symmetrical face
- Competent lips
- Slightly convex profile
- Accentuated labio-mental fold
- Normally functioning temporomandibular joints
- Maximum opening 42 mm without deviation

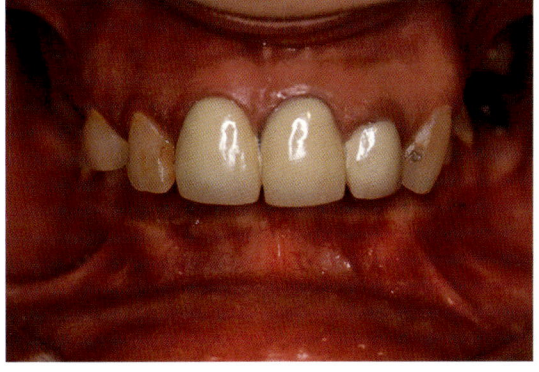

Figure 12.1

Anterior teeth—labial view

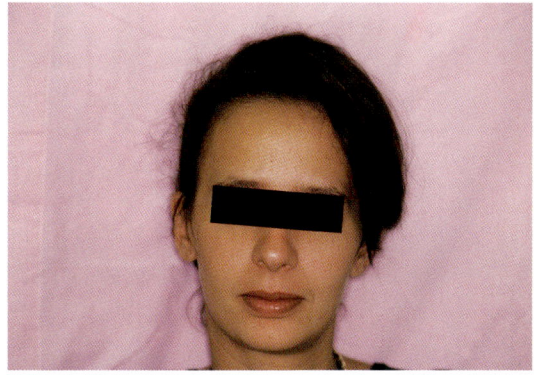

Figure 12.2

Face—frontal view

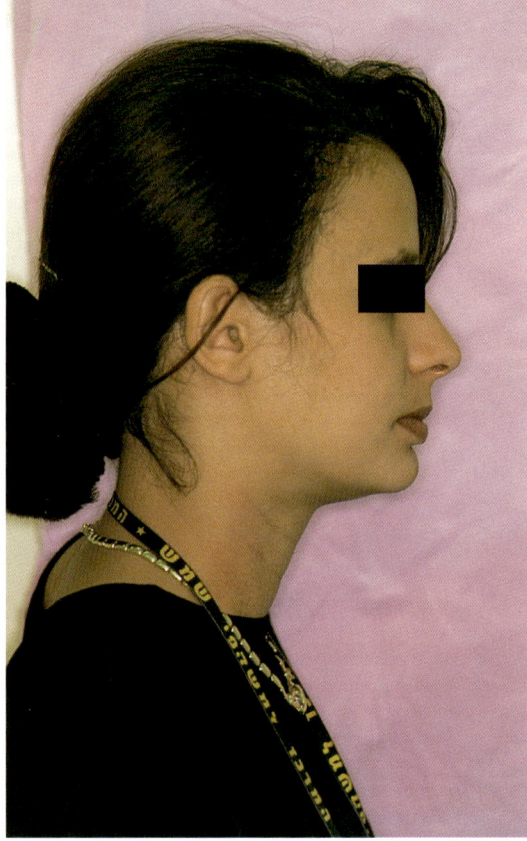

Figure 12.3

Face—side view

INTRA-ORAL EXAMINATION

Maxilla (Figure 12.4):

- Discrepancy between dental and facial midlines
- Parabolic asymmetric arch form
- Evidence of previous sores in the anterior palate
- Maxillary right premolars lacking coronal elements due to severe caries
- Caries
- Porcelain fused to metal crowns on the right central and both left incisor teeth

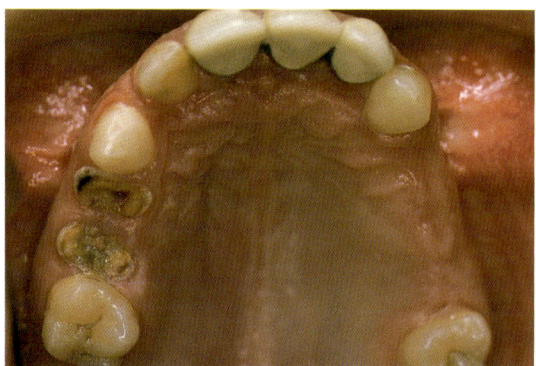

Figure 12.4

Maxillary arch—palatal view

- Missing teeth:

$$\underline{8\ 7} \mid \underline{4\ 5\ 6\ 8}$$

Mandible (Figure 12.5):

- Oval arch shape
- Anterior crowding
- Primary and secondary caries
- Defective large restorations
- Destroyed coronal structure
- Rotated and lingually inclined cuspids and premolars
- Missing teeth:

$$\overline{7\ 6} \mid \overline{6}$$

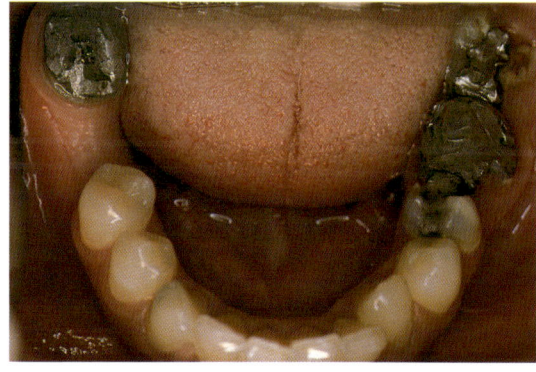

Figure 12.5

Mandibular arch—lingual view

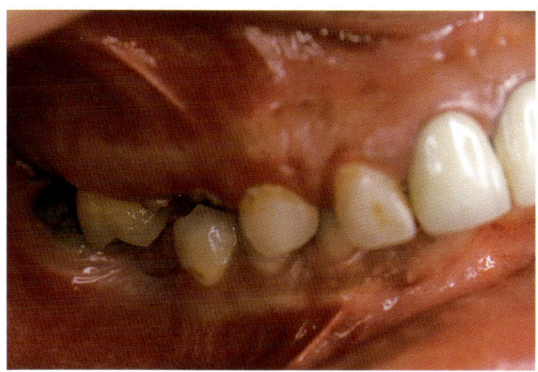

Figure 12.6

Occlusion—right side

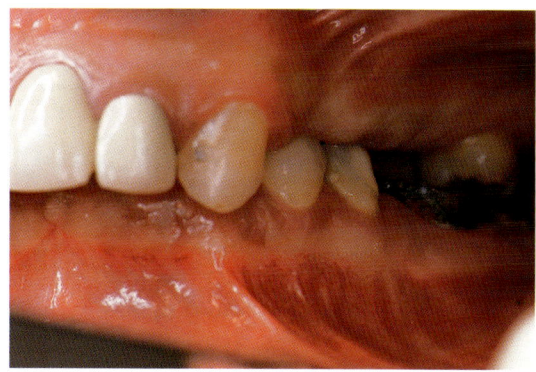

Figure 12.7

Occlusion—left side

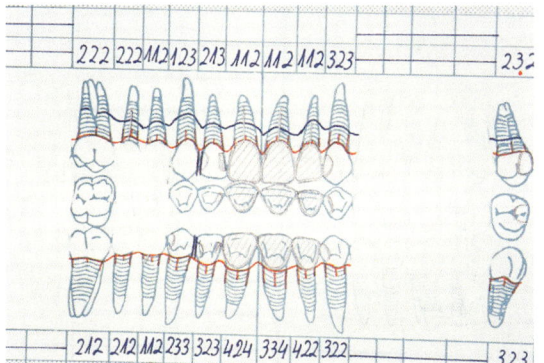

Figure 12.8

Periodontal chart—pre-treatment, maxilla

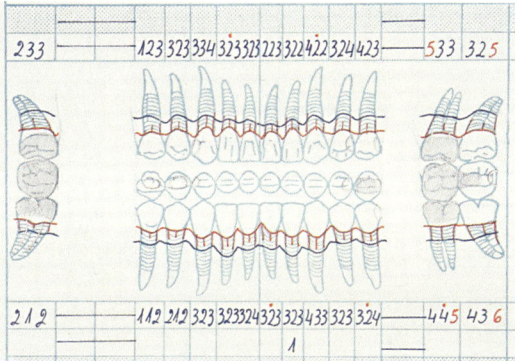

Figure 12.9

Periodontal chart—pre-treatment, mandible

An occlusal examination revealed that the patient was Angle class II division I, with deep impinging bite (Figures 12.1, 12.6 and 12.7). There was an overbite of 8.0 mm with tissue impingement and an overjet of 6.0 mm. The interocclusal rest space was 1.0 mm. Centric occlusion (CO) was concentric to centric relation (CR). Fremitus in centric occlusion:

$$
\begin{array}{c|c}
\text{I II} & \text{I} \\
3\ 2\ 1 & 1\ 2\ 3
\end{array}
$$

Periodontal examination (Figures 12.8 and 12.9) revealed poor oral hygiene with plaque and calculus. Probing depths of up to 4.0 mm on the maxillary teeth and up to 4.0 mm on the mandibular teeth were found, with bleeding on probing on some of the mandibular teeth. Inflamed tissue was noted.

FULL MOUTH PERIAPICAL RADIOGRAPHIC EXAMINATION
(Figures 12.10 and 12.11)

- Defective root canal therapy
- Periapical radiolucent areas

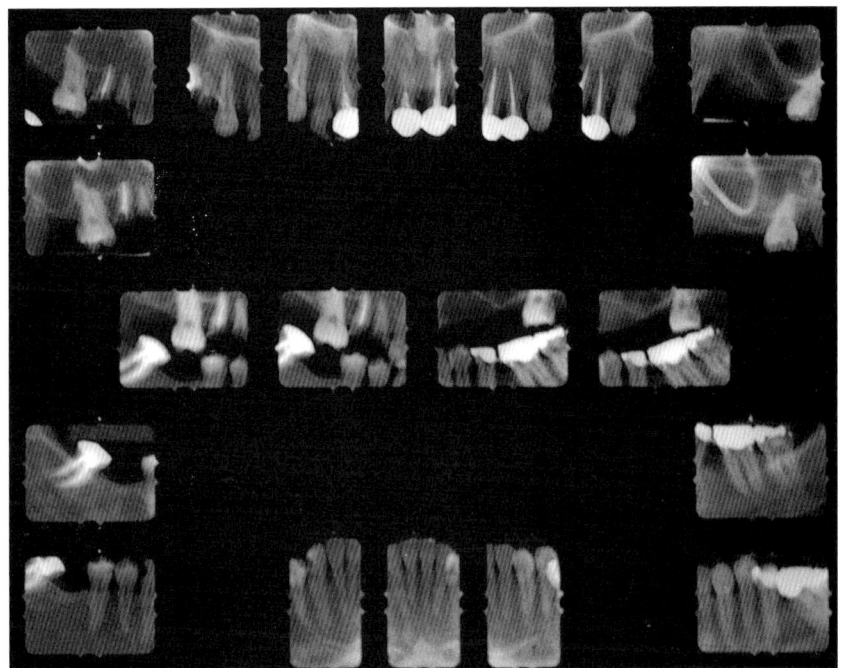

Figure 12.10

Radiographs of maxilla and mandible—pre-treatment, periapical

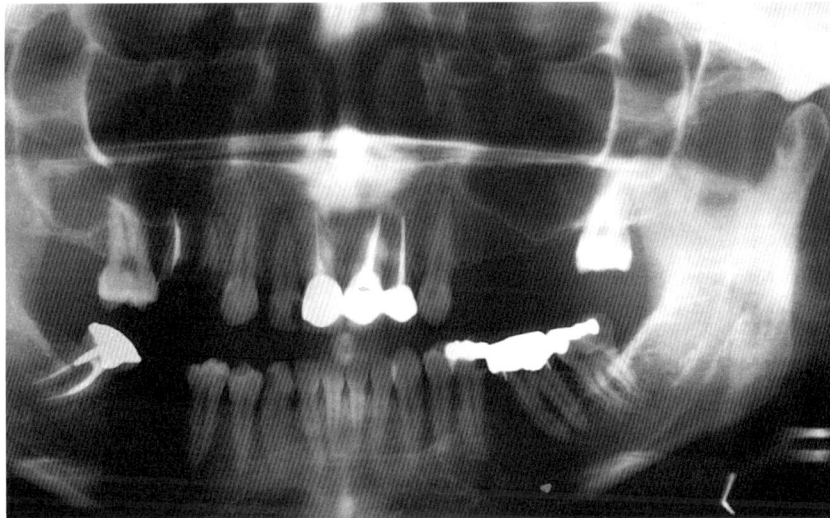

Figure 12.11

Radiographs of maxilla and mandible—pre-treatment, panoramic

- Good bone support on all remaining teeth
- Rampant caries
- Destroyed coronal structure
- Low maxillary sinus floor on both sides of maxilla

ESTHETIC EVALUATION AND PROBLEMS (Figure 12.12)

- High lip line
- Anterior maxillary gingival margins non-continuous

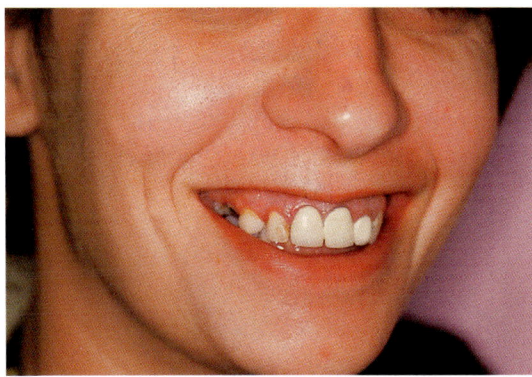

Figure 12.12

Anterior teeth—labial view, esthetic problem

- The maxillary incisor teeth were large and stuck out
- Discrepancy between maxillary and mandibular midlines
- The maxillary incisors did not contact the lower lip
- A wide smile exposed the gingival tissues in the maxilla

INDIVIDUAL TOOTH PROGNOSIS

- Hopeless:

$$\frac{5\,4\,\Big|}{\Big|}$$

- Poor:

$$\frac{\Big|}{\Big|\,8}$$

- Fair:

$$\frac{1\ \Big|\ 1\ 2}{8\ \Big|\ 5\ 7}$$

- Good:

$$\frac{6\,3\,2\ \Big|\ 3}{5\,4\,3\,2\,1\ \Big|\ 1\,2\,3\,4}$$

DIAGNOSIS

- Angle class II division I, with deep impinging bite

- Faulty occlusal relationship, and faulty occlusal plane
- Rampant carious lesions
- Defective restorations and endodontic treatment (periapical lesions)
- Missing teeth
- Poor esthetics
- Gingivitis
- Reduced posterior support
- Reduced vertical dimension
- Primary occlusal trauma
- Loss of tooth structure

ABOUT THE PATIENT

The patient was a young woman with a large amount of coronal tooth structure loss due to rampant caries. She was very apprehensive but had finally overcome her fear of dentists and, after visiting many dental clinics, decided on having her dental treatment as soon as possible. She had high expectations from her dental treatment. She wanted to improve her esthetic appearance and would have preferred fixed restorations, but understood the difficulty involved.

POTENTIAL TREATMENT PROBLEMS

A deep bite accompanied by loss of vertical dimension and an increased overjet, along with the great difference in jaw size and tooth position, made it very difficult to achieve good occlusal relationships which enabled the inclusion of the anterior segments in occlusal support. By restoring lost vertical dimension, needed for the rehabilitation, the jaw relations would be made worse. To utilize implants for posterior support would improve the situation, but would require pre-implant surgery. The problem of the rampant caries had to be overcome before any permanent restorations were undertaken.

TREATMENT POSSIBILITIES

Maxilla:

- Fixed and removable partial prostheses
- Fixed partial prosthesis supported by remaining teeth and implants (would necessitate pre-implant surgery)
- Fixed prosthesis
- Orthognathic surgery, orthodontic treatment and fixed prosthesis

Mandible:

- Fixed partial prosthesis
- Fixed partial prosthesis supported by remaining teeth and implant

TREATMENT PLAN

INITIAL PREPARATION

- Dietary changes
- Oral hygiene instruction
- Fluoride rinses and gel application
- Changing the vertical dimension to relieve the palatal tissue impingement
- Caries removal
- Referral for endodontic therapy
- Evaluation of patient cooperation
- Referral for computerized tomography (CT) radiographs to determine implant possibility
- Restorative treatment with restorations and provisional fixed acrylic restorations for the teeth with a sizeable loss of tooth structure

- Orthodontic treatment for uprighting and realigning teeth
- Re-evaluation and planning of pre-prosthetic periodontal surgery
- New provisional fixed acrylic restorations at the new vertical dimension of occlusion in order to check patient adaptation
- Re-evaluation
- Fixed partial prostheses for both the maxilla and the mandible

TREATMENT

Initial preparation included oral hygiene instruction, scaling, and curettage. Canine platforms were then built on the lingual surfaces of the maxillary cuspid teeth opening the vertical dimension of occlusion by approximately 2.5 mm (Figure 12.13). This allowed healing of the palatal gingiva by preventing impingement of the mandibular anterior teeth on the palate (Figure 12.14).

Endodontic treatment was performed on the maxillary left third molar and the mandibular left second molar. Caries removal and provisional restorations were done where indicated. At this time the anterior maxillary splint was sectioned and removed (Figure 12.15). Transitional acrylic crowns were then made for these teeth (Figure 12.16). CT radiographs were then taken of the maxilla to determine the amount and quality of bone available for implant placement (Figures 12.17 and 12.18). After extraction of the maxillary right premolars, the remaining maxillary teeth were then prepared for full crowns and transitional fixed partial prostheses constructed (Figures 12.19 and 12.20).

Re-evaluation at this time showed that the bucco–lingual jaw relationships on the

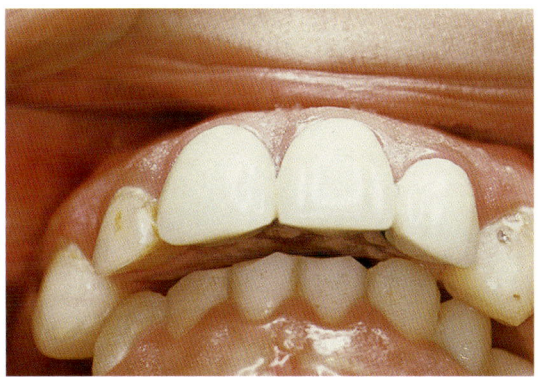

Figure 12.13

Canine platform to open vertical dimension

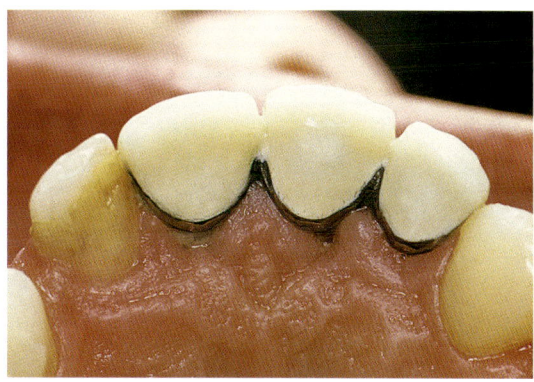

Figure 12.14

Healing of the palatal gingiva

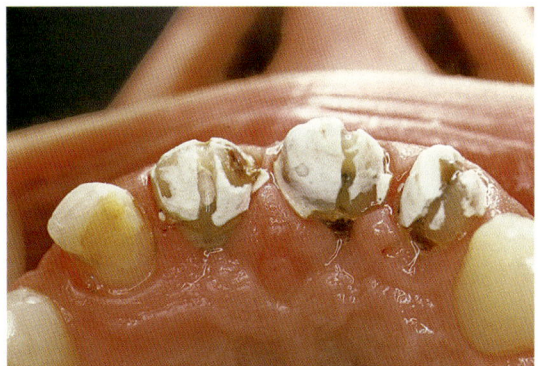

Figure 12.15

Removing existing crowns

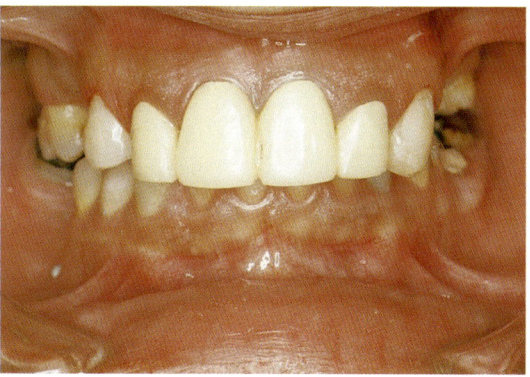

Figure 12.16

Transitional prosthesis—maxilla

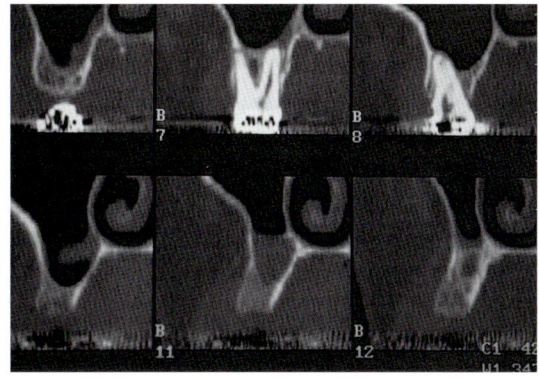

Figure 12.17

CT scan, maxilla—right side

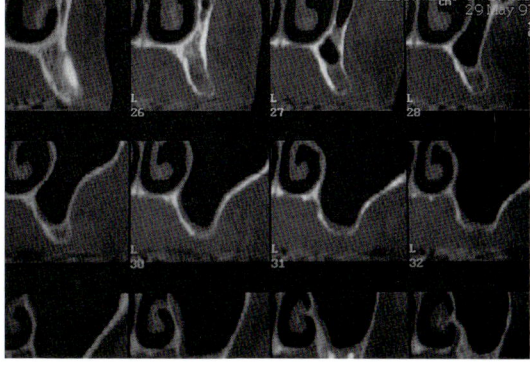

Figure 12.18

CT scan, maxilla—left side

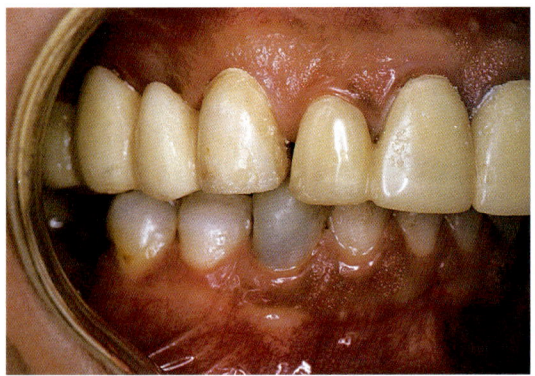

Figure 12.19

New transitional prosthesis—maxilla, right side

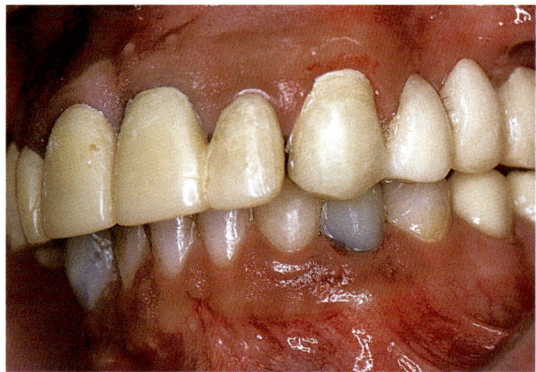

Figure 12.20

New transitional prosthesis—maxilla left side

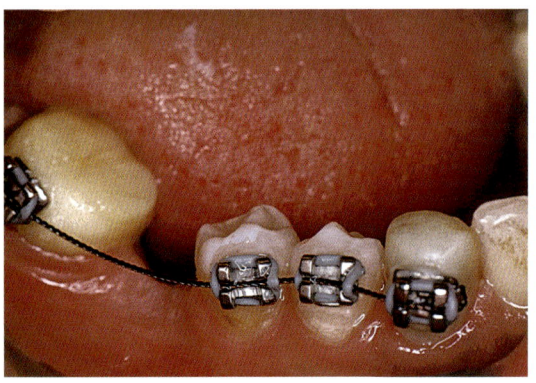

Figure 12.21

Orthodontic treatment—uprighting right mandibular third molar

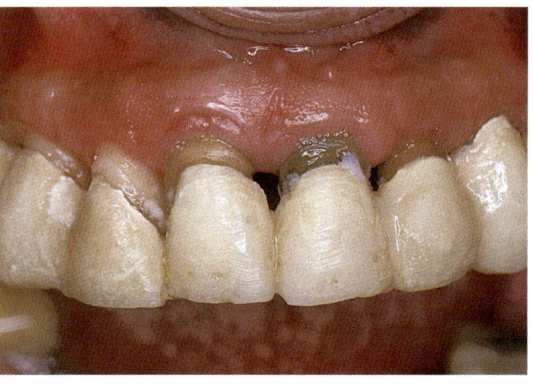

Figure 12.22

Periodontal surgery—anterior maxilla, after healing

right side had worsened with the opening of the vertical dimension. Therefore there remained two options for restoring the mandible on the right side. The first option was orthodontic uprighting of the mandibular third molar and then a fixed partial prosthesis from the second premolar to the third molar to replace the missing molar teeth. The second option would be to implant a single wide body implant in the area of the mandibular right first molar and then do a fixed restoration on it, thus not involving the third molar in posterior support.

The first option was chosen and orthodontic treatment was instituted to upright the mandibular third molar (Figure 12.21). At this time, a further re-evaluation was done. It was decided that due to the relatively young age of the patient (26), the fact that she did not want implants, and that there was only a relatively small span to be restored on the mandibular right side, a fixed partial prosthesis was chosen.

Periodontal surgery was performed in the anterior segment of the maxilla in order

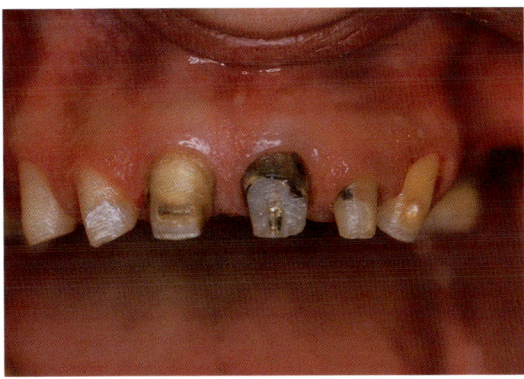

Figure 12.23

Final preparation of maxillary teeth

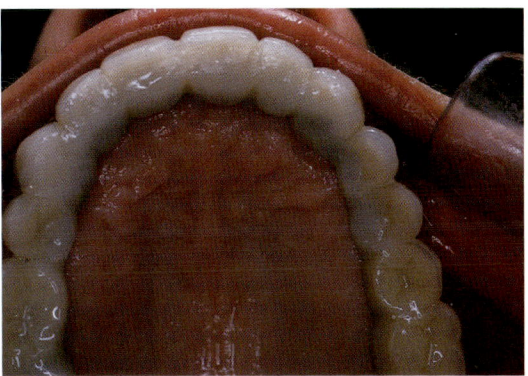

Figure 12.24

Final transitional prosthesis—maxilla

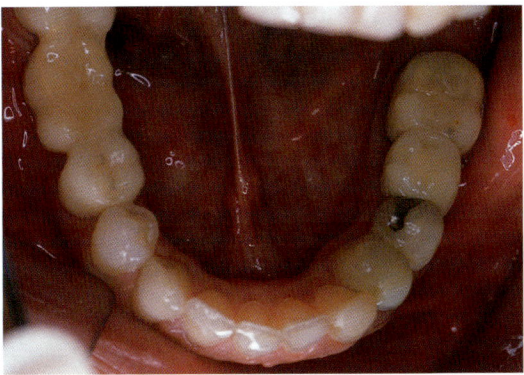

Figure 12.25

Final transitional prosthesis—mandible

to even up the gingival margins and provide additional tooth structure for retention of the fixed prosthesis (Figure 12.22).

At completion of orthodontic and periodontal treatment the teeth were reprepared and new provisional restorations were made to maintain the new vertical dimension and to stabilize the teeth after the orthodontic treatment. These transitional restorations also enabled the dentist to evaluate the patient's adaptation to the new occlusal jaw relations (Figures 12.23–12.25).

During a period of 3 months with the provisional restorations at the new vertical dimension of occlusion, the patient exhibited no temporomandibular joint or muscular problems. Copper band elastomeric impressions were taken and stone dies were fabricated from the individual impressions. On these dies, Pattern resin copings were made and fitted in the mouth. Polyether pick-up impressions were done for the working models. The individual dies were placed into the impression and the model was made. Centric relation was recorded at the new proven vertical dimension using Pattern resin (Figures 12.26 and 12.27). This was done by leaving the provisional restorations in place on the left side while fitting the Pattern resin copings and recording the centric relation record on the copings on the right side. The provisional restorations were then removed on the left side and the Pattern resin copings placed on the supporting teeth (Figure 12.28).

Metal copings were then cast and fitted in the mouth, and the copings connected for soldering. The copings were soldered and checked again for proper fit in the mouth and a new centric registration record was done in Pattern resin material.

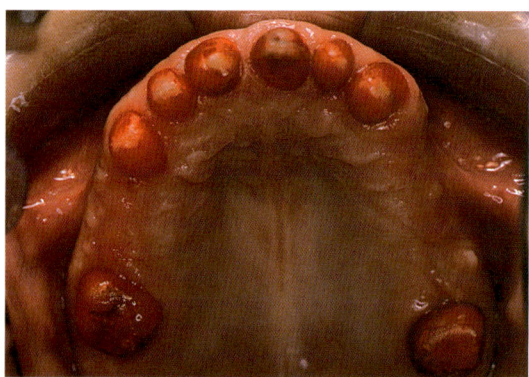

Figure 12.26

Pattern resin coping try-in—maxilla

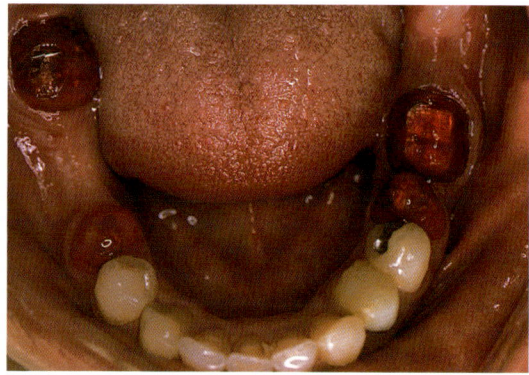

Figure 12.27

Pattern resin coping try-in—mandible

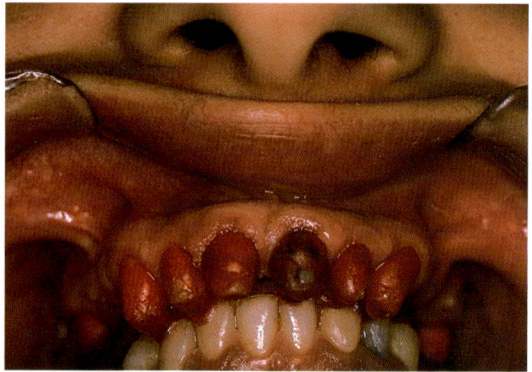

Figure 12.28

Centric relation record on pattern resin copings at new vertical dimension

Full arch polyether impressions were made for tissue detail. The models were then mounted on a Hanau articulator with the aid of a face bow registration, and the porcelain was baked.

The final and minute adjustments of the biscuit bake porcelain were carried out in the mouth. The final glaze was applied to the prostheses, and the prostheses were cemented with Temp-Bond for a period of 2 weeks. They were then cemented with zinc oxyphosphate cement for permanent cementation (Figures 12.29–12.32).

SUMMARY

The patient presented with a severe problem of Angle class II deep bite with impingement of the palatal tissues by the mandibular anterior teeth. She had missing and malpositioned teeth. There was a loss of vertical dimension and malocclusion complicated by rampant caries. All these factors made it mandatory to open the vertical dimension in order to restore the patient to a healthy and physiological occlusion. This would worsen the occlusal relationship and prevent anterior occlusal support. By means of limited orthodontic treatment and modification of the occlusal relationships, we were able to give the patient a fixed restoration that included the support of many of the remaining teeth, thus giving the patient a functional and esthetic solution to her dental problems.

CASE DISCUSSION
AVINOAM YAFFE

The patient presented to our clinic with a complicated situation of missing teeth, rampant caries, loss of the coronal tooth

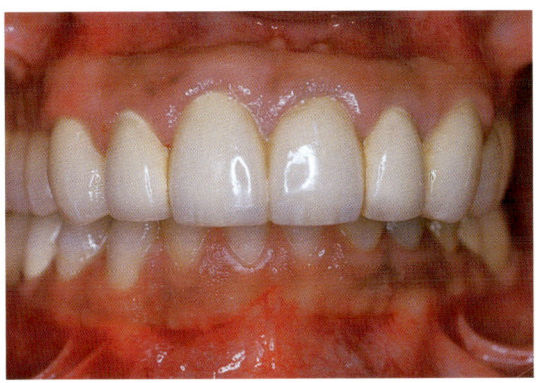

Figure 12.29

Treatment completed—permanent treatment completed, anterior view

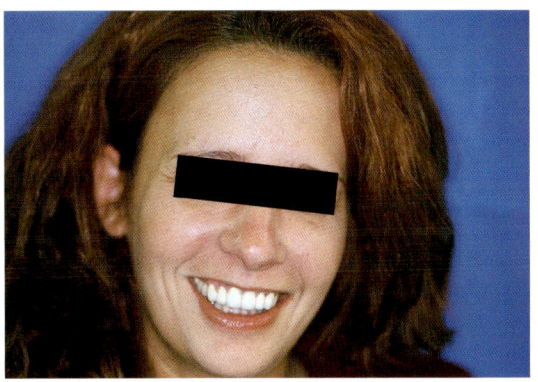

Figure 12.30

Treatment completed—patient smiling

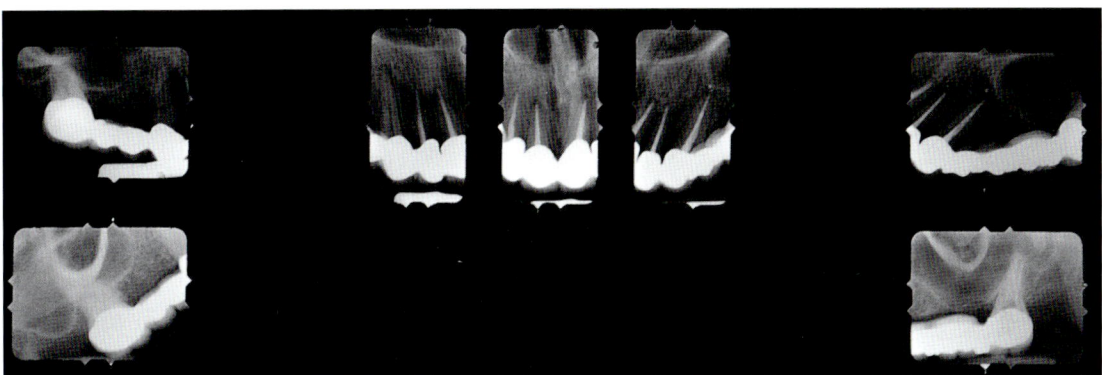

Figure 12.31

Treatment completed—radiographs, maxilla

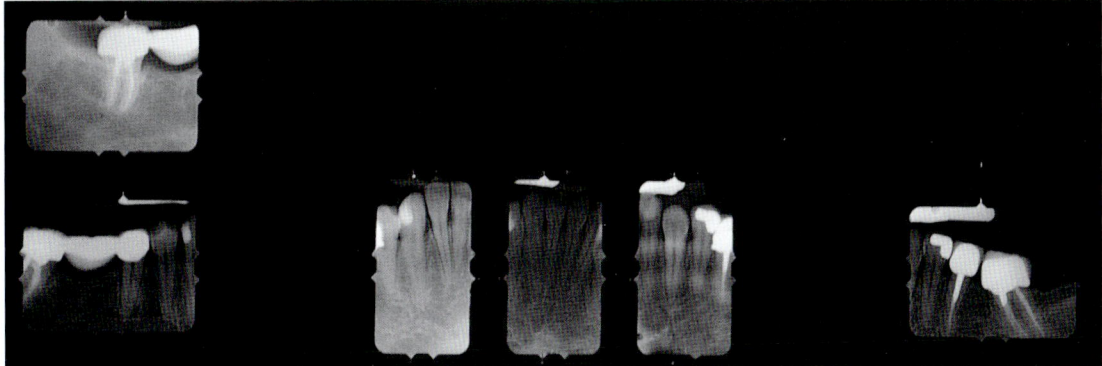

Figure 12.32

Treatment completed—radiographs, mandible

structure in most of the remaining teeth, loss of vertical dimension and soft tissue impingement causing suppuration. The treatment of choice should have been orthognathic surgery, but the patient refused to undergo this. This situation presented us with a challenge, which would be difficult to cope with. By using the canine platform as a tool, and guide, we changed the vertical dimension to a workable situation and worked out the occlusal relationships and occlusal scheme to this pre-determined scheme. We aimed at including as many teeth as possible to participate in occlusal support using adjunctive orthodontics and including the canine teeth in support and guidance by the placement of platforms on both the maxillary and mandibular canine teeth.

The periodontal surgery performed to reach both sound tooth structure and a pleasant appearing smile in the anterior region was successful. In this patient, the almost impossible has been achieved without orthognathic surgery and implants that would have required pre-prosthetic surgery, to which the patient objected. She received a functional physiologic and esthetic solution to an almost impossible problem.

CASE DISCUSSION
HAROLD PREISKEL

The management of this patient's treatment demonstrates what can be achieved using conventional periodontal and prosthodontic therapy when orthognathic surgery is contraindicated or unwanted by the patient. The key to rebuilding the occlusal scheme appeared to rest with the clever use of the upper canines as a platform. Of course without the patient's motivation, the endodontic therapy, and the periodontal therapy, nothing would have been of avail. The combination of motivation, clever planning, and meticulous execution of relatively conventional techniques appears to have produced a good-looking and functional occlusion that I hope will last for years.

PATIENT 13   TREATMENT WITH LIMITED FINANCIAL RESOURCES

Treatment by Tzachi Lehr

THE PATIENT

The patient, a 40-year-old male came to the clinic for dental treatment. His chief complaints were (Figures 13.1 and 13.2):

'I have no teeth to chew with.'
'Food packs between my teeth.'
'I can't smile.'
'I have a bad taste in my mouth.'

PAST MEDICAL HISTORY

The patient's medical history was non-contributory.

PAST DENTAL HISTORY

Since 1982, the patient had most of his dental treatment done at Hadassah. There he had a transitional mandibular removable partial denture made, but did not use it. His dental file revealed that the left maxillary third molar was extracted in 1985, the mandibular right first molar in 1992, and the mandibular left second premolar in 1995. He said he had no specific habit patterns, although until recently he ate lots of sweets. Recently he has refrained from eating sweets, due to the severe pain that occurs whenever he does. His esthetic appearance greatly concerns him and he noticed that he hardly ever smiles anymore.

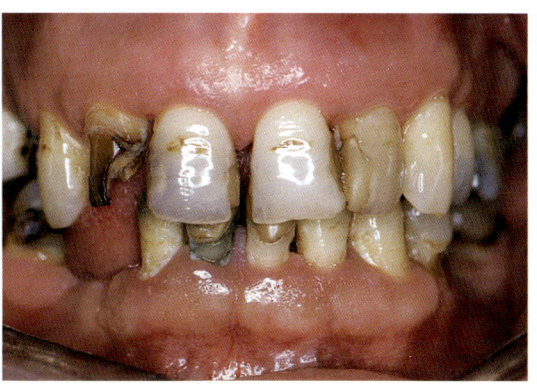

Figure 13.1

Anterior teeth—labial view

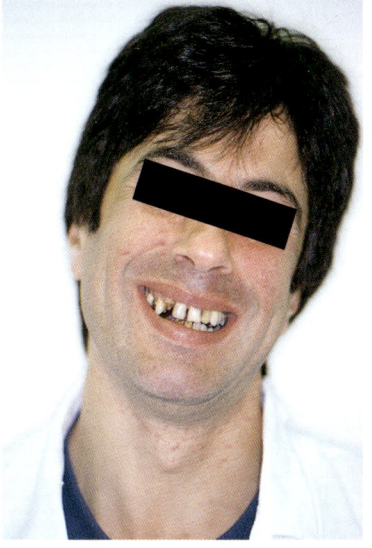

Figure 13.2

Face—frontal view

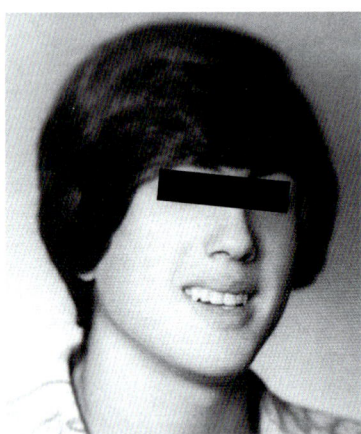

Figure 13.3

Face—frontal view (from 23 years ago)

He showed pictures of himself when he was younger, showing a large smile and healthy teeth (Figure 13.3).

EXTRA-ORAL EXAMINATION
(Figures 13.2 and 13.4)

- Symmetrical face
- Straight profile

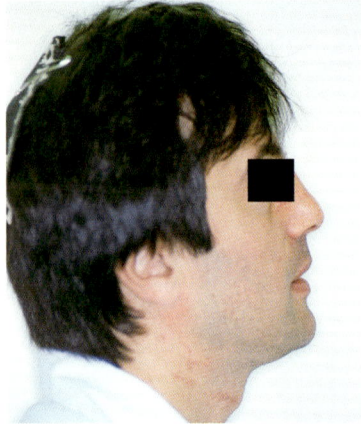

Figure 13.4

Face—side view

- Temporomandibular joint was normal
- Mandibular motions were within normal limits
- Normal facial musculature
- Maximum opening of 45 mm
- Incompetent lips
- Trapped lower lip

INTRA-ORAL AND FULL-MOUTH PERIAPICAL RADIOGRAPH EXAMINATION

Maxilla (Figure 13.5):

- Parabolic arch
- Caries
- Spacing between the anterior teeth
- Missing left third molar tooth
- Right lateral incisor and right first premolar prepared for full coverage but without provisional restorations
- Large amalgam restorations on the left premolars and molars
- Left second molar and right third molar with large caries in the crown section, extending into the root
- Missing right first molar with anterior drifting of the second and third molars

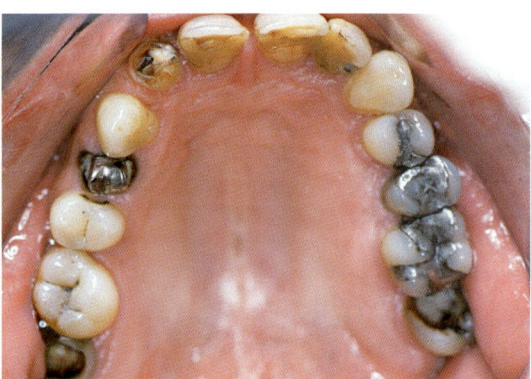

Figure 13.5

Maxillary arch—palatal view

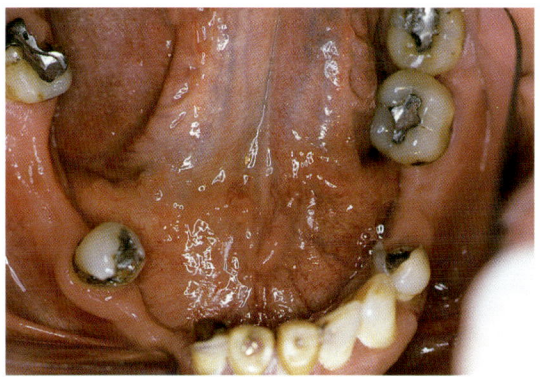

Figure 13.6

Mandibular arch—lingual view

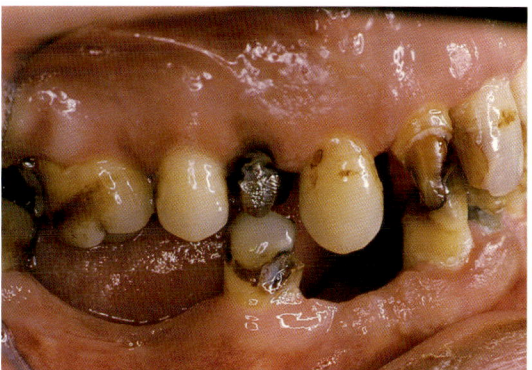

Figure 13.7

Occlusion—right side

Mandible (Figure 13.6):

- Parabolic arch
- Mesial inclination of the left second and third molars
- Amalgam restorations on the posterior teeth
- Missing teeth:

$$\frac{|}{7\,6\,4\,3\,|\,5\,6}$$

- Provisional acrylic crowns on the central incisors
- Deep caries:

$$\frac{|}{8\,5\,2\,|\,4\,7}$$

Occlusal examination (Figures 13.7 and 13.8) revealed that the patient was Angle class I. The interocclusal rest space was 3.0–4.0 mm. Overjet was 2.0 mm and overbite was 3.0 mm. There was no difference between centric relation and centric occlusion. There was a midline discrepancy. There was spacing between the maxillary incisor teeth and the left lateral incisor and left cuspid were slightly rotated. Non-working side interferences were noted between the mandibular right third molar and the maxillary right second molar.

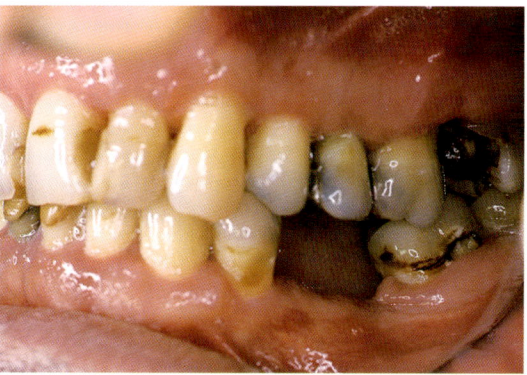

Figure 13.8

Occlusion—left side

Fremitus:

- Maxillary right central incisor—grade I in closing and right working jaw movements
- Maxillary left central incisor, left lateral incisor, and right lateral incisor—grade I in centric occlusion and protrusive jaw movements

The periodontal examination (Figures 13.9 and 13.10) revealed calculus and plaque, probing depths of up to 10.0 mm on most of the maxillary teeth and up to

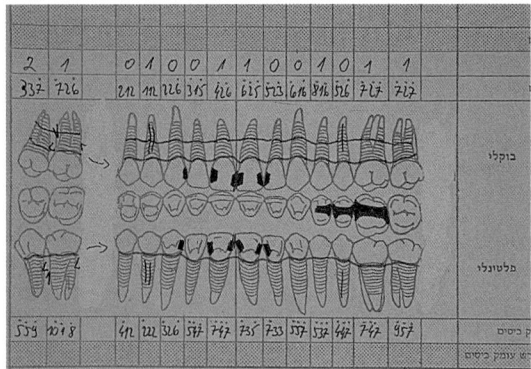

Figure 13.9

Periodontal chart—pre-treatment, maxilla

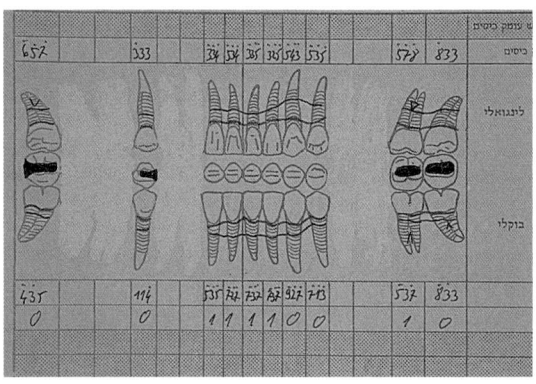

Figure 13.10

Periodontal chart—pre-treatment, mandible

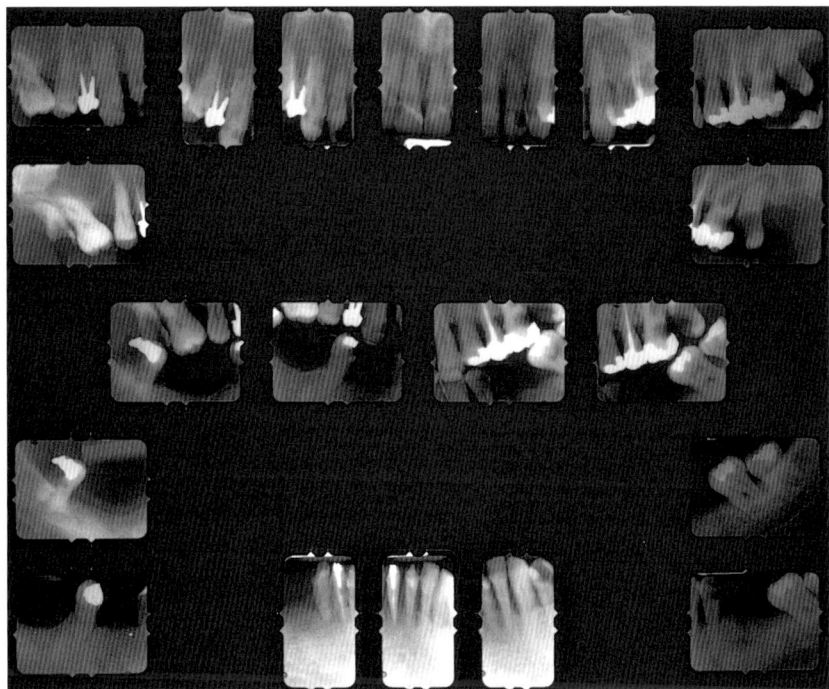

Figure 13.11

Radiographs of maxilla and mandible—pre-treatment

8.0 mm on many of the mandibular teeth. There was bleeding of the gingiva on probing on all the teeth. There was slight gingival recession around some of the teeth. Class 1 mobility was found on the mandibular incisor teeth. The maxillary molars had class I–II furcation involvement on the mesial and distal surfaces. The maxillary first premolar had both class III mesial and lingual furcation involvement. The mandibular molars had class I furcation involvement on the buccal surfaces.

FULL-MOUTH PERIAPICAL SURVEY (Figure 13.11)

- Endodontic treatment:

$$\frac{4\ |\ 5}{1\ |}$$

- Perio-endo lesion on left maxillary first molar
- Periapical lesion on left maxillary second molar
- Recent extraction site—mandibular left second premolar
- Rampant caries and secondary caries around cast post in maxillary right central incisor
- Extensive horizontal and vertical bone loss around most of the remaining teeth

INDIVIDUAL TOOTH PROGNOSIS

- Hopeless:

$$\frac{8\ 4\ |\ 7}{\ \ \ |}$$

- Questionable:

$$\frac{7\ |\ 4\ 6}{\ \ |\ 7}$$

- Poor:

$$\frac{\ \ \ \ |\ 3}{2\ 1\ |\ 1\ 2}$$

- Fair:

$$\frac{5\ 2\ 1\ |\ 1\ 2\ 3\ 5}{4\ |\ 8}$$

- Good:

$$\frac{3\ |}{\ \ |}$$

SUMMARY OF FINDINGS

The patient, a 40-year-old male in good health, came to the clinic complaining of difficulty in eating, poor esthetics, food packing between his teeth and a bad taste in his mouth. He had poor oral hygiene, plaque and calculus, and severe inflammation accompanied by deep probing depths and furcation involvements. Some of the teeth were mobile.

DIAGNOSIS

- Advanced adult periodontitis
- Missing teeth
- Loss of posterior support
- Decreased vertical dimension of occlusion
- Rampant primary and secondary caries
- Faulty restorations
- Periapical lesions
- Faulty occlusal planes
- Shifting of teeth
- Primary occlusal trauma (due to trapped lower lip)
- Secondary occlusal trauma with primary origin of trauma (due to trapped lower lip)
- Deep bite
- Poor esthetics

ABOUT THE PATIENT

The patient was highly motivated for treatment. He requested a fixed rather than a removable restoration, but his financial capabilities were limited.

TREATMENT PLAN

PHASE 1: INITIAL PREPARATION

Initial treatment including:

- Oral hygiene instruction
- Scaling and root planing
- Diet counseling regarding cariogenic food

- Topical fluoride treatment with Elmex gel (GABA Ltd; Basel, Switzerland)
- Caries excavation
- Maxillary left second molar—distal buccal root resection
- Mandibular right third molar—distal root resection
- Extractions:

$$\frac{8\ 4\ \big|\ 7}{7}$$

- Endodontic treatment:

$$\frac{6\ 2\ \big|\ 2\ 6}{8\ 2\ \big|\ 4}$$

PHASE 2: POSSIBILITIES

Maxilla:

- Fixed prosthesis
- Fixed and partial removable prostheses if maxillary left first premolar and molar could not be saved

Mandible:

- Complete overdenture
- Fixed and partial removable prostheses

- Fixed prosthesis supported by natural teeth and implants (rejected by the patient due to cost)

TREATMENT

Initial treatment consisted of oral hygiene instruction, scaling and root planing. The maxillary right lateral incisor was repre-pared, the caries excavated, and a provisional crown made. Endodontic treatment was done on the maxillary lateral incisors and the maxillary left second premolar, and left first molar. At this point, a re-evaluation was done and even though the patient's oral hygiene had greatly improved, bleeding on probing and the probing depths had only been slightly reduced (Figures 13.12 and 13.13).

In the mandible where pocket depths and mobility also had not been significantly reduced, and considering the limited financial means of the patient, and the poor prognosis of the remaining teeth, it was decided to make a removable prosthesis rather than a fixed one. The mandibular left second molar, central incisors, and left lateral incisor were extracted and the

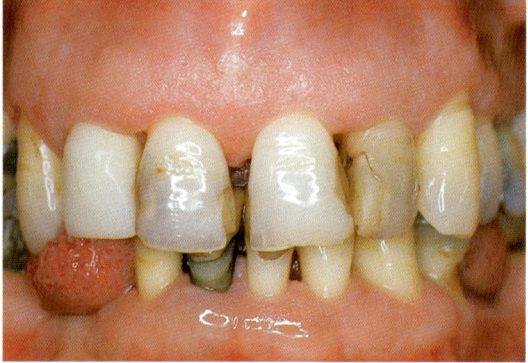

Figure 13.12

Anterior teeth—labial view, after initial preparation

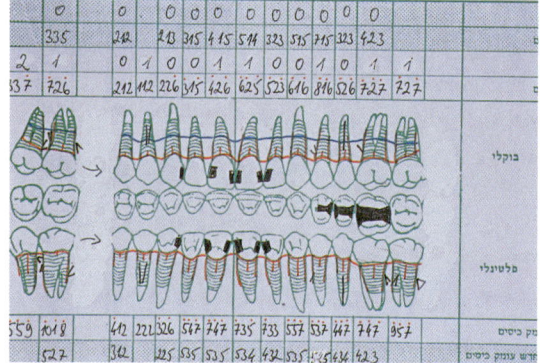

Figure 13.13

Periodontal chart—first re-evaluation

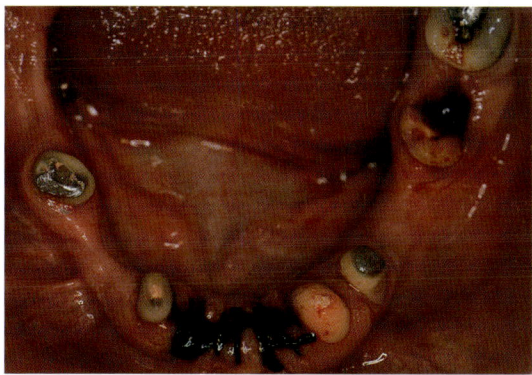

Figure 13.14 a

Mandibular anterior teeth—occlusal view after extractions and endodontic treatment

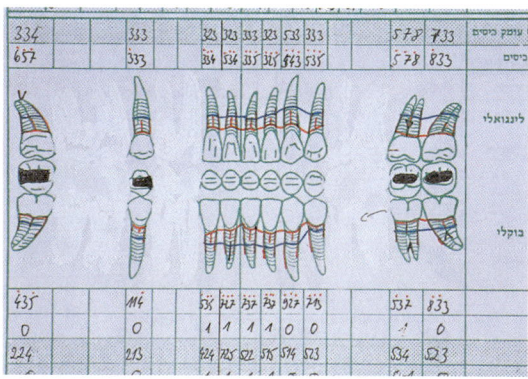

Figure 13.14 b

Periodontal chart—re-evaluation of mandible

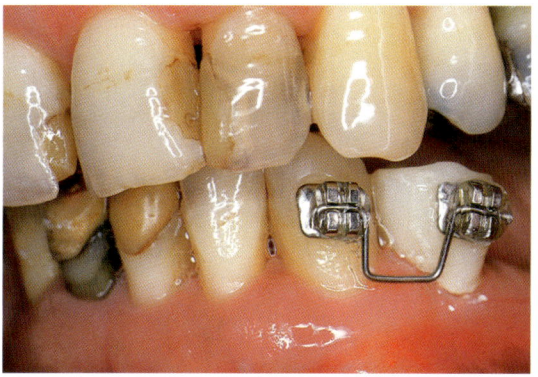

Figure 13.15

Anterior teeth—orthodontic treatment to close spaces and retract teeth

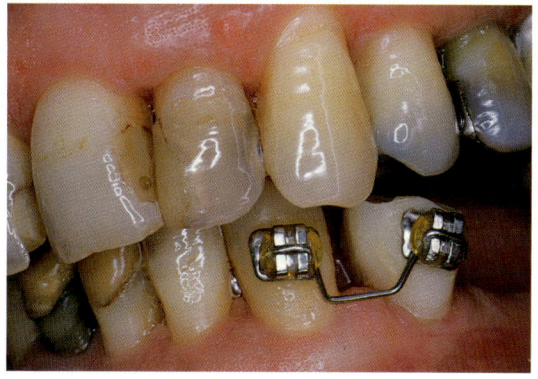

Figure 13.16

Anterior teeth—orthodontic treatment completed

remaining teeth were endodontically treated (Figure 13.14). Due to crown proximity, orthodontic treatment was performed to separate the left cuspid from the first premolar (Figures 13.15 and 13.16). The remaining teeth were then prepared, provisional acrylic copings were made and a transitional removable partial overdenture was made (Figures 13.17 and 13.18).

Periodontal surgery (open flap curettage) in order to reduce pocket depths as well as to determine the prognosis of the left first premolar was then performed in the maxilla. During the surgery, it was decided to extract the maxillary left first premolar due to the extensive furcation involvement (class III).

The second re-evaluation was now done and revealed that the probing depths had greatly diminished and the bleeding on probing had disappeared. Except for the mandibular right lateral incisor (class I mobility), there was no mobility of the teeth (Figures 13.19 and 13.20).

The disto-buccal roots of the maxillary first molars were amputated and the

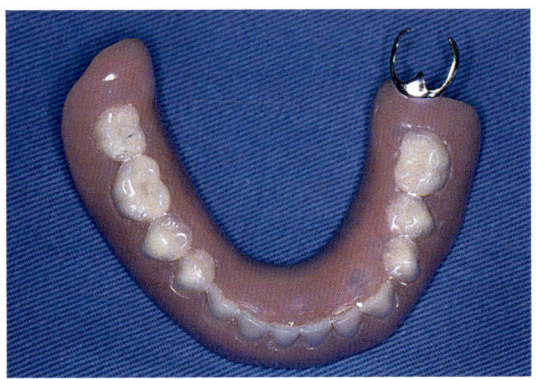

Figure 13.17

Mandibular removable partial denture

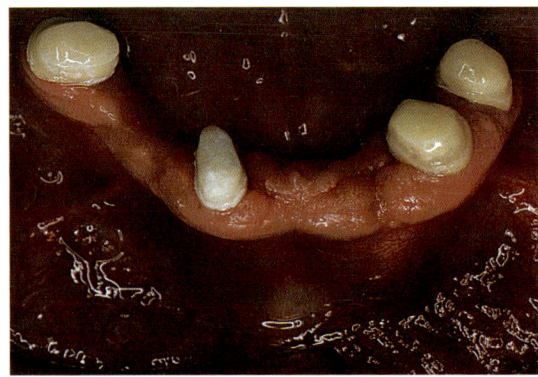

Figure 13.18

Mandible—provisional acrylic copings for overdenture

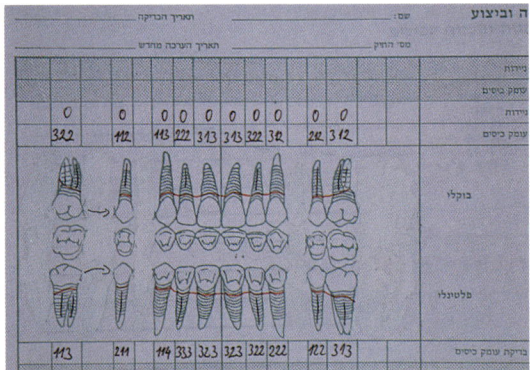

Figure 13.19

Periodontal chart—maxilla, re-evaluation

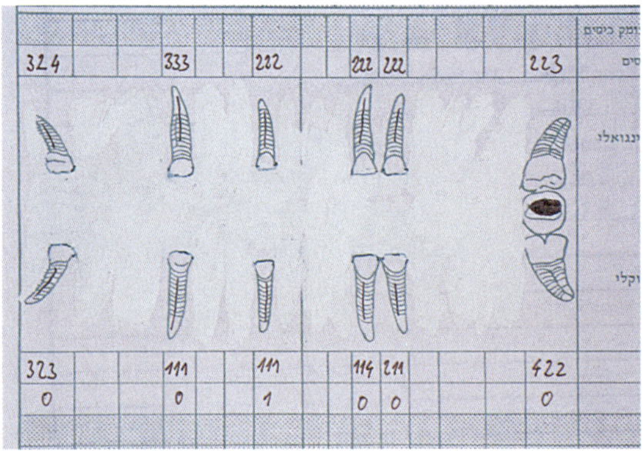

Periodontal chart—mandible, re-evaluation

Figure 13.20

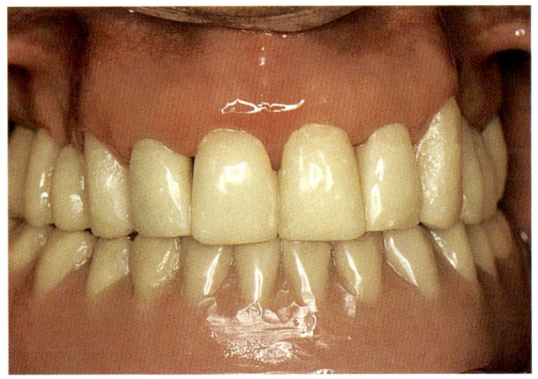

Figure 13.21

Transitional restorations—maxilla and mandible

remaining maxillary teeth were prepared for full coverage and a provisional acrylic restoration was made (Figure 13.21):

$$ 6\text{-}5\text{-}X\text{-}3\text{-}2\text{-}1 \mid 1\text{-}2\text{-}3\text{-}X\text{-}5\text{-}6 $$

In the maxilla, copper band elastomeric impressions were made of all the prepared teeth and Pattern resin copings made to fit the stone dies. These copings were fitted in the mouth and a polyether full arch impression was then taken of the maxilla and the master model made. The copings were

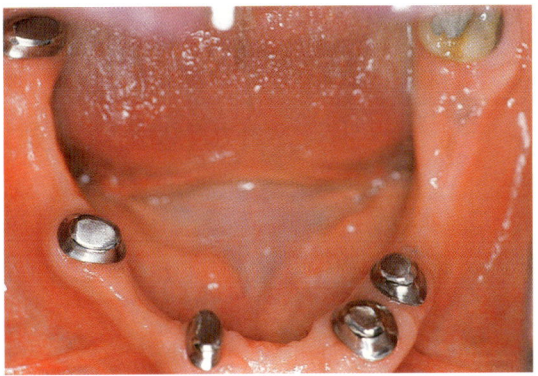

Figure 13.22

Mandible—magnetic copings for overdenture

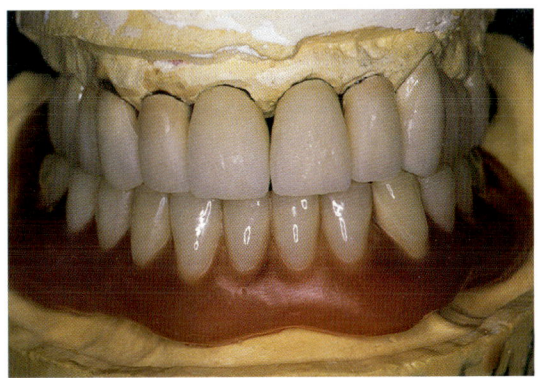

Figure 13.23

Maxillary bisc-bake and mandibular overdenture set up on Hanau articulator

also then used for a centric relation record at the vertical dimension of occlusion of the provisional restorations. This was done by cutting the provisional bridge between the central incisors and leaving one side in place, while recording the centric relation in Pattern resin on the copings on the other side. The provisional remaining bridge was then removed and the vertical dimension recorded on the Pattern resin copings while on the contralateral side, the Pattern resin copings maintained the vertical dimension of occlusion. A polyether full arch impression was then taken of the maxilla, the master model was poured and mounted to the mandibular model of the transitional removable partial denture by means of the Pattern resin centric record.

Metal copings were then cast and fitted in the mouth and connected by Pattern resin for soldering. These were soldered together, refitted and a new centric relation record made. A polyether impression was then undertaken for tissue detail and a pick-up of the fixed prosthesis in order to make a final master model. This was mounted on a Hanau articulator by means of a facebow registration and the Pattern

resin registration on the soldered metal prosthesis. The shade was chosen and porcelain baked to the metal. This was fitted in the mouth and the occlusion adjusted to the lower jaw.

At this point, impressions were done to make magnetic copings for the remaining lower teeth. These were fitted and cemented into place (Figure 13.22). A final impression in a custom tray was taken of the mandible and cast in albastone. A chrome cobalt metal framework was then cast and fitted in the mouth.

An acrylic and wax bite tray was then made on this model over the metal framework and fitted in the mouth. The centric relation record was then taken at the established vertical dimension of occlusion. This model was then mounted on the articulator by means of the bite tray with the centric record. The mandibular teeth were then set up (Figure 13.23) and checked in the mouth. The denture teeth were made of porcelain in order to match the material in the fixed prosthesis in the maxilla.

The mandibular removable partial denture was processed and inserted. The maxillary fixed prosthesis was glazed and

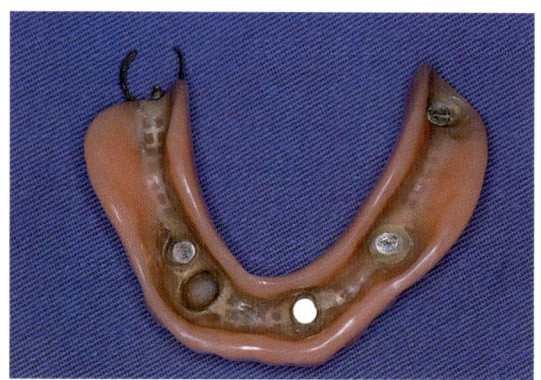

Figure 13.24

Completed mandibular partial denture—tissue view

cemented, with Temp-bond cement. After one week, the magnets were cold cured with acrylic into the denture and the maxillary prosthesis permanently cemented. Magnets were not used in all the areas, only opposite the right third molar, second premolar, lateral incisor, and left first premolar. The left cuspid area did not have a magnet (Figures 13.24–13.27).

SUMMARY

This patient presented with a very deteriorating situation in his mouth. In spite of

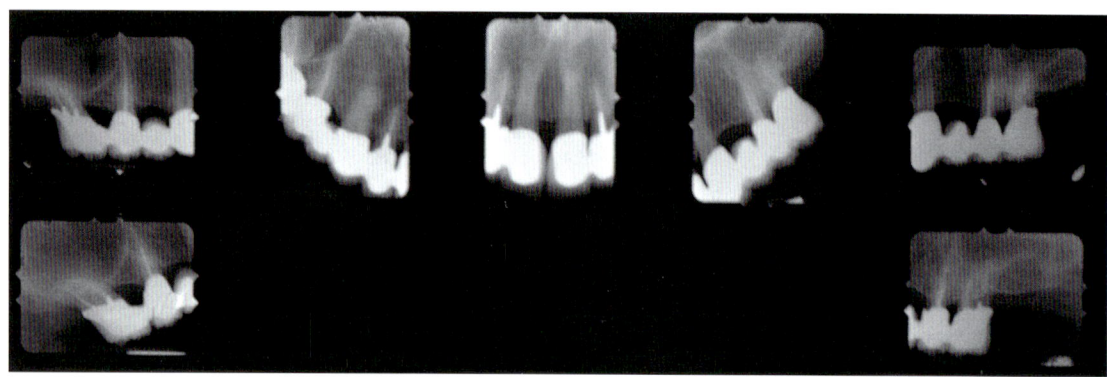

Figure 13.25

Radiographs of completed treatment, maxilla

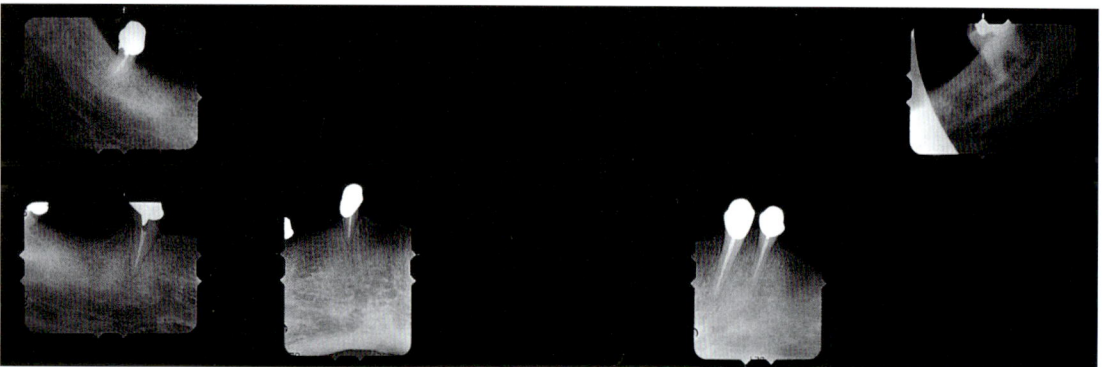

Figure 13.26

Radiographs of completed treatment, mandible

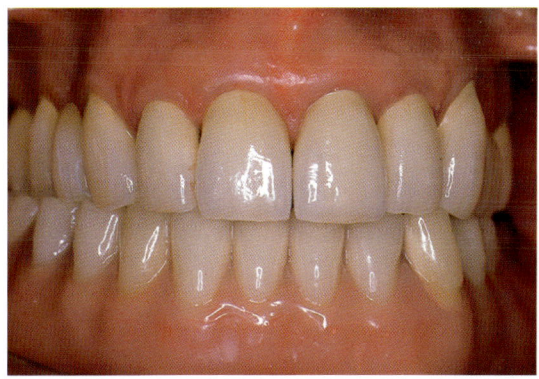

Figure 13.27

Treatment completed—permanent resorations, anterior view

restoration with the greatest possible prognosis. For obvious esthetic reasons the maxillary fixed restoration was made of porcelain fused to metal restoration. In order to cope with the attrition that would take place, porcelain teeth were installed in the removable, magnet-supported, fixed partial denture. It can be concluded that with the economic restriction we faced the young patient received an esthetic and functional solution.

his general good health, he had rampant caries and severe advanced periodontitis, many missing teeth, the majority in the mandible, and severe bone loss. There were tipped, malposed, and extruded teeth. There were many hopeless and questionable teeth among his few remaining teeth, yet the patient wanted a fixed prosthesis. Due to the patient's financial condition, this could not be achieved. However, an esthetic and functional solution was found for his dental problems.

CASE DISCUSSION
AVINOAM YAFFE

This case presentation describes a young patient with a severe caries problem aggravated by neglect, and complicated by periodontal condition and a poor economic situation. The patient was treated with the idea of supplying the best cost-efficient

CASE DISCUSSION
HAROLD PREISKEL

If the implant option is to be excluded, then the amount of dental support available effectively dictates a removable lower prosthesis opposing an upper fixed restoration. Such an approach dictates meticulous planning of the occlusal surfaces and, naturally, assumes that the supporting structures are not only healthy but that the patient can maintain them in this state. It might be argued that as a telescopic approach was used on most of the lower abutments then a telescopic retainer could have been included on the left molar rather than employing a conventional clasp. Using more than two magnets and porcelain teeth for the denture involves a possibility that during chewing the leverages may disengage one of the magnets from its keeper and produce a clicking sensation. The other problem is simply finding room for the underlying substructure while providing retention for the artificial teeth. The operator appears to have produced a functional and good-looking restoration.

Treatment by Irit Kupershmidt

THE PATIENT

The patient, a 44-year-old man, had been assaulted with an ax about 6 months before visiting the Hadassah School of Dental Medicine Graduate Prosthodontic Clinic. His injuries included scalp wounds, fracture of the right side of his skull, fracture of the left mandible, left maxillary sinus hemorrhage, lacerations of the cheek, and many broken teeth (Figure 14.1). His main complaints were the following:

'I have no sensations in my upper and lower lips on the left side and it gives me a bad feeling.'
'It hurts when I eat on my left side.'
'The missing teeth bother me when chewing, but not so much during speech.'

'The esthetics doesn't bother me that much.' (Figure 14.2)

PAST MEDICAL HISTORY

A year and a half prior to his coming for treatment, the patient had a myocardial infarct, and after undergoing an angiogram, was treated with angioplasty. He suffered from high blood pressure and was being treated with Cartia (aspirin 100 mg), Normiten (altenolol), and Cordil (isosorbide dinitrate).

PAST DENTAL HISTORY

For 10 years previous to his assault, he had not seen a dentist and could not recall

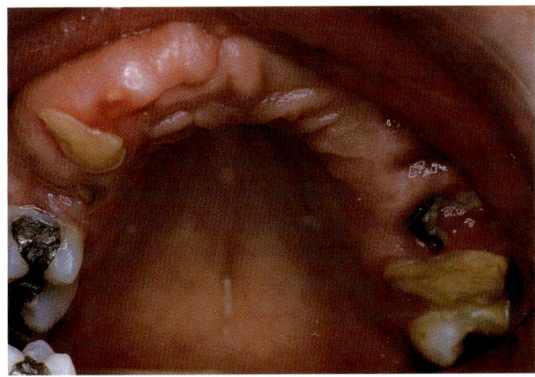

Figure 14.1

Maxillary teeth—palatal view

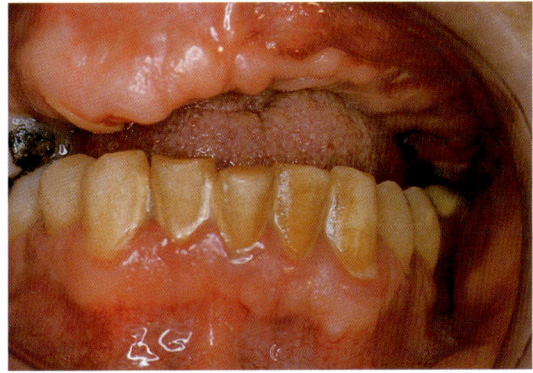

Figure 14.2

Anterior teeth—labial view

the condition of his teeth before the assault, but thought that some of them had crowns. Following his assault, his mandible was fixated with a titanium mesh and intra-arch wiring for one month at the Department of Oral and Maxillofacial Surgery at Hadassah. After removal of the wiring, he was not able to open his mouth more than 26 mm as measured at the maxillary and mandibular central incisor teeth. Physiotherapy brought about gradual improvement of the condition.

EXTRA-ORAL EXAMINATION
(Figures 14.3 and 14.4)

- Facial asymmetry, with a large scar on the left side
- Normally functioning muscles of mastication

- The temporomandibular joints were asymptomatic but the patient had limited mandibular movements
- There was a deviation to the left at the end of the jaw opening movement
- The maximum opening between the incisors was 50 mm, measured from the mandibular incisal edge to the incisal papillae
- Straight profile

INTRA-ORAL AND FULL-MOUTH PERIAPICAL RADIOGRAPH EXAMINATION
(Figures 14.1, 14.2, 14.5–14.9)

- Missing teeth
- All the maxillary teeth were fractured, most of them beneath the gum line, except for the right molars, the right

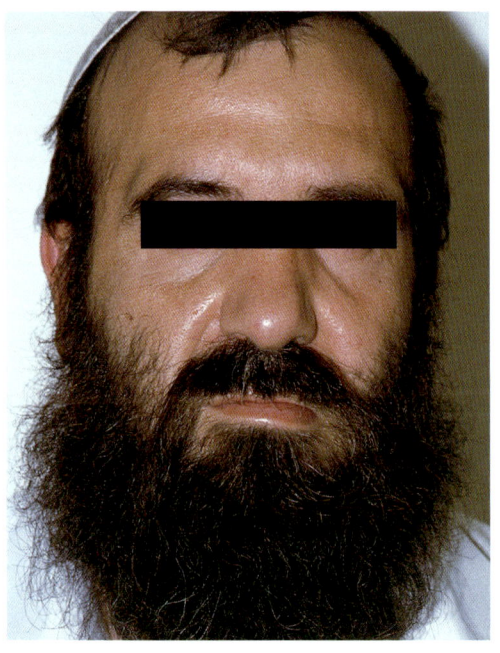

Figure 14.3

Face—frontal view

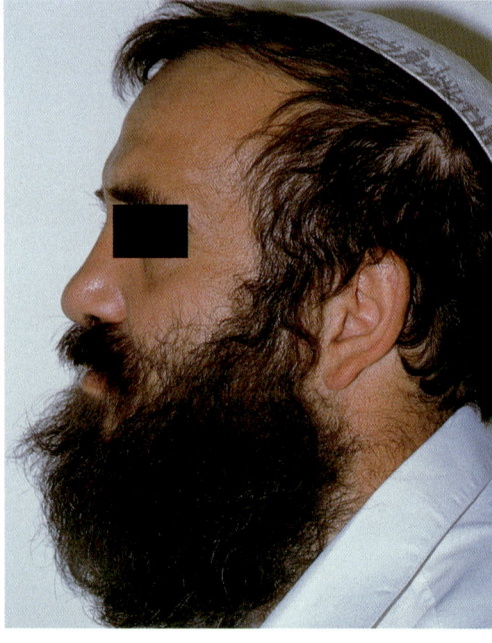

Figure 14.4

Face—left profile view

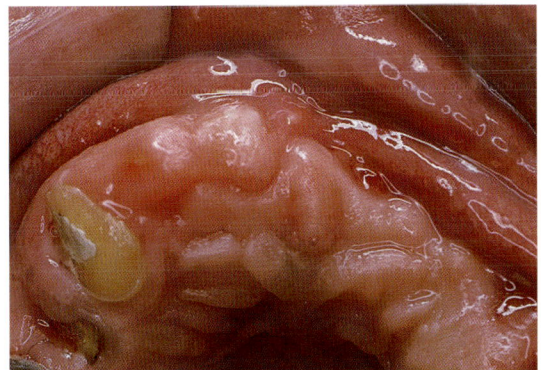

Figure 14.5

Anterior maxillary teeth—palatal view, close-up

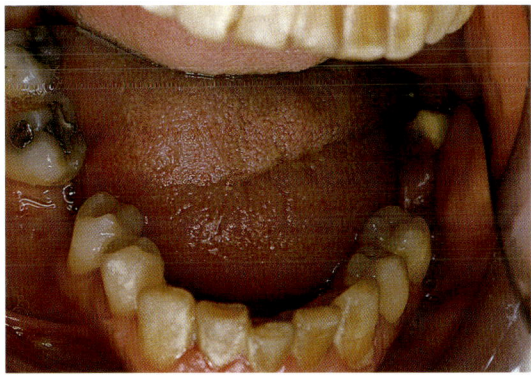

Figure 14.6

Mandibular arch

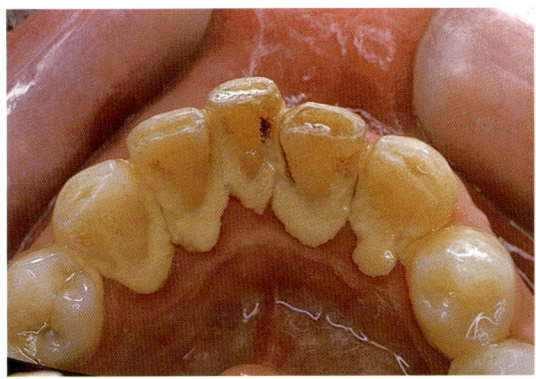

Figure 14.7

Anterior mandibular teeth—lingual view, close-up

second premolar, and the left second and third molars
- The large scar on the inner left side of the cheek severely limited the opening of his mouth
- High palate and loss of soft tissue and bone in the anterior part of the maxilla (Figure 14.5)
- Mandibular left second and third molar, right first molar, and the right central incisor teeth were missing
- The anterior teeth were rotated and crowded. The lower left third molar was covered by soft tissue (Figure 14.6)

- Caries
- Extensive bone loss around some teeth
- Titanium mesh in the left mandible
- Tipping and rotation of some teeth
- Nasopalatine duct cyst
- Periapical abscesses around some maxillary teeth
- The interocclusal rest space was 3.0 mm
- Restricted mandibular movements
- Discrepancy between centric occlusion (CO) and centric relation (CR) of 0.5 mm, with an anterior slide
- In all lateral excursions, contact was on the right side, on the maxillary and mandibular premolars and molars
- In protrusive movements, contacts were between the maxillary and mandibular right molars

Periodontal examination revealed poor oral hygiene accompanied by large amounts of plaque and calculus (Figure 14.7), probing depths of up to 4.0 mm on the maxillary teeth and up to 5.0 mm on the mandibular teeth (mandibular left third molar), with bleeding of the gingiva on probing on some of the teeth (Figure 14.8).

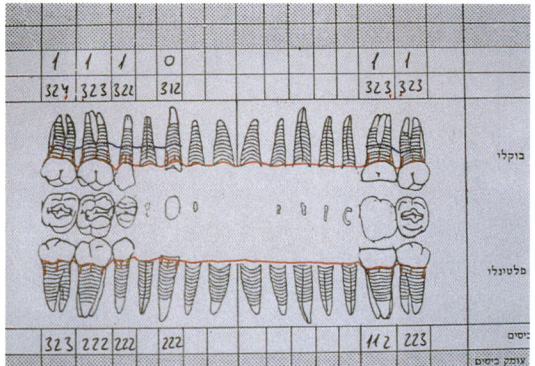

Figure 14.8a

Periodontal chart

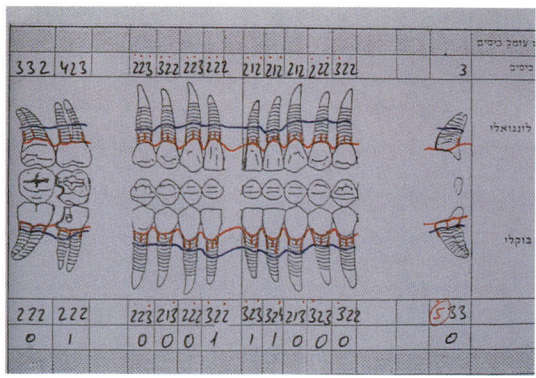

Figure 14.8b

Periodontal chart

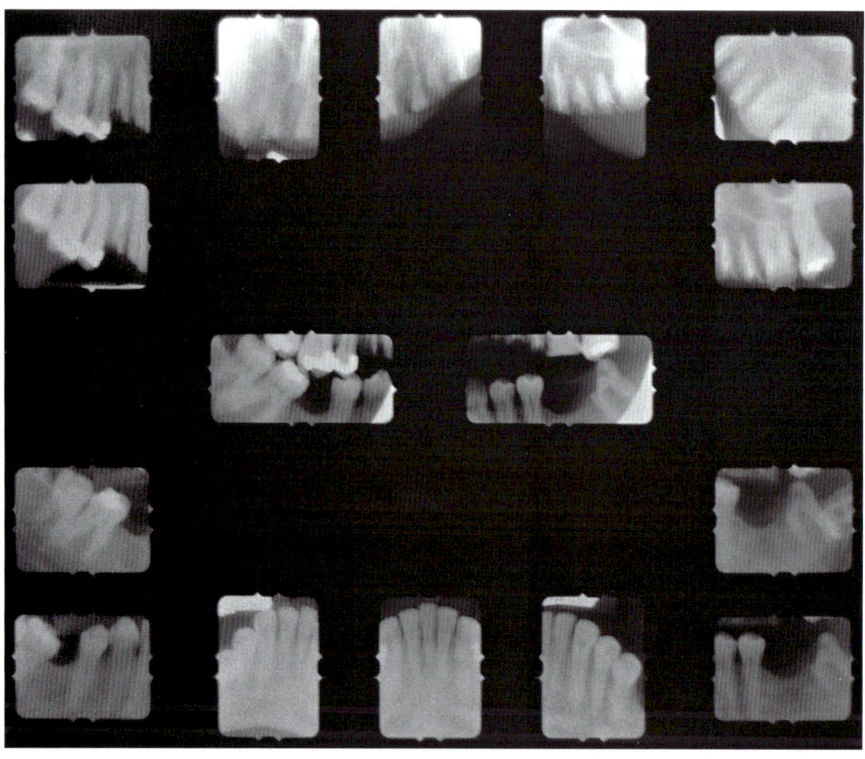

Figure 14.9

Radiographs of maxilla and mandible—pre-treatment

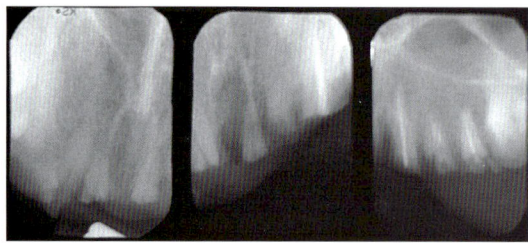

Figure 14.10

Radiographs of maxilla—anterior teeth, pre-treatment

INDIVIDUAL TOOTH PROGNOSIS

The prognosis for the remaining teeth was the following:

- Very poor (Figure 14.10):

$$\frac{4\ 2\ 1\ |\ 1\ 2\ 3\ 4\ 5}{8}$$

- Fair:

$$\frac{3\ 2\ |\ 6}{}$$

- Good: the rest of teeth

DIAGNOSIS

- Multiple fractured teeth, status post-trauma
- Loss of bony and soft tissue support in the maxilla status post-trauma
- Reduced occlusal support
- Shallow vestibulum space
- Loss of sensation in the lips on the left side
- Status post-mandibular fracture
- Caries and faulty restorations
- Poor esthetics
- Periapical changes
- Decreased vertical dimension
- Nasopalatine duct cyst
- Gingivitis

ABOUT THE PATIENT

The patient, who suffered from poor health, had had a severe traumatic experience that, due to his injuries, would still require additional extensive medical treatment. In an instant, he went from a full dentition to a condition where he felt that most of his maxillary teeth were missing. The patient wanted a fixed prosthesis, but was willing to accept a removable prosthesis as a temporary solution to his problems.

POTENTIAL TREATMENT PROBLEMS

- Widespread fractured maxillary teeth due to trauma, accompanied by loss of bone and soft tissue support, complicating a full mouth rehabilitation
- Reduced vestibulum space due to the scarring, limiting movement
- A nasopalatine duct cyst that might jeopardize implant placement for prosthetic support

TREATMENT ALTERNATIVES

Maxilla:

- Removable partial denture
- Removable partial denture supported by natural teeth and implants
- Fixed partial prosthesis or prostheses supported by implants and remaining teeth

Mandible:

- Removable tooth-supported partial prosthesis
- Fixed partial prosthesis, each either tooth- or implant-supported

TREATMENT PLAN

The final treatment plan was then chosen which consisted of pre-prosthetic surgery to prepare the site in the maxilla for implants, a fixed anterior maxillary prosthesis supported by the maxillary right second premolar, the maxillary right cuspid and the maxillary right

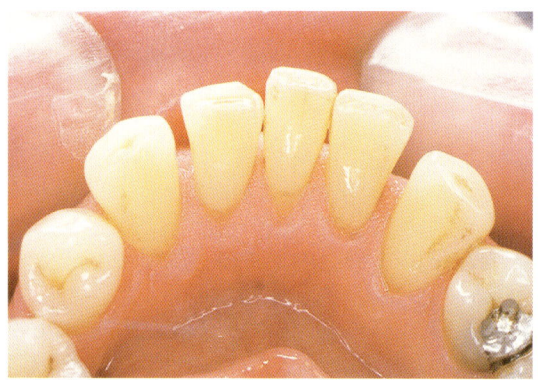

Figure 14.11

Mandibular arch—lingual view, after initial treatment

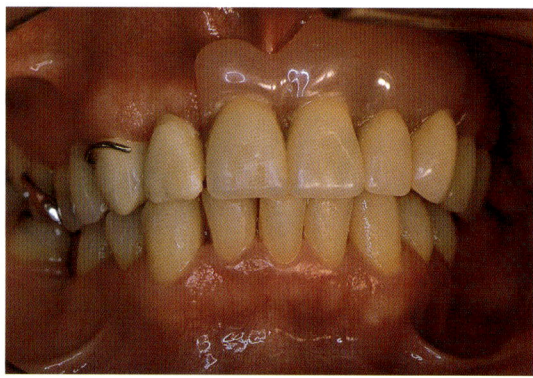

Figure 14.12

Anterior teeth after initial treatment

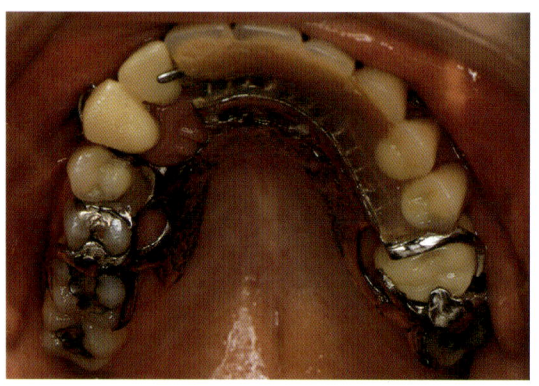

Figure 14.13

Transitional crowns and maxillary removable partial denture

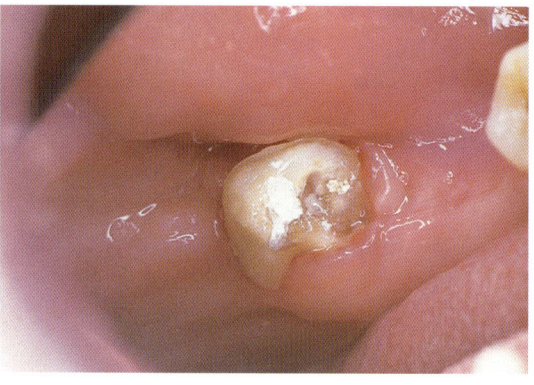

Figure 14.14

Mandibular left third molar after periodontal surgery

lateral incisor, and a maxillary fixed partial prosthesis supported by implants from the right maxillary central incisor to the left maxillary second premolar. A crown was also to be fabricated for maxillary left first molar tooth. The missing mandibular right first molar would not be replaced.

TREATMENT

Initial preparation included scaling, curettage, root planing and oral hygiene instruction. At the end of this stage, significant improvement of the soft tissue could be discerned (Figures 14.11 and 14.12). At this time, periodontal re-charting and evaluation demonstrated that the pockets depths had diminished greatly and that the bleeding on probing had disappeared.

Endodontic therapy was performed on the maxillary right cuspid and maxillary left first molar. The mandibular left first premolar and right third molar and left second molar were restored with amalgam restorations. The maxillary right lateral incisor,

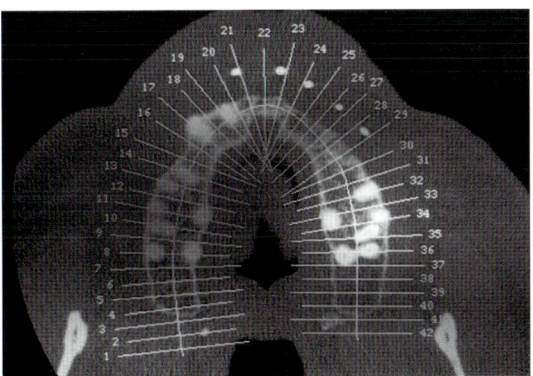

Figure 14.15

CT scan—maxilla

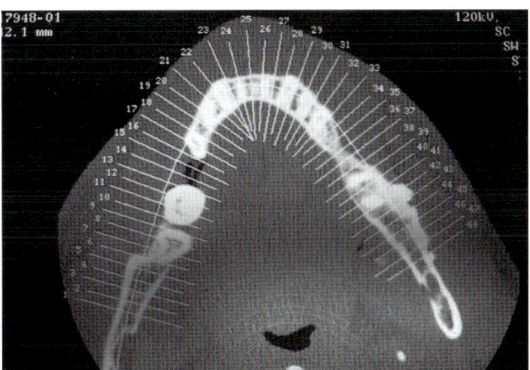

Figure 14.16

CT scan—mandible

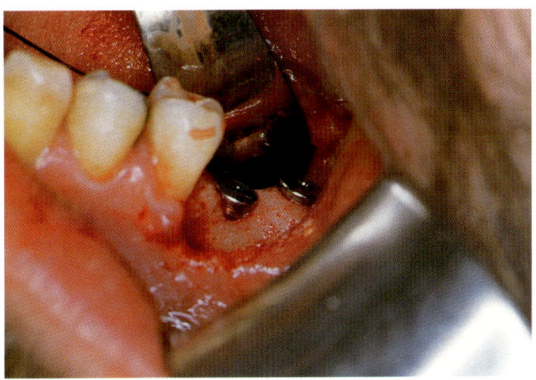

Figure 14.17

Implant insertion—left mandibular molar area

which was fractured and buried under the gingival tissue, was exposed with a crown lengthening procedure, followed by endodontic therapy.

A transitional removable maxillary partial denture was then made to replace the missing anterior teeth (even though the roots were not yet extracted) to stabilize the occlusion and push back the vestibulum as much as possible in the scarred area (Figure 14.13). Crown lengthening was then performed on the mandibular third molar to expose it in order to perform endodontic

therapy (Figure 14.14). The prognosis was not favorable, but it was decided to keep the tooth as it was the only tooth in the mandible maintaining occlusal support on the left side.

A CT radiograph of the maxilla (Figure 14.15) revealed a large radiolucent area which, at surgery, was confirmed as a nasopalatine cyst. It was then decided to place an autogenous bone implant on the pre-maxilla to provide bone support for future implant placement. The bone was taken from the chin area and checked for integration after 6 months.

A CT radiograph of the mandible (Figure 14.16) showed that there was room for two implants in the left mandibular molar area, but this required removal of the mesial root of the mandibular third molar. The mesial root was extracted and two implants were placed (Figure 14.17). The distal root was left in place, temporarily, to maintain occlusal support for a transitional fixed partial prosthesis during implant placement and healing.

The treatment for the maxilla was then commenced. It was planned to consist of fixed partial prostheses supported by both natural teeth and implants. A fixed partial

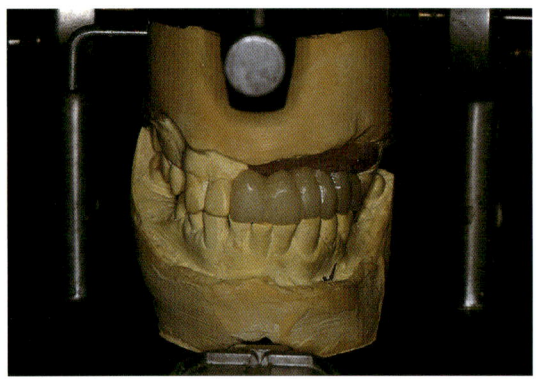

Figure 14.18

Wax-up of maxillary anterior crowns—frontal view

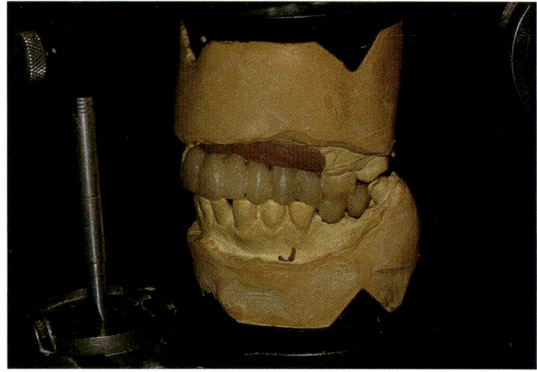

Figure 14.19

Wax-up of maxillary anterior crowns—left side

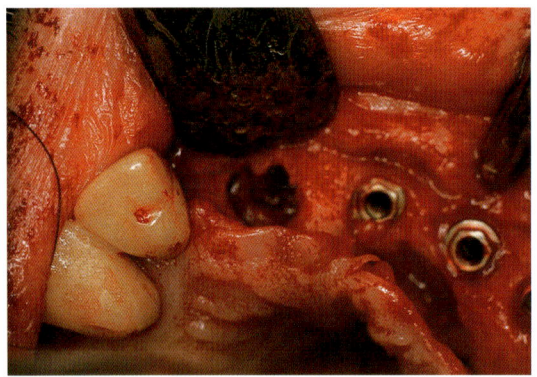

Figure 14.20

Implant insertion—maxillary anterior area

prosthesis would extend from the maxillary right second premolar to the right lateral incisor, replacing the missing right first premolar. A single crown for the maxillary left first molar and a six-unit fixed partial prosthesis supported by five implants from the maxillary right central incisor area to the maxillary left second premolar area were to be constructed.

In the mandible, an implant-supported fixed partial prosthesis was proposed to replace the missing left molars. The missing right first molar tooth was not to be

replaced as the occlusion had been stable in the area despite the tooth being missing for many years. There were no gingival or caries problems in the area, and to replace the missing tooth with an implant-supported fixed partial prosthesis would require orthodontic therapy to upright the second and third molar teeth. To replace the tooth with a fixed prosthesis would necessitate preparing the second premolar, which had no restorations or caries.

Following successful bone implantation in the area of the nasopalatine cyst, a wax-up was done to determine the ideal location of the maxillary and mandibular teeth that were to be replaced by the implant supported fixed prosthesis (Figures 14.18 and 14.19). Five implants were inserted in the maxilla (Figure 14.20). In the mandible two implants were inserted. When the implants were uncovered, it was discovered that the implant in the maxillary central incisor area had failed and, due to the extensive bone loss, it would be impossible to replace it with a wide-body type implant (Figure 14.21).

Following a re-evaluation, it was decided to make an anterior maxillary fixed prosthesis supported by only four implants, with

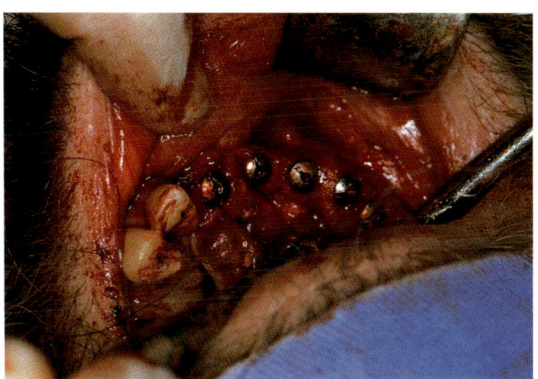

Figure 14.21

Stage two surgery—exposure of maxillary implants

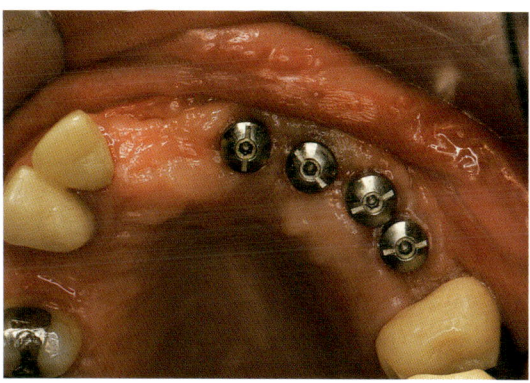

Figure 14.22

Maxillary implants after healing after second stage surgery

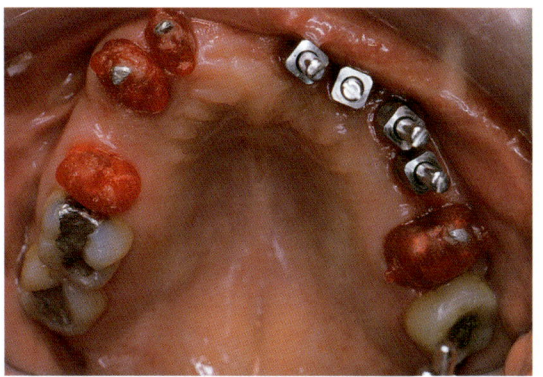

Figure 14.23

Duralay and abutment impression copings fitted—maxilla

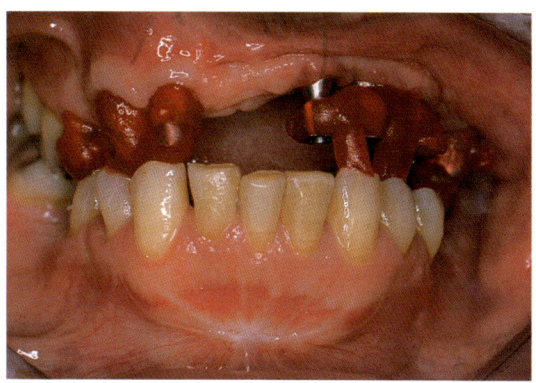

Figure 14.24

Duralay copings fitted—centric relation record

the central incisor as a cantilever (Figure 14.22). The implants had been placed in a curve and thus provided resistance to multidirectional forces.

During the course of treatment, it was discovered that the maxillary right cuspid had a periapical lesion. The tooth was asymptomatic, was not sensitive to percussion, and did not have deep probing depths. An exploratory surgical procedure revealed granulation tissue around the root apex, which was enucleated. It was thought at that time that the periapical area

was an extension of granulation tissue from the failed implant in the maxillary right central incisor area.

Copper band elastomeric impressions were made of all the prepared teeth and Duralay copings were constructed. These copings were used for the final impression for the master model and to record centric relation at the vertical dimension of the temporary restorations (Figures 14.23 and 14.24).

Unfortunately, at the metal coping fitting stage, a fistula was noticed round the maxillary right cuspid and a 10 mm probing

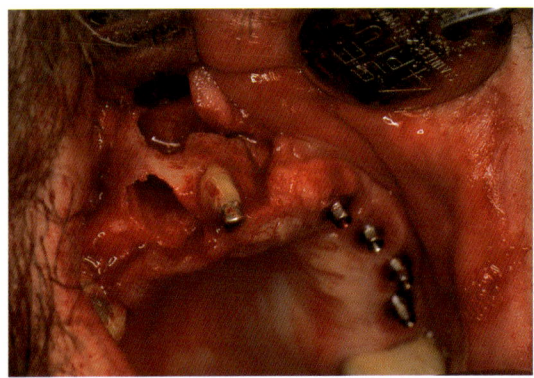

Figure 14.25

Maxilla after extraction of right cuspid

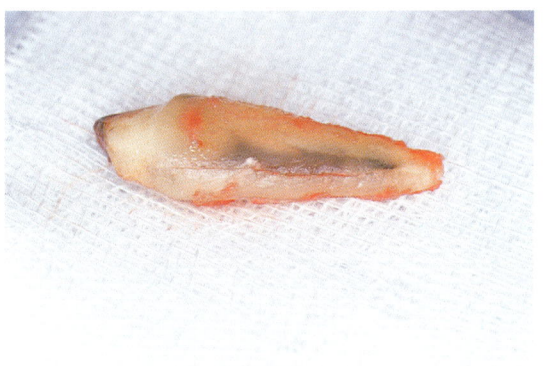

Figure 14.26

Extracted right cuspid—showing fracture

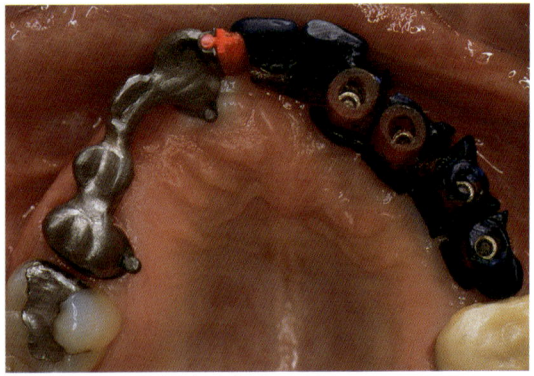

Figure 14.27

Metal copings try-in maxilla—after soldering and showing semi-precision attachment connecting tooth- and implant-supported prostheses

depth was found on the palatal aspect of the tooth. A second exploratory surgical procedure was then performed, which revealed massive bone loss on the palatal aspect of the tooth (Figure 14.25). The tooth was extracted and a longitudinal fracture of the root was discovered (Figure 14.26).

The treatment plan was again modified, to a fixed partial prosthesis from the right maxillary second premolar to the right maxillary lateral incisor. These teeth had

excellent bone support. A semi-precision attachment was made to connect this prosthesis and the anterior and left posterior prosthesis supported by the four implants. The implants would help support the fixed prosthesis in lateral jaw movements, and the attachment would also allow the teeth to move apically within the limits of the periodontal membrane in centric occlusion.

The metal copings were soldered and, after try-in of the soldered metal framework (Figure 14.27), another elastomeric impression was made for the tissue reproduction model. These models were mounted on a semi-adjustable articulator (Hanau) using a facebow registration, and centric records were taken at the vertical dimension of occlusion using Duralay with a Neylon technique.

The porcelain was baked and the occlusion checked at the biscuit bake stage in the mouth and all adjustments needed were then made. The porcelain was then glazed. The crowns and bridges were cemented with Temp-Bond. After one month the crowns and bridges were cemented with zinc oxyphosphate cement for permanent cementation (Figures

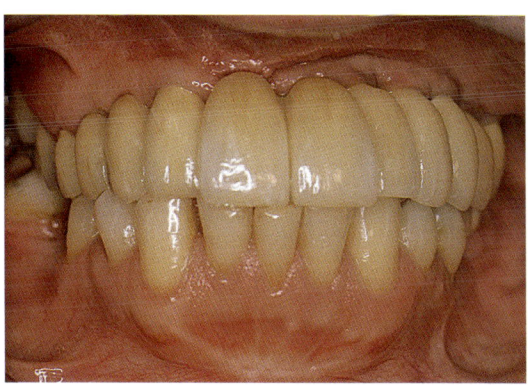

Figure 14.28

Treatment completed—anterior view

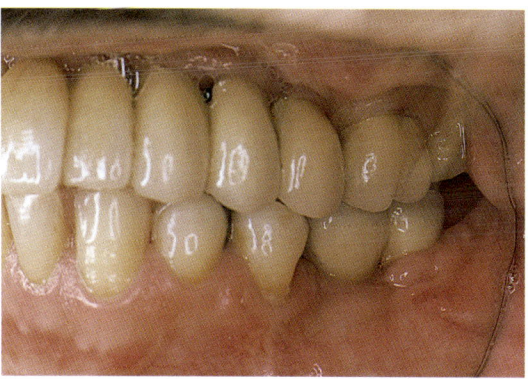

Figure 14.29

Treatment completed—left side

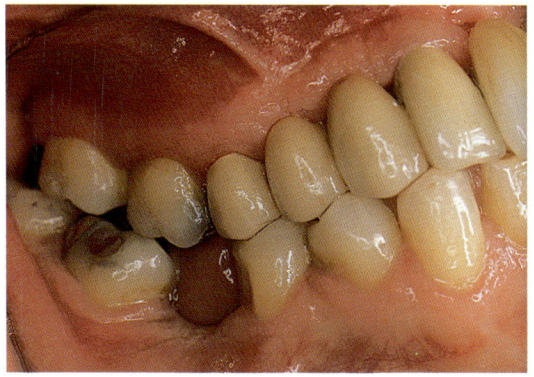

Figure 14.30

Treatment completed—right side

14.28–14.30). A complete series of radiographs was taken after completion of treatment (Figure 14.31).

SUMMARY

The patient presented with a variety of problems. Due to his unfortunate accident, he had been left with scalp wounds, fractures of the right side of his skull and the left mandible, left maxillary sinus hemorrhage, lacerations of the cheek, and many broken teeth. Though he had large amounts of calculus and plaque, he was periodontally resistant. The attack left him with scarred tissue, and also limited ability to open his mouth. He had many broken teeth and was also missing hard and soft tissue in the maxilla. A year previous to the attack, he had a myocardial infarct and was still being treated with assorted medication. The patient requested a fixed prosthesis even though he was prepared to accept a removable prosthesis during treatment, but only on a temporary basis. During treatment many unsuspected problems arose and the treatment had to be constantly adjusted to the new circumstances. In spite of all these problems, an excellent result was achieved using a combination of natural teeth and implant-supported fixed prostheses.

CASE DISCUSSION
AVINOAM YAFFE

The patient, a 44-year-old male, was referred for treatment at the Graduate Clinic following a traumatic injury that changed overnight his general well-being and

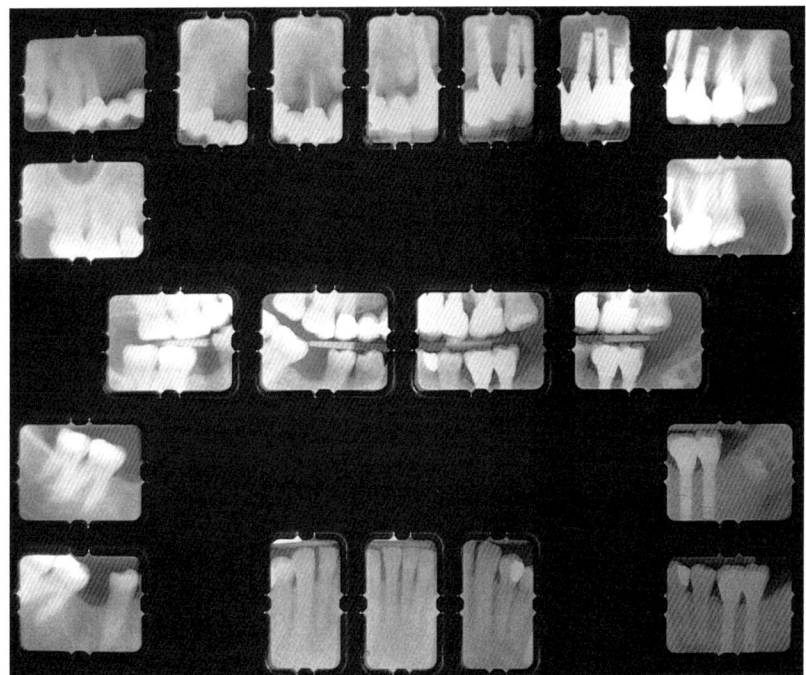

Figure 14.31

Post-treatment radiographs

primarily affected his masticatory system. He was a very pleasant and accommodating patient who adjusted easily to the constant changes in his treatment plan. He did, however, insist on having a fixed restoration, and was willing to go through whatever procedures were needed to achieve this goal. The treatment plan had to be modified during treatment and even at a final stage, due to unexpected complications. In the final treatment, a fixed prosthesis was fabricated and special emphasis was placed on the occlusal scheme to protect both the natural teeth and the implants. A non-working contact that existed on the right side during lateral jaw movements was adjusted to a situation that maintained contact there, while at the same time kept working contacts on the implants on the left side. The semi-precision attachment between the implant and tooth-supported bridges was intended

to provide some fixation for the bridge during lateral movements.

The restorations were monitored very carefully during the last 2 years and it is our hope that the customized restoration, along with meticulous planning of the occlusion, will provide many years of lasting service. It was also planned that, in the future, if the teeth supporting the maxillary prosthesis on the right side were to fail, additional implants would be implanted and their prosthesis would be connected to the existing implant-supported prosthesis.

CASE DISCUSSION
HAROLD PREISKEL

A particularly interesting facet of this patient's treatment represents his reaction to the appalling physical injuries he received. It is apparent that before the attack the state of his dentition was not of particular interest to him. One might have expected the inevitable psychological reaction to his experience to have made him even less interested in looking after his teeth. Quite the reverse happened, and I am confident that the team treating him had a significant influence upon his attitude: they are to be congratulated.

It is also intriguing to note that the patient insisted on a fixed maxillary prosthesis despite the fact that such an approach both complicated and lengthened the treatment, compromised the esthetics (although not by very much), and made maintenance far more difficult. The step-by-step approach employed provided versatility that was put to good use to overcome a few unexpected events. In a long and complex course of treatment, we all receive the occasional surprise.

I quite understand why a premature onlay graft was not employed, since this would have complicated the treatment still further and obliged the patient to be without his removable prosthesis for some time. The net result was that the implants were positioned slightly palatal to the ideal position, but in a perfectly acceptable relationship. The price to pay was the need to construct the facial surfaces of the restorations considerably labial to the implant which, in turn, leads to a maintenance problem. It is encouraging that so far the patient has maintained a good level of plaque control and his motivation has not waned.

Connecting the maxillary-implant-supported section to the tooth-supported prosthesis by means of a semi-precision retainer is not universally accepted. There have been suggestions that there is a serious risk of intrusion of the tooth-supported section. Only time will tell and I look forward to an update. From every point of view, the operators are to be congratulated on the outcome of this patient's treatment.

PATIENT 15   A NEW VERTICAL OCCLUSION

Treatment by Shaul Gelbard

THE PATIENT

The patient, a 43-year-old woman, presented herself for examination and consultation with the following complaints:

'My teeth are disappearing.' (Figure 15.1)
'When I brush my teeth, the gums bleed.'

PAST MEDICAL HISTORY

The patient suffered from hyperostosis corticalis generalista, a bone disease characterized by thickening of the face due to the formation of cortical bone, usually in the mandible. The patient suffered from Worth's disease, which in her case was arrested at the age of 20. About 24 years ago, due to this condition, she had surgery to decrease the size of her chin (Figures 15.2 and 15.3).

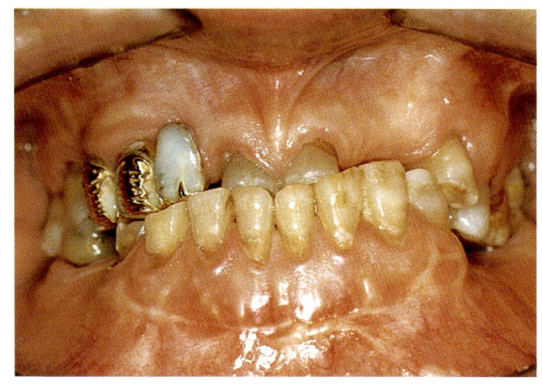

Figure 15.1

Anterior teeth—labial view

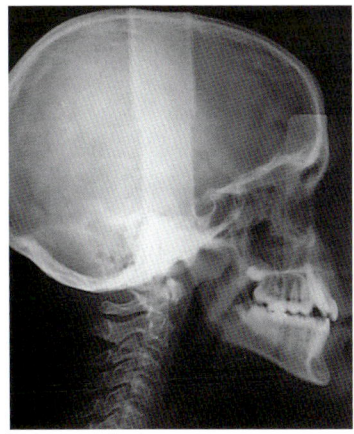

Figure 15.2

Cephalometric radiograph of normal patient

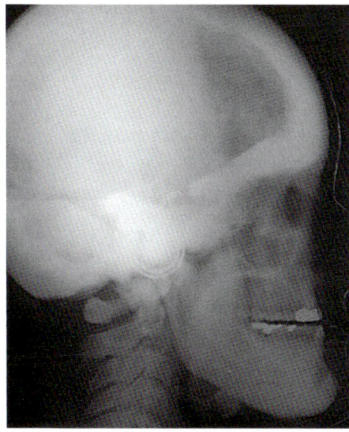

Figure 15.3

Cephalometric radiograph of the patient

163

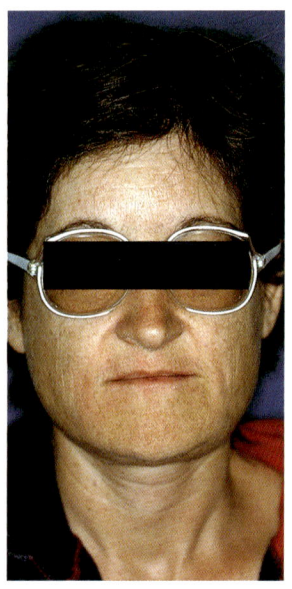

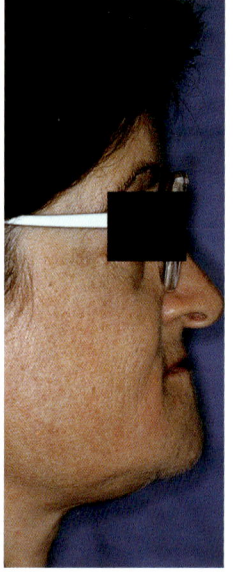

Figure 15.4

Face—frontal view

Figure 15.5

Face—profile

EXTRA-ORAL EXAMINATION
(Figures 15.4 and 15.5)

- Asymmetric and wide face
- Drooping eyes
- Narrow lips
- Enlarged lower third of the face
- Straight profile
- Protruding chin with a wide mandible
- Wide smile, without showing any teeth
- Maximum opening was 38.0 cm

INTRA-ORAL EXAMINATION
(Figures 15.6 and 15.7)

- Anterior cross bite (see Figure 15.1)
- Distorted occlusal plane
- Extrusion of the maxillary left posterior and mandibular anterior teeth (Figures 15.8 and 15.9)
- Amalgam restoration on maxillary right second molar

- Faulty fixed partial prosthesis of gold and acrylic:

$$\dfrac{4\ 3\ \mathrm{X}\ \big|}{\phantom{4\ 3\ \mathrm{X}}\big|}$$

- Missing teeth:

$$\dfrac{8\ 5\ 2\ \big|\ 2\ 3}{8\ 7\ 5\ \big|\ 5\ 6\ 8}$$

- Extreme wear of the teeth accompanied by chipping of the enamel and cupping of the dentine
- Rounded arch form, with broad ridges

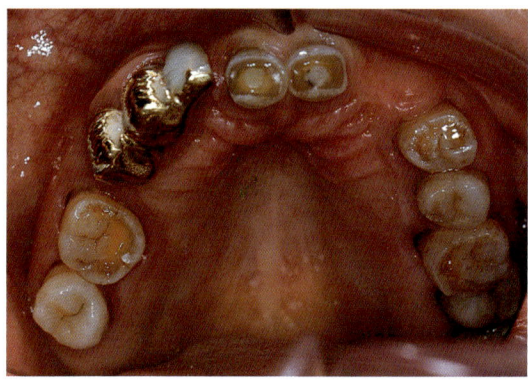

Figure 15.6

Maxillary arch—palatal view

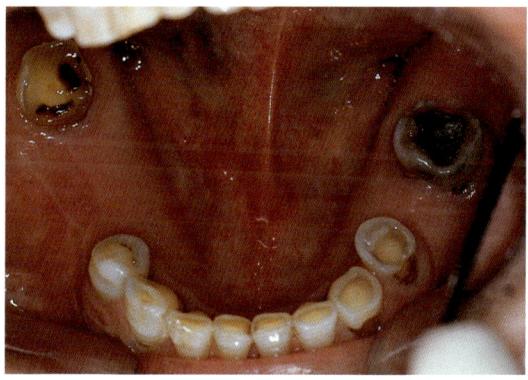

Figure 15.7

Mandibular arch—lingual view

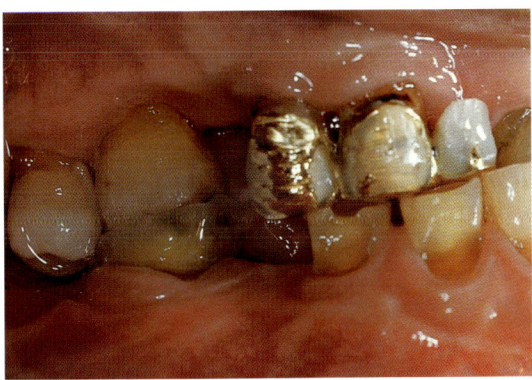

Figure 15.8

Occlusion—right side

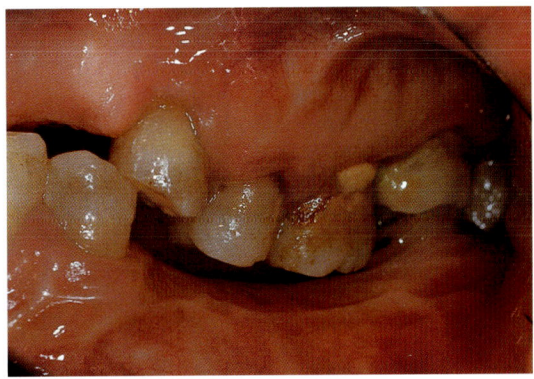

Figure 15.9

Occlusion—left side

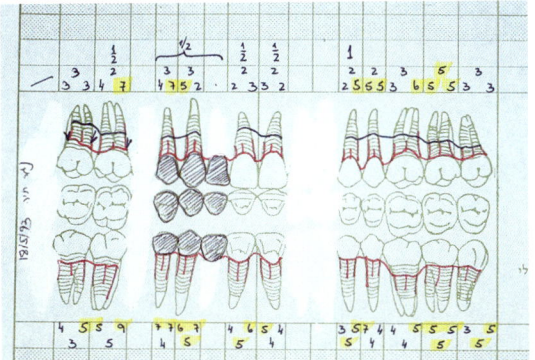

Figure 15.10

Periodontal chart—maxilla

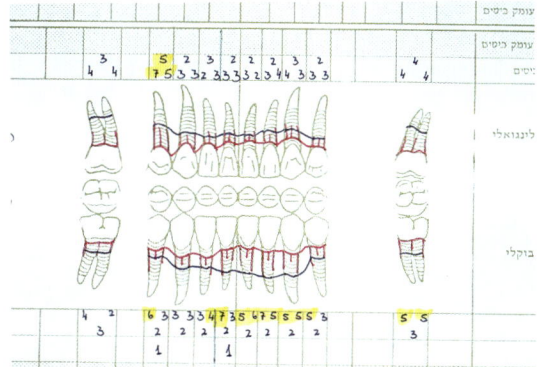

Figure 15.11

Periodontal chart—mandible

• Scarring of the tissue from the surgery to decrease the size of the chin

An occlusal examination revealed that the patient was Angle class III modification 2 according to Ross (Figures 15.8 and 15.9). There was a reversed overbite of 1.0 mm and an overjet of 1.0 mm. The interocclusal rest space was 8.0 mm and the maximum opening between the incisors was 46 mm, with an 'S' deviation in opening or closing movements. There was a 2.0 mm discrepancy between centric occlusion (CO) and centric relation

(CR). The lateral jaw movements were in group function. In protrusive movements, there was complete balance. There were balancing side interferences in lateral movements. There was fremitus class I on the maxillary incisor teeth, and a faulty occlusal plane.

The periodontal examination revealed plaque, calculus, inflammation around most of the teeth, probing depths of up to 9.0 mm on the maxillary teeth and up to 7.0 mm on the mandibular teeth, with bleeding on probing on some teeth (Figures 15.10 and 15.11).

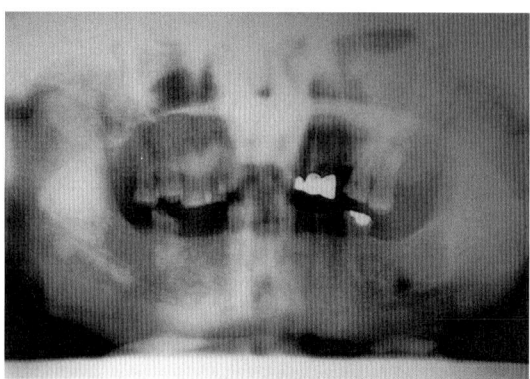

Figure 15.12

Panoramic radiograph—pre-treatment

FULL-MOUTH PERIAPICAL SURVEY (Figure 15.12)

A complete series of X-rays revealed the following findings:

- Missing teeth:

$$\frac{8\,5\,2\;|\;2\,3}{8\,7\,5\;|\;5\,6\,8}$$

- Endodontic treatment:

$$\frac{1\;|\;1}{\;|\;7} \qquad \frac{1\;|\;1}{\;|\;7}$$

- Small caries lesion in the mandibular right first molar tooth
- Thickening and condensation of the bone to such an extent that it was very difficult to differentiate between the roots of the teeth and the surrounding bone
- Hyperostosis corticalis generalista

INDIVIDUAL TOOTH PROGNOSIS

- Hopeless: none

- Poor:

$$\frac{7\,6\,4\,3\;|\;4\,5\,6\,7}{6\;\;\;|}$$

- Fair:

$$\frac{1\;|\;1\,8}{4\,3\,2\,1\;|\;1\,2\,3\,4\,7}$$

SUMMARY OF FINDINGS

The 43-year-old patient with Angle class III modification 2 occlusion, status post-surgery, and suffering from hyperostosis corticalis generalista, came to the clinic complaining of extreme wear of her teeth and the fear that her teeth would soon disappear. She also noticed that her gums bled when she brushed her teeth. She exhibited extreme wear of her teeth, extrusion of many teeth, plaque, calculus, missing teeth, and faulty restorations.

DIAGNOSIS

- Hyperostosis corticalis generalista
- Moderate with localized advanced adult type periodontitis
- Excessive tooth wear
- Occlusal disharmony with reduced occlusal support
- Missing teeth
- Faulty restorations
- Poor esthetics
- Reduced vertical dimension
- Caries

ABOUT THE PATIENT

The patient was very cooperative; her main desire was to have an esthetic and fixed restoration. Within a short period of time, she improved her oral hygiene, and her periodontal condition improved.

POTENTIAL TREATMENT PROBLEMS

The patient presented with a variety of problems:

- Poor occlusal relationships
- Loss of vertical dimension
- Lack of occlusal posterior support
- Extreme wear
- Moderate with localized advanced periodontitis

POSSIBLE TREATMENT SOLUTIONS

For the poor occlusal relationships:

- A sliding surgical osteotomy procedure in which a block of bone including the teeth is removed and reset in a more favorable position. This was rejected because the patient refused to undergo any extensive surgical procedure.
- Orthodontic treatment to intrude the teeth to acquire a physiological occlusion. This option was also rejected because of the fear of root resorption due to the patient's unique bone condition.
- Crown lengthening periodontal surgery to enable the teeth to be reduced in occlusal height in order to achieve a physiological occlusion and expose sound tooth structure for the margins of the restorations. This option was also rejected as it was felt that the surgery would cause bifurcation and trifurcation involvement of the premolar and molar teeth.
- Gradual selective equilibration of the teeth and the addition of acrylic to the transitional restorations in the opposing jaws in order to improve the occlusal plane.

For the loss of vertical dimension:

- After the occlusal equilibration, the optimum vertical dimension for an esthetic result would be determined and, according to that, the vertical dimension would be opened by means of an occlusal appliance.

For the extreme wear:

- The teeth that were very worn would receive crown restorations to replace the lost tooth structure.

For the moderate to advanced periodontitis:

- Most of the probing depths were due to 'pseudo pockets', and it was felt that after initial preparation, these would diminish in size. If not, the problem would be solved with periodontal surgery.

TREATMENT PLAN

Before treatment was started, a diagnostic wax-up was done on study models mounted on a Hanau articulator with a facebow registration and a centric relation record in order to evaluate the esthetic and occlusal solutions (Figure 15.13).

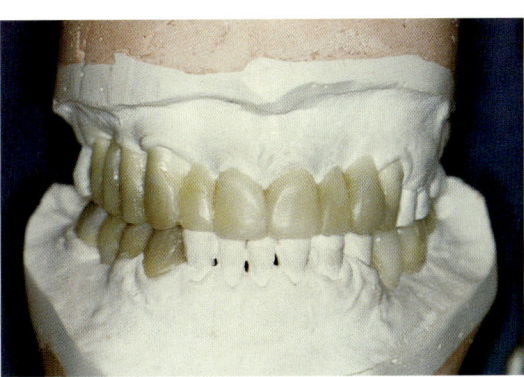

Figure 15.13

Diagnostic wax-up on Hanau articulator

TREATMENT ALTERNATIVES

Maxilla:

- Fixed partial prosthesis
- Fixed and removable partial prosthesis

Mandible:

- Fixed partial prosthesis
- Fixed and removable partial prosthesis
- Fixed partial prosthesis with implants support

TREATMENT

Initial preparation included scaling, root planing, curettage, and oral hygiene instruction (Figures 15.14 and 15.15), caries removal, and a mandibular diagnostic appliance due to the class III occlusion to evaluate the change in vertical dimension, followed by transitional restorations. At the completion of this stage, a clinical re-evaluation was done to determine whether there had been periodontal, esthetic and occlusal improvement. The occlusal appliance was observed for 8 weeks. At that time, an obvious improvement in the periodontal supporting tissue could be seen, pockets depths had diminished greatly and bleeding on probing had disappeared. It also was evident that the patient had completely adjusted to the new vertical dimension (Figures 15.16 and 15.17).

At this time, transitional restorations were made at the new vertical dimension (Figure 15.18). Implants were also done in the left mandibular posterior quadrant as it was felt that the mandibular left first premolar and second molar did not provide enough support for a fixed partial prosthesis (Figure 15.19).

Due to the faulty plane of occlusion on the left side, the maxillary premolars and molars were gradually selectively equilibrated and acrylic was added to the transitional mandibular restorations to prevent overeruption of the equilibrated teeth. In this manner, an optimal plane of occlusion was achieved.

Once the transitional restorations fulfilled all the esthetic, physiological and functional expectations of the patient and the dentist, the teeth were reprepared and individual

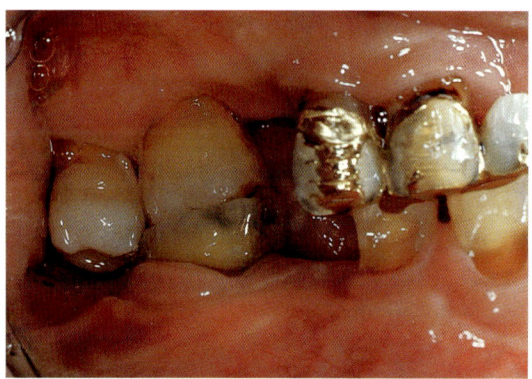

Figure 15.14

Teeth—right side, after initial preparation

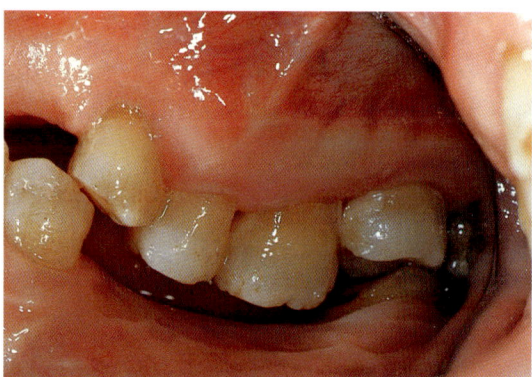

Figure 15.15

Teeth—left side, after initial preparation

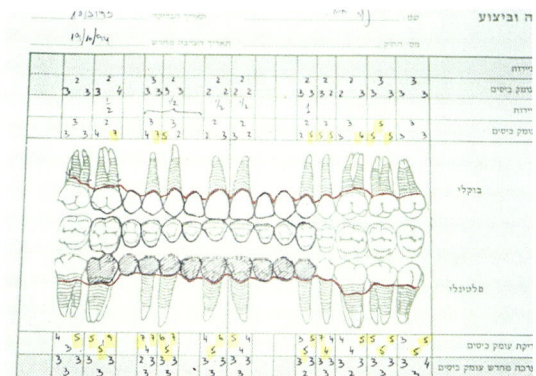

Figure 15.16

Periodontal chart—maxilla, re-evaluation

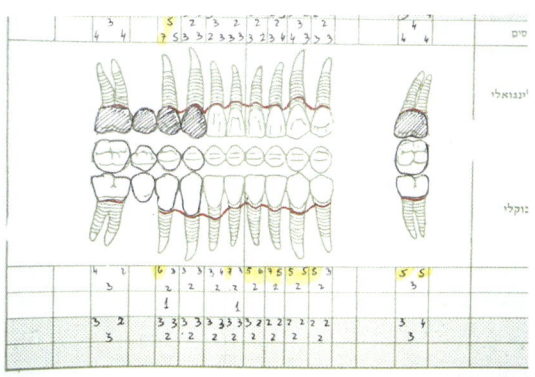

Figure 15.17

Periodontal chart—mandible, re-evaluation

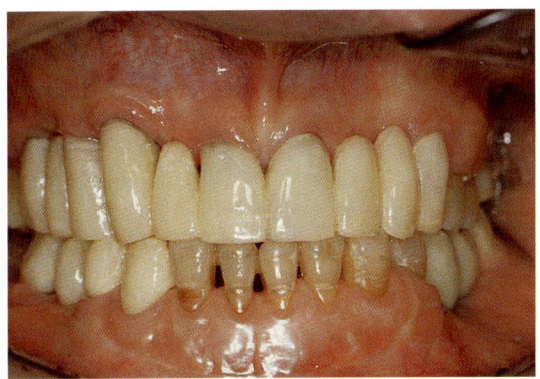

Figure 15.18

Transitional restorations

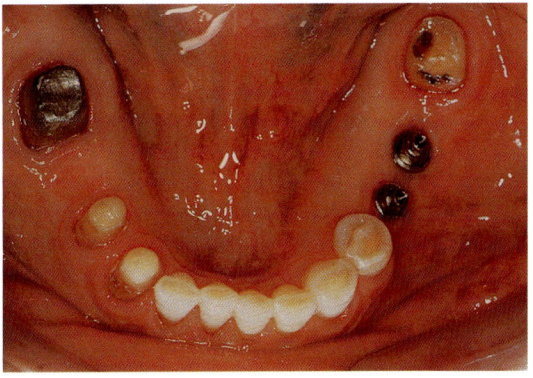

Figure 15.19

Implants—mandible, left posterior region

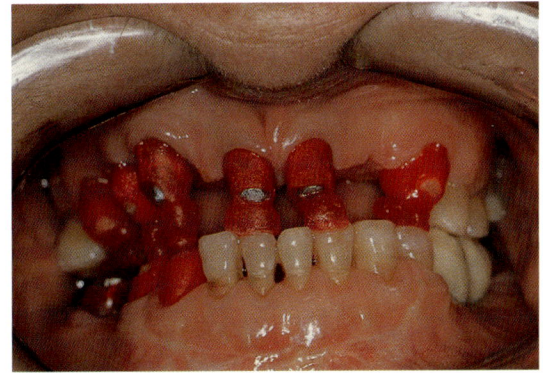

Figure 15.20

Centric relation record in Duralay

copper band impressions were made of all the prepared teeth. Duralay copings were then made and the vertical dimension of occlusion was recorded with these copings (Figure 15.20). An elastomeric impression (Impergum) was then done to provide a working model which included the dies and the implant analogues (Figure 15.21). A facebow registration was taken to facilitate mounting the maxillary cast on a semi-adjustable articulator (Hanau). The metal copings were cast and fitted. They were connected with Duralay for soldering.

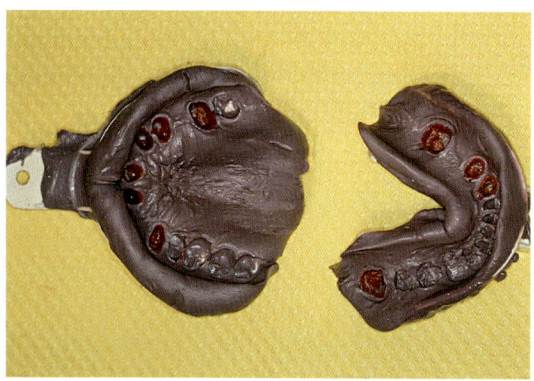

Figure 15.21

Elastomeric impressions

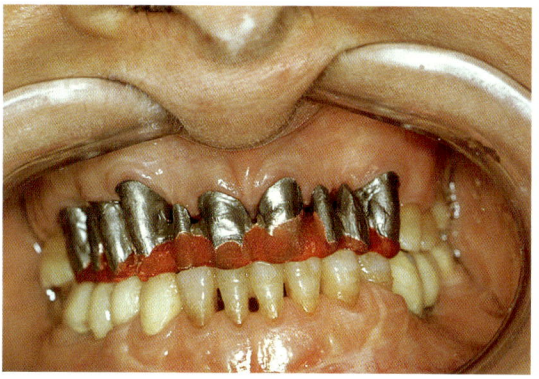

Figure 15.22

Soldered coping try-in and centric relation registration

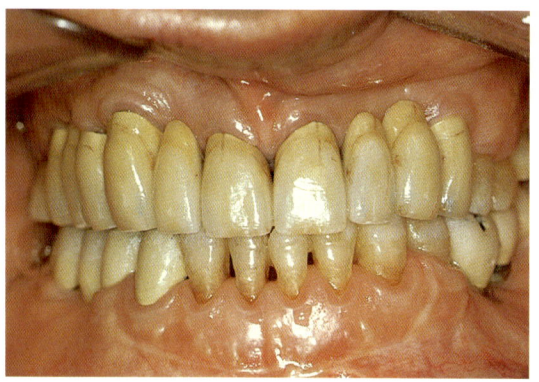

Figure 15.23

Treatment completed—permanent restorations

Centric relation was recorded in Duralay (Figure 15.22), and another elastomeric impression was made for tissue detail. The models were then mounted on a Hanau articulator, again with the aid of a facebow registration, and the porcelain was baked. Models of the transitional restorations provided a buccal key for the position and shape of the porcelain, thus copying the transitional restorations. The biscuit bake porcelain was checked and adjusted in the mouth. After the occlusion was finalized, the final glaze was applied to the prostheses. The prostheses were cemented with

Temp-Bond for a period of 2 weeks. They were then cemented with zinc oxyphosphate cement for permanent cementation (Figure 15.23).

The patient has been returning for follow-up and maintenance twice a year since then and has not had any problems (Figure 15.24).

SUMMARY

The patient presented with a severe problem of extreme wear on many teeth and a reduced vertical dimension of occlusion. She also had a pathologic occlusion with serious balancing side and protrusive premature contacts during mandibular movements. In addition to these problems, she suffered from a severe periodontal problem and was very concerned about her esthetics. The treatment consisted of changing the vertical dimension of occlusion by selective grinding and addition of restorative material, where needed, in order to provide a physiological occlusion. The final restorations thus provided a physiological, functional and esthetic solution for her problems.

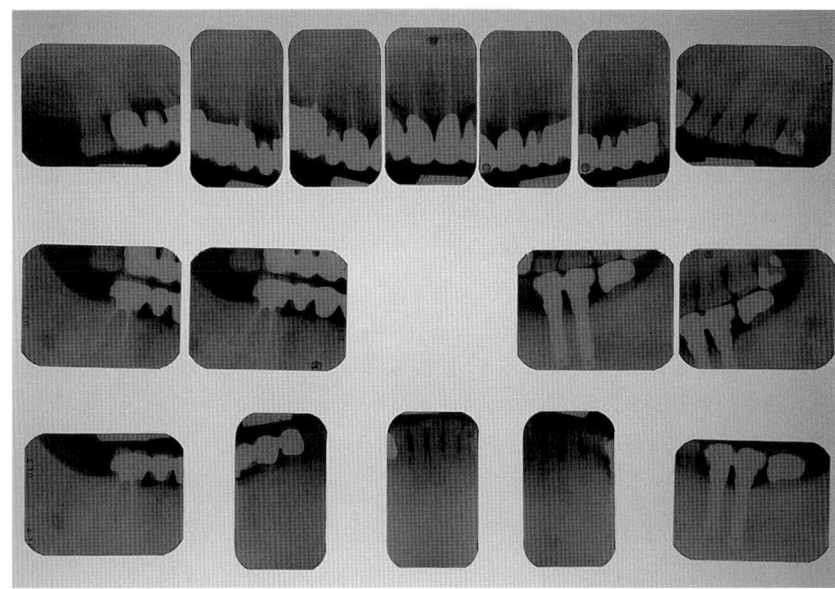

Figure 15.24

Post-treatment radiographs

CASE DISCUSSION
AVINOAM YAFFE

The patient presented in the clinic with a complicated situation: missing teeth, severe wear, overeruption of posterior teeth, combined with advanced periodontal disease aggravated by a class III malocclusion with occlusal interferences. The situation necessitated a dramatic change in the vertical dimension that had a negative as well as a positive effect. The positive effect was in the relationship between the anterior teeth, changing a class III relation to an almost class I relation, thus facilitating involvement of the anterior teeth in guidance and support. It also facilitated restoration of the posterior quadrants that had undergone severe overeruption. The negative effect was the change in the crown-to-root ratio. This, however, was minimal due to the compensatory eruption of the teeth during the retrograde wear. In summary, a 43-year-old patient was treated successfully and the pathological occlusion that was on a course of self destruction was changed to a long-lasting therapeutic, physiological occlusion.

CASE DISCUSSION
HAROLD PREISKEL

This patient presented an interesting treatment planning problem. Apart from the unusual medical complication, the operator had to assess a new vertical dimension of occlusion. A combination of tooth loss and tooth wear, possibly accentuated by a forward mandibular posture, have all led to a class III incisor relationship. By how much was it safe to increase the vertical dimension of occlusion? His treatment appears to have followed a logical pattern with alternative avenues considered at the outset. Apart from the all important periodontal and endodontic therapy, the use of transitional restorations is mandatory with problems like these. The planning of the occlusal scheme is to be commended and the overall result is gratifying.

PATIENT 16   ADVANCED PERIODONTAL DISEASE

Treatment by Ayal Tagari

THE PATIENT

The patient, a 70-year-old male, retired school principal, presented at the dental clinic in 1989 requesting treatment. His main complaint was 'I don't have enough teeth to chew with.' (Figure 16.1).

PAST MEDICAL HISTORY

- 1938: Surgical removal of a growth under the left ear, followed by radiotherapy when the growth recurred.
- 1948: Second surgical removal of the growth, which had again recurred.
- 1962: Third surgical removal of the growth, this time with a diagnosis of pleomorphic adenoma.

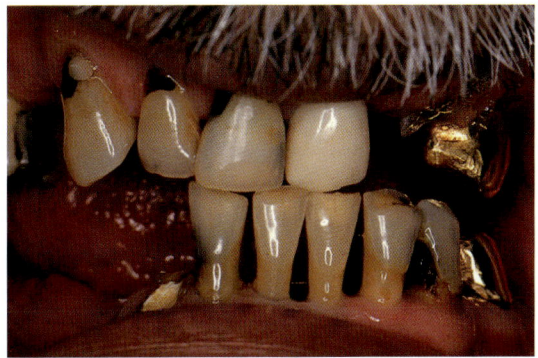

Figure 16.1

Frontal view of teeth

- 1977: With further recurrence of the growth, accompanied by paralysis of the seventh cranial nerve on the left side, new surgery was performed to remove the growth and the parotid salivary gland, leaving the patient with permanent damage to the left seventh cranial nerve. A gold leaf weight was then placed in the left eyelid to enable it to open and close in a normal manner.

PAST DENTAL HISTORY

Prior to his appearance at the dental clinic in 1989, the only treatments he remembered receiving were extractions. The patient could not remember exactly when the teeth were treated. His dental history also included periods of diminished saliva flow and the inability to adjust to a removable prosthesis.

EXTRA-ORAL EXAMINATION

- Hypotonicity of the facial muscles on the left side caused facial asymmetry (Figure 16.2).
- The temporomandibular joints were normal
- Maximum opening was 55 mm without any deviation on opening and closing

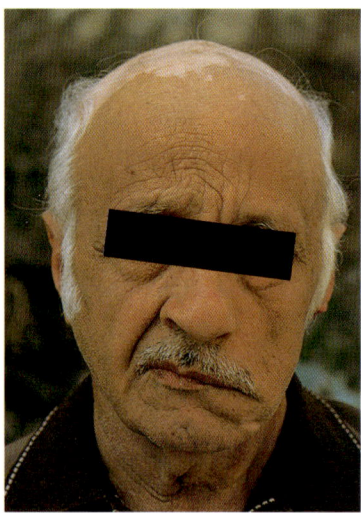

Figure 16.2

Frontal facial view

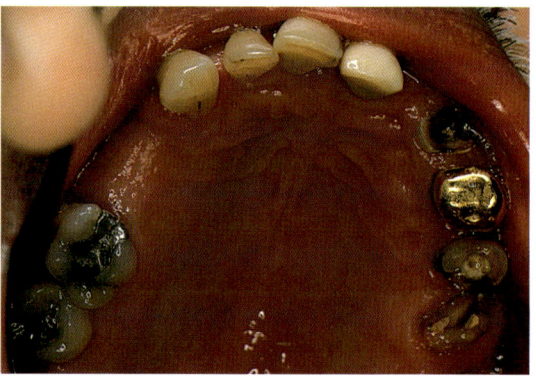

Figure 16.3

Mandibular arch

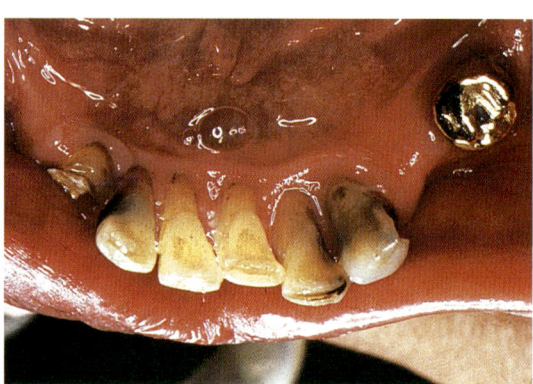

Figure 16.4

Maxillary arch

INTRA-ORAL AND FULL-MOUTH PERIAPICAL RADIOGRAPH EXAMINATION
(Figures 16.1–16.9)

Maxilla (Figure 16.3):

- The left cuspid and first molar were fractured beneath the gingival tissue; the left central incisor had a provisional restoration
- There was class 1 mobility on the left central incisor, the left premolars, and the left second molar teeth

Mandible (Figure 16.4):

- The right cuspid was fractured beneath the gingival tissue
- There was class 3 mobility on all the incisor teeth and class 2 mobility on the left second premolar
- The left cuspid had class 1 mobility
- There were faulty restorations and extensive caries on most of the remaining teeth

- Missing teeth:

$$\frac{8\;5\;4\;\;\;\big|\;\;2}{8\;7\;6\;5\;4\;\;\big|\;\;4\;6\;7\;8}$$

- Extensive caries and loss of crown structure
- 50% bone loss around the mandibular anterior teeth
- Periapical abscess maxillary central incisor tooth
- Radio-opacity in the periapical area of the left mandibular first premolar

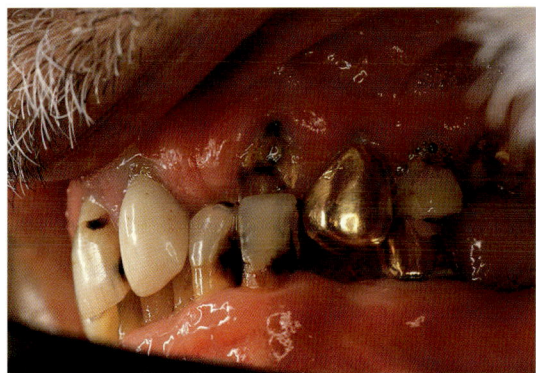

Figure 16.5

Occlusion—left side

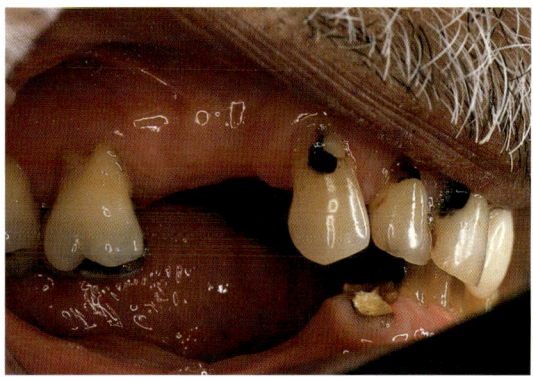

Figure 16.6

Occlusion—right side

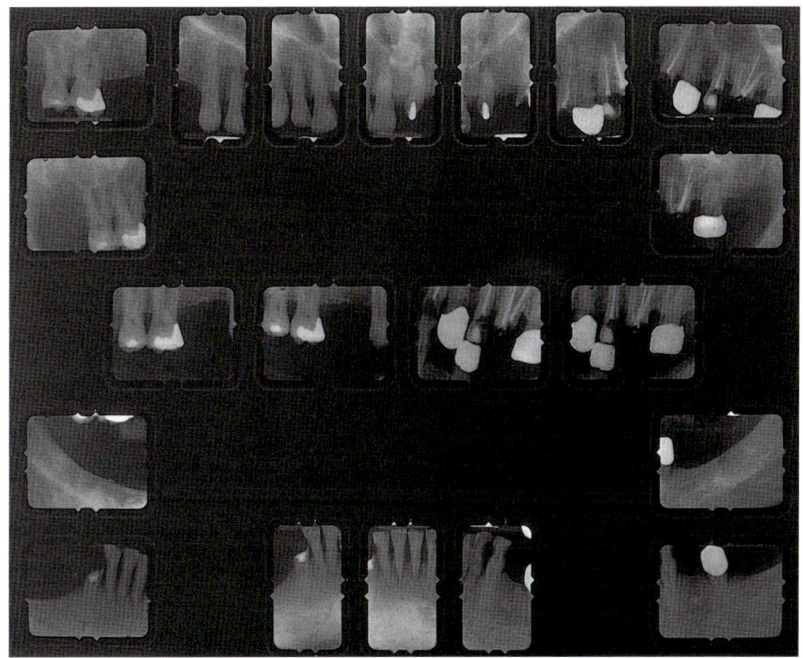

Figure 16.7

Radiographs of maxillary and mandibular teeth

An occlusal examination revealed extrusion of many teeth, a faulty plane of occlusion, vertical overbite of 8.0 mm, and horizontal overjet of 4.0 mm (Figures 16.5 and 16.6). The patient had difficulty executing lateral and protrusive movements of the mandible. The only occlusal contacts were between the left second premolars. The mandibular anterior teeth occluded with the palatal gingival tissue (see Figure 16.5).

The periodontal examination revealed gingival recession, but with minimal probing depths—up to 3.0 mm at the maximum (Figures 16.8 and 16.9).

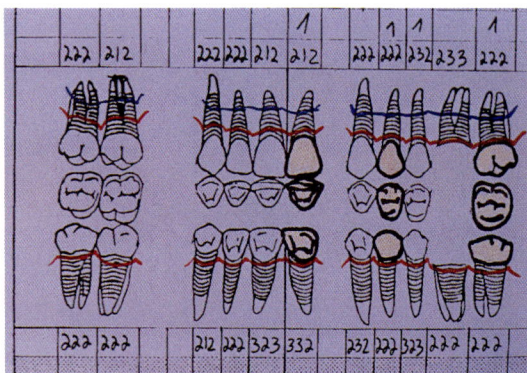

Figure 16.8

Mandibular periodontal chart

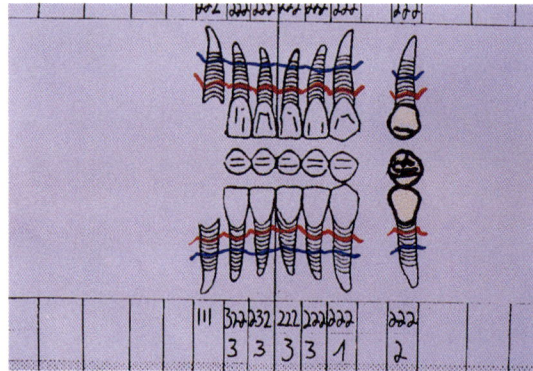

Figure 16.9

Maxillary periodontal chart

INDIVIDUAL TOOTH PROGNOSIS

The prognosis for the remaining teeth was the following:

* Very poor:

$$\frac{\quad\quad|\ 1\ 4\ 5\ 6\ 7}{3\ \ \ |\ 5}$$

* Poor:

$$\frac{\quad\quad\quad|}{2\ 1\ \ \ |\ 1\ 2}$$

* Fair: the rest of the teeth

In the past, the patient had difficulty adjusting to a removable partial denture and had discarded it.

DIAGNOSIS

* Missing teeth
* Extruded teeth
* Reduced occlusal support
* Loss of vertical dimension
* Occlusal trauma
* Mobile teeth
* Rampant caries
* Faulty restorations

* Periapical lesions
* Resorbed alveolar ridges
* Anterior traumatic overbite
* Adult type periodontitis
* Peripheral seventh cranial nerve damage

ABOUT THE PATIENT

The patient understood that his dental treatment would be complex and extend over a long period of time. He agreed to the need to try and save as many teeth as possible. He also voiced his preference for a fixed prosthesis rather than a removable one.

POTENTIAL TREATMENT PROBLEMS

* The patient had many missing teeth
* Due to rampant caries, some of the remaining teeth were almost totally destroyed
* There was reduced alveolar bone support in the anterior part of the mandible and increased mobility in the mandibular incisor teeth

- The patient was in occlusal trauma and biting on the maxillary palatal tissues during chewing
- Due to the fact that the patient objected to a removable prosthesis, the treatment might have to be compromised

TREATMENT PLAN ALTERNATIVES

Maxilla:

- Fixed partial prosthesis
- Fixed and removable partial prostheses
- Fixed telescopic prosthesis

Mandible:

- Fixed and removable partial prostheses
- Removable telescopic prosthesis
- Overdenture

TREATMENT

The treatment was divided into five phases:

PHASE 1

After initial treatment consisting of oral hygiene instruction, scaling and root planing, the patient showed a marked improvement in his home care and the periodontal tissues exhibited great improvement. It was then decided to splint the anterior mandibular teeth with orthodontic ligature for stabilization. Following re-evaluation, a final treatment plan was discussed. This would then be a fixed partial prosthesis in the maxilla, and a fixed anterior partial prosthesis with a removable clasp retained posterior partial prosthesis in the mandible.

PHASE 2

In the second phase, the priority was treatment of pain and infection, stabilizing the occlusion, and obtaining occlusal support. After completion of the initial preparation. The right mandibular cuspid and the left maxillary central incisor were treated endodontically. The left maxillary second molar was extracted. The faulty crown on the maxillary left second premolar was removed and the tooth was treated endodontically. Excavation of caries and restoration of the left maxillary cuspid and premolars was then done. The mandibular anterior teeth were shortened in height and splinted with orthodontic wire (Figures 16.10 and 16.11).

At this time a transitional fixed prosthesis was made, extending from the maxillary right lateral incisor to the left first premolar tooth. The mandibular right cuspid was then orthodontically separated from the mandibular right lateral incisor, and this was added to the anterior mandibular splint. A transitional crown was made for the maxillary left second premolar tooth and a transitional fixed prosthesis was made from the mandibular left cuspid to the left second premolar (Figure 16.11). The periodontal re-evaluation revealed that the pockets depths had diminished greatly and that bleeding on probing had disappeared.

PHASE 3

At this point, after the periodontal evaluation, additional occlusal support was established by means of a transitional, mandibular, removable partial prosthesis (Figure 16.12). Periodontal surgery on the maxillary left first molar revealed a perforation. The disto-buccal root was removed.

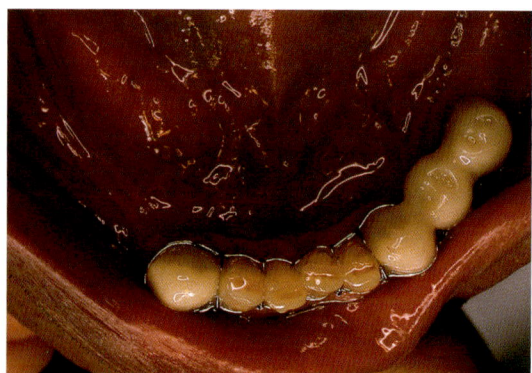

Figure 16.10

Lingual view of anterior mandibular teeth

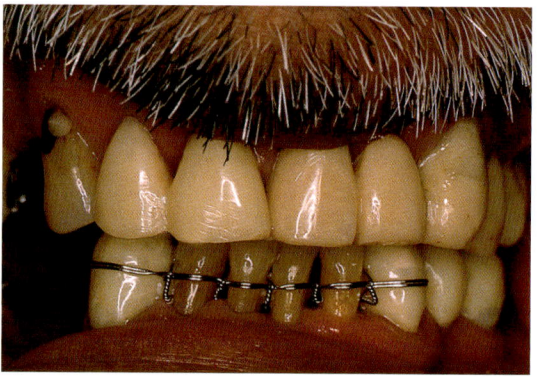

Figure 16.11

Frontal view of teeth

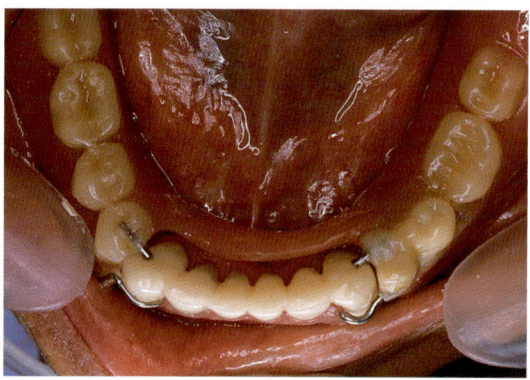

Figure 16.12

Lingual view of mandibular temporized teeth

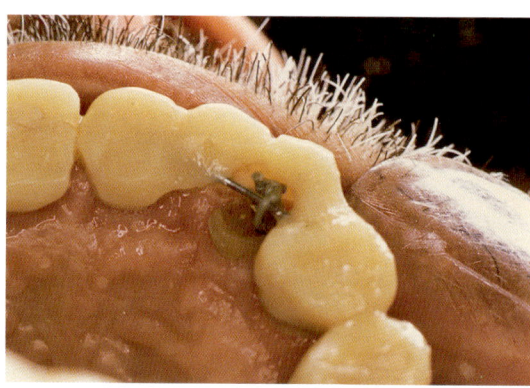

Figure 16.13

Forced eruption of maxillary cuspid

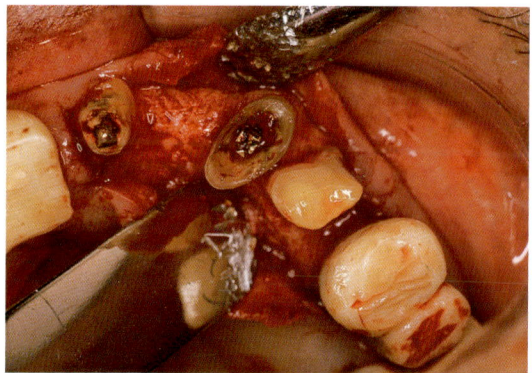

Figure 16.14

Crown lengthening procedure—maxillary cuspid

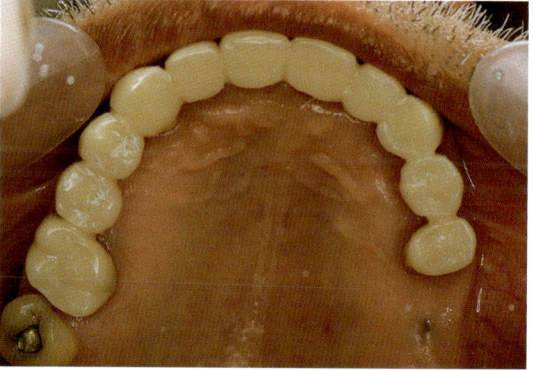

Figure 16.15

Maxillary transitional prosthesis

During caries excavation, additional necessary endodontic treatments were done. Orthodontic treatment, which consisted of forced eruption of the maxillary left cuspid, was then performed (Figure 16.13). In preparation for the crown, a crown lengthening periodontal surgical procedure (CLP) was done to gain sound tooth structure (Figure 16.14).

PHASE 4

At the completion of orthodontic and periodontal treatment, a transitional fixed partial prosthesis was made, extending from the maxillary right first molar to the maxillary left second premolar (Figure 16.15). Endodontic treatment on the mandibular right cuspid and the mandibular left second premolar was then done. Due to continual infection, and pocketing, the two remaining roots of the maxillary left first molar were extracted. Due to severe pain, the mandibular left cuspid was then endodontically treated.

PHASE 5

At completion of initial preparation and re-evaluation, the final phase of treatment was carried out. Copper band elastomeric impressions were taken of all the prepared teeth and Duralay copings were made. These copings were used for the final impression for the master model and to record centric relation at the vertical dimension of the temporary restorations. The metal copings were then fitted and soldered. After try-in of the soldered metal framework (Figure 16.16), another elastomeric impression was done to reproduce an accurate tissue transfer. These

models were mounted on a semi-adjustable articulator (Hanau) using a facebow registration and centric records taken at the vertical dimension of occlusion in Pattern resin using the Neylon technique. In the mandible, the porcelain was baked, and the occlusion checked in the mouth at the biscuit bake stage; all adjustments needed were then made (Figure 16.17).

The removable partial denture framework was constructed. It was fitted and an altered cast impression was then made for soft

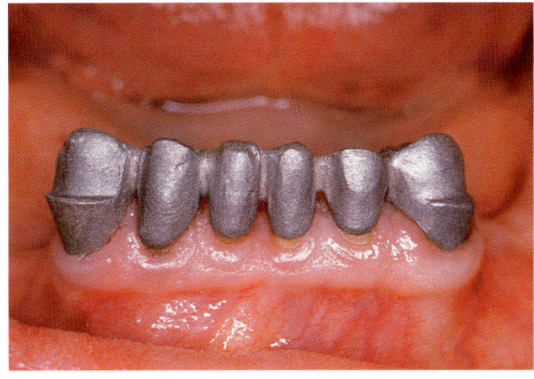

Figure 16.16

Soldered metal copings being fitted—mandible

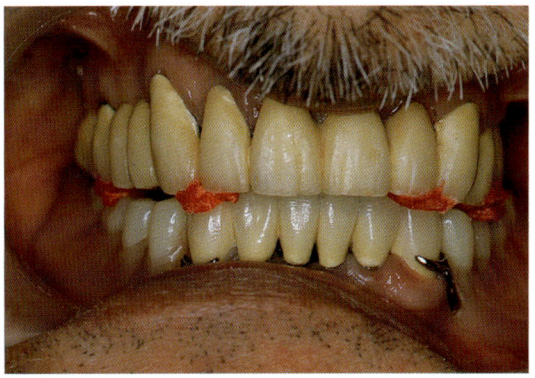

Figure 16.17

Biscuit bake try-in

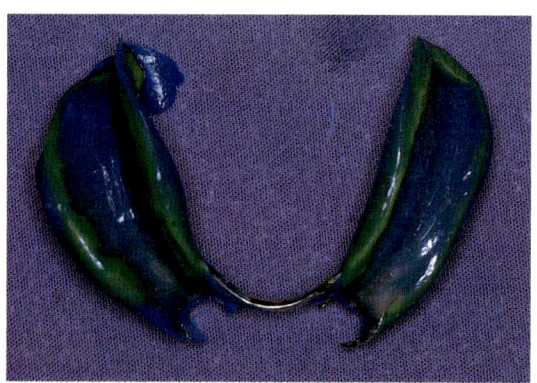

Figure 16.18

Altered cast impression

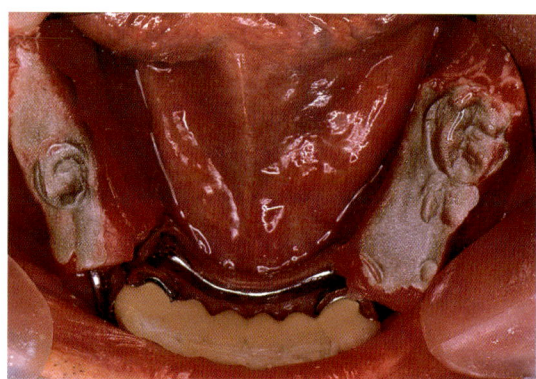

Figure 16.19

Centric occlusion recording in wax

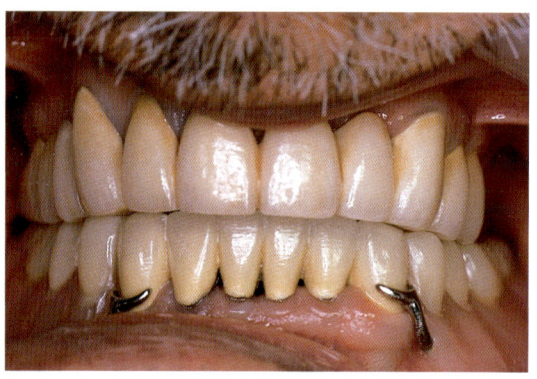

Figure 16.20

Treatment completed—post-treatment anterior view

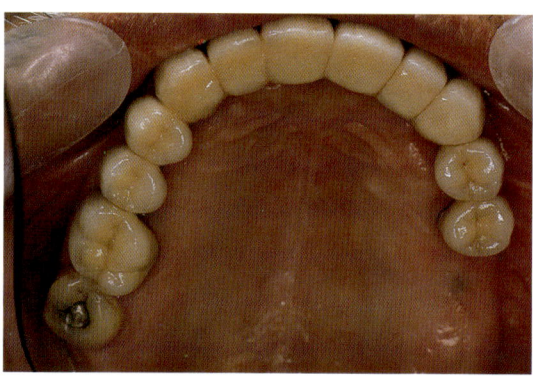

Figure 16.21

Treatment completed—maxilla

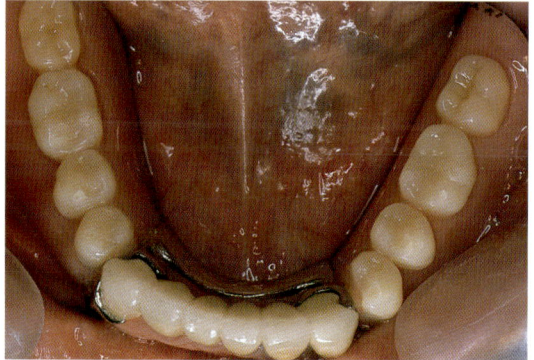

Figure 16.22

Treatment completed—mandible

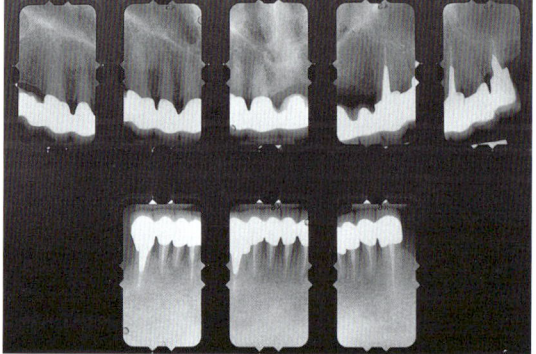

Figure 16.23

Treatment completed—radiographs, anterior teeth

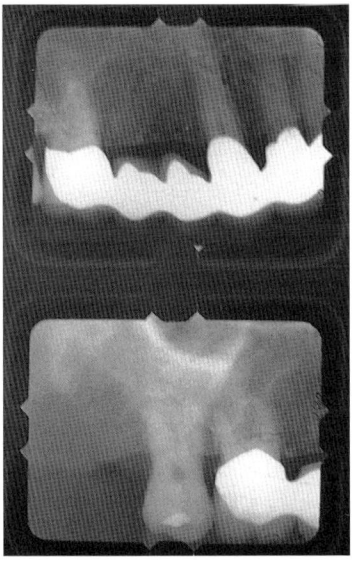

Figure 16.24

Treatment completed—radiographs, right side

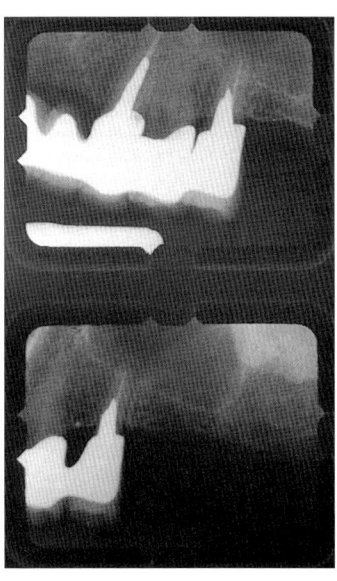

Figure 16.25

Treatment completed—radiographs, left side

tissue duplication (Figure 16.18). At the same time, a soft wax occlusal record was taken to mount the model on the articulator (Figure 16.19). Teeth were set up on the partial denture and fitted in the mouth. The porcelain was then glazed. The crowns and bridges were cemented with Temp-Bond and the removable mandibular partial prosthesis inserted. The crowns and bridges were then cemented with zinc oxyphosphate cement for permanent cementation (Figures 16.20–16.22). A complete series of radiographs was done after completion of treatment (Figures 16.23–16.25).

SUMMARY

The patient, a 70-year-old retired school principal, presented with many varied problems. He had undergone a number of surgical procedures to remove a pleomorphic adenoma, which left him with permanent facial nerve damage and loss of the left parotid gland. His face drooped, and was asymmetrical. The mandibular anterior teeth exhibited class 3 mobility, which gave a poor prognosis for their long-term retention. He had rampant caries, related to his medical history, and many broken teeth. His vertical dimension of occlusion was overclosed and he was traumatizing the anterior palatal tissue when closing his mouth. The patient requested a fixed prosthesis, even though during treatment he agreed to accept a removable prosthesis. In the course of treatment many problems arose, and his treatment had to be adjusted to the new circumstances. In spite of all these problems, an excellent result was achieved using a combination of fixed and removable prostheses.

CASE DISCUSSION
AVINOAM YAFFE

The patient, a 70-year-old male, presented to the clinic for treatment. He had many missing teeth, loss of occlusal support, and anterior traumatic overbite aggravated by advanced periodontal disease. His condition was complicated by status post-pleomorphic adenoma of the left parotid gland, that left him with facial asymmetry and paralysis of the seventh cranial nerve. The treatment was started in 1989, when the use of dental implants was just beginning in Israel, and they were mainly placed in the anterior region of the mandible. At that time, a great effort was made to save the patient's remaining teeth. His vertical dimension was changed, and his mandibular anterior teeth were shortened to improve the crown-to-root ratio, while creating an incisal platform for the maxillary transitional restoration. The aim of his treatment was to join tooth support for vertical dimension to posterior occlusal support by means of the removable partial denture. In order to cope with his problem of severe caries, fluoride rinses were administered as well as the use of artificial saliva. The restorations that were made restored function, esthetics, and occlusal support to the complete satisfaction of both the patient and the treatment team.

CASE DISCUSSION
HAROLD PREISKEL

The treatment team demonstrated their ability to take the failing dentition of a 70-year-old patient with a compromised medical history and to transform it into healthy, functional, and good-looking units. To achieve this, most of the specialities within dentistry were involved. Forced eruption and other orthodontic treatment, endodontic treatment, and, naturally, periodontal therapy are all involved in this well thought out plan. I was pleased to note that the mandibular bilateral distal extension removal prosthesis was made with an altered cast technique. Since the anterior teeth were splinted crowns, a better looking restoration might have been achieved using attachments, albeit at the cost of increased complexity to manufacture and to maintain. This treatment was commenced well over a decade ago.

Professor Yaffe has intimated that today it is just possible that the use of implants might realize the patient's dream of fixed prostheses in both jaws. Naturally, this may be feasible. However, what is for sure is that the principle of treatment carried out in the previous decade is just as sound today as it was then, and will probably be good for many years to come.

IV CONGENITAL DISORDERS

PATIENT 17   SEVERE UNILATERAL CLEFT LIP AND PALATE

Treatment by Miriam Calev

THE PATIENT

The patient, a 27-year-old builder, presented himself for examination and consultation. His complaints were as follows:

'I have difficulties in eating and breathing because of the hole in my palate.' (Figure 17.1)
'Sometimes my teeth hurt.'
'My scar is ugly but it will be fixed soon.'

PAST MEDICAL HISTORY

The patient suffered from a peptic ulcer for which he was taking medication (Gastro 40 mg daily) and congenital unilateral cleft lip and palate. He only had one kidney, having donated a kidney to his father for transplantation.

PAST DENTAL HISTORY

In the past, a general dentist had treated him in his village and had referred him for orthodontic treatment at Hadassah Dental School.

EXTRA-ORAL EXAMINATION
(Figures 17.2 and 17.3)

* Asymmetrical face on right side due to unilateral cleft lip and palatal scar, and nose deformity

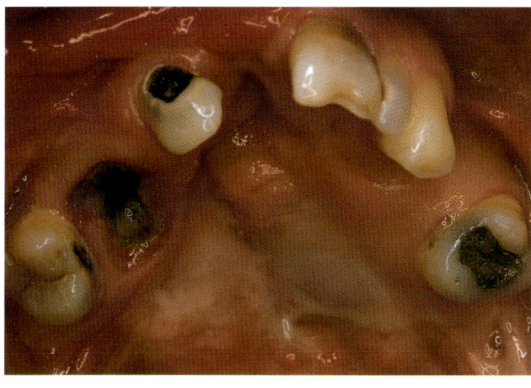

Figure 17.1

Maxillary arch—palatal view

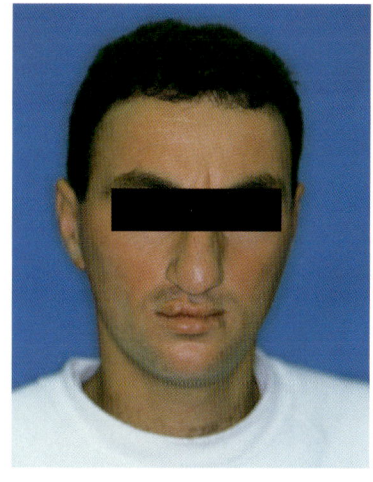

Figure 17.2

Face—frontal view

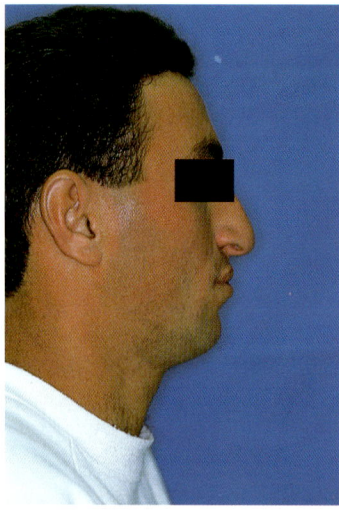

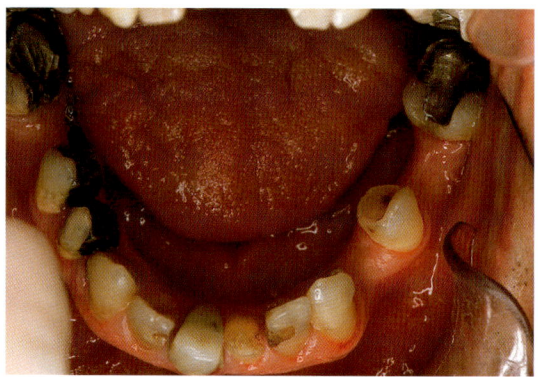

Figure 17.4

Mandibular arch—lingual view

Figure 17.3

Face—side view

- Competent lips
- Straight profile with slight concavity and depression of the nose
- Normally functioning temporomandibular joint, with bilateral clicking on opening
- Maximum opening 38 mm, with a slight deviation to the left upon opening
- Negative overbite of 8.0 mm
- Enlarged lower third of the face

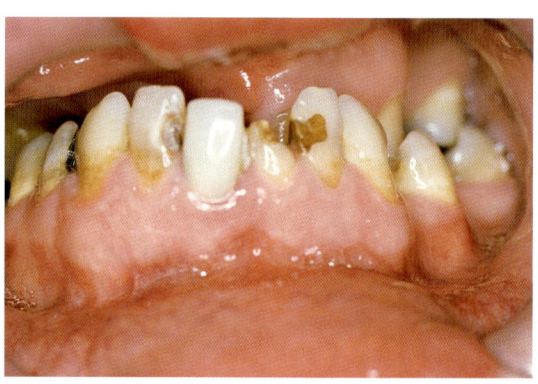

Figure 17.5

Anterior teeth—labial view

INTRA-ORAL EXAMINATION
(Figures 17.1, 17.4 and 17.5)

Maxilla:

- Small and underdeveloped jaw
- Triangular arch form
- Oronasal-palatal fistula close to the midline
- Plaque
- Gingivitis
- Caries
- Residual roots
- Purulent exudate from the right first molar

- Missing teeth:

$$\frac{8\ 5\ 4\ 2\ 1\ \ \big|\ \ 4\ 5\ 6\ 8}{}$$

- Malposition of maxillary right cuspid

Mandible:

- Large parabolic arch shape
- Plaque
- Gingivitis
- Anterior crowding
- Primary and secondary caries
- Defective large restorations
- Missing teeth:

$$\frac{}{7\ 6\ \ \big|\ \ 4\ 6\ 7}$$

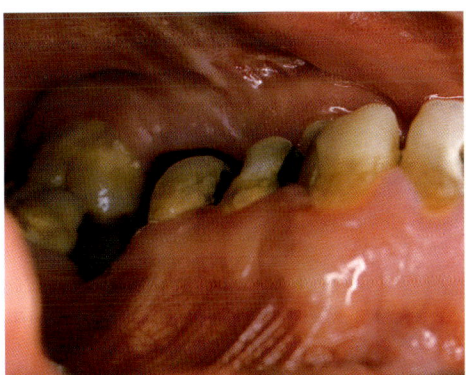

Figure 17.6

Occlusion—right side

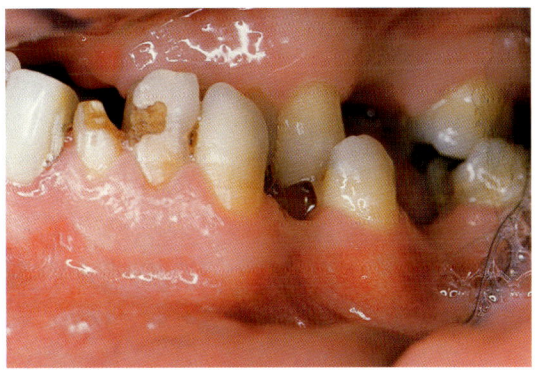

Figure 17.7

Occlusion—left side

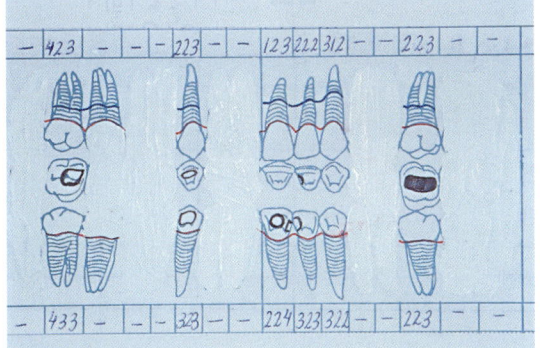

Figure 17.8

Periodontal chart—pre-treatment, maxilla

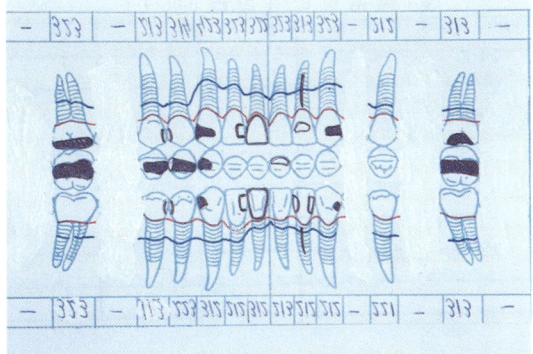

Figure 17.9

Periodontal chart—pre-treatment, mandible

Occlusal examination revealed that the patient was Angle class III (Figures 17.5–17.7), with a reverse overbite of 8.0 mm and a reverse overjet of 3.0 mm. There were wear facets on the right second premolar and second molars. The interocclusal rest space was 3.0 mm, measured between the incisors. There was a slight discrepancy between centric occlusion (CO) and centric relation (CR). Anterior and bilateral posterior cross-bite was found. Centric occlusal contacts were found on the right second molars, right maxillary cuspid to right mandibular first premolar, left

cuspids, and left second molars. Occlusal balancing side and protrusive premature contacts during lateral and protrusive mandibular movements were noted.

Periodontal examination (Figures 17.8 and 17.9) revealed unsatisfactory oral hygiene with plaque and calculus. Probing depths were found of up to 4.0 mm on the maxillary teeth and up to 3.0 mm on the mandibular teeth, with bleeding on probing on some teeth. There was inflammation around most of the teeth.

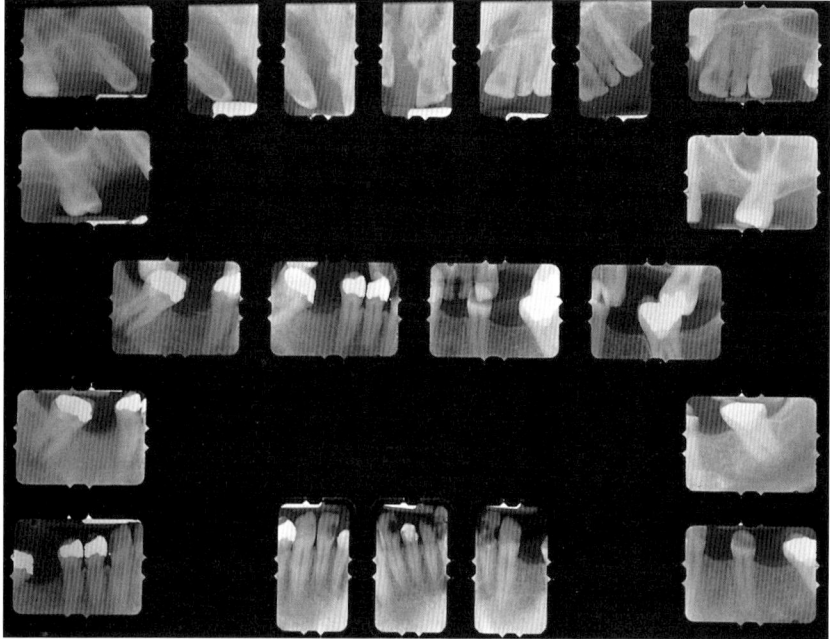

Figure 17.10

Radiographs of maxilla and mandible—pre-treatment

FULL MOUTH PERIAPICAL RADIOGRAPHIC EXAMINATION
(Figure 17.10)

- Endodontic treatment—mandibular right lateral incisor with poor condensation
- Periapical radiolucent areas around the right mandibular third molar and lateral incisor, and the left lateral incisor and third molar
- Good bone support of all remaining teeth
- Caries
- Lateral maxillary right alveolar and palatal cleft
- Short roots of the maxillary anterior teeth
- Residual roots—maxillary right first molar

INDIVIDUAL TOOTH PROGNOSIS

- Hopeless:

$$\dfrac{6\ |}{|}$$

- Poor:[1]

$$\dfrac{|}{7\ |\ 2}$$

- Fair:[1]

$$\dfrac{3\ |\ 1\ 2}{5\ 4\ 2\ 1\ |\ 1\ 7}$$

- Good:

$$\dfrac{7\ 3\ |\ 7}{3\ |\ 3\ 5}$$

SUMMARY OF FINDINGS

The patient, a 27-year-old man, suffering from a peptic ulcer and status post-surgery for congenitally unilateral cleft lip and palate, and complaining of difficulty in eating, bleeding gums, and esthetic problems, came to the clinic for treatment.

[1] Teeth $\overline{8}|\overline{8}$ are listed in the periodontal chart as $\overline{7}|\overline{7}$. As determined by radiographic evaluation, they really are third molar teeth that have shifted mesially to the second molar position.

He presented with poor oral hygiene, plaque, gingival inflammation, and shallow and intermediate probing depths. He had deep caries, residual roots, crowded anterior mandibular teeth, defective endodontic treatment and restorations. There were periapical lesions around four mandibular teeth and occlusal interferences during lateral and protrusive mandibular movements.

DIAGNOSIS

- Cleft lip and palate (oronasal fistula) (status post surgery)
- Angle class III with anterior and bilateral posterior cross-bite accompanied by severe interarch discrepancy
- Faulty occlusal relationship, and faulty occlusal plane
- Carious lesions
- Defective restorations and endodontic treatment (periapical lesions)
- Crowded anterior mandibular teeth
- Poor esthetics
- Gingivitis
- Reduced anterior and posterior support
- Reduced vertical dimension
- Residual root

ABOUT THE PATIENT

The patient was very conscientious, and willing to cooperate in spite of his physical handicaps (scar, limited mouth opening). He had high expectations from his dental treatment and even more so from the planned plastic surgery procedures. He wanted to improve his appearance but did not have any preferences for fixed versus removable restorations. He did not appreciate the significance of proper oral hygiene and its importance in his treatment.

POTENTIAL TREATMENT PROBLEMS

Cleft lip and palate:
- Scarred lip
- Esthetic problems
- Limited opening

Oronasal fistula:
- Breathing problems
- Eating problems
- Phonetic problems

Underdevelopment of the maxilla:
- Missing teeth
- Jaw discrepancy
- Failure of osseous union

Arch level
Maxilla:

- Few remaining teeth with unfavorable distribution and malposition of the right cuspid
- Open oronasal fistula

Mandible:

- Remaining teeth had poor prognosis due to caries and defective restorations.

Inter-arch level
Cross-bite and Angle class III jaw relationship

- Large interarch discrepancy
- Limited mouth opening and limited mandibular movements
- The need to change the vertical dimension in order to restore the mouth
- The small difference between centric relation and centric occlusion

TREATMENT ALTERNATIVES

Maxilla:

- Telescopic, removable partial denture
- Fixed partial prosthesis and small obturator
- Fixed and removable partial prostheses

Mandible:

- Fixed partial prosthesis

TREATMENT PLAN

Phase 1: initial preparation

- Oral hygiene instruction
- Scaling and curettage
- Dietary changes
- Fluoride rinses and gel application
- Extraction of residual roots
- Caries removal
- Evaluation of patient cooperation

Phase 2

- Orthodontic and surgical consultations
- Endodontic therapy where indicated
- Restorative treatment with restorations and provisional fixed acrylic restorations for the teeth with ample loss of tooth structure

Phase 3

- Orthodontic treatment for uprighting and realigning teeth
- Re-evaluation and planning of pre-prosthetic periodontal surgery
- New provisional fixed acrylic restorations at the new vertical dimension of occlusion in order to check patient adaptation
- Re-evaluation

Phase 4

- Fixed partial prostheses for both the maxilla and the mandible

TREATMENT

Initial preparation included oral hygiene instruction, scaling, and curettage. Caries removal and provisional restorations were done where indicated. The maxillary right first molar roots were extracted. Endodontic therapy was performed on the mandibular right premolars, the mandibular right third molar, the maxillary left central and lateral incisors, and all the mandibular incisors.

At this point, it was determined that the patient was actively participating in his treatment, as his oral hygiene was greatly improved (Figures 17.11–17.14).

Upon completion of the endodontic treatment, the right mandibular third molar was restored with an amalgam post and core, and the other endodontically treated teeth were prepared for cast post and cores and provisional restorations.

After consultation with the plastic surgery and oral and maxillofacial surgery departments, the decision was made by all concerned that additional surgery would not contribute to the success of the treatment, and would probably only traumatize the patient. Periodontal surgery (vestibulum deepening), due to the lack of attached gingiva, was performed upon the maxillary right cuspid, including a soft tissue graft from a donor site in the palate, and the

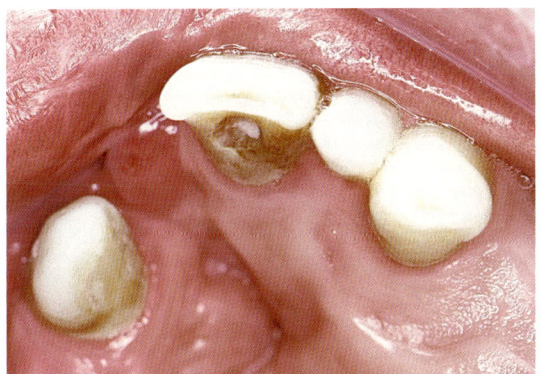

Figure 17.11

Anterior maxillary teeth—palatal view, after initial preparation

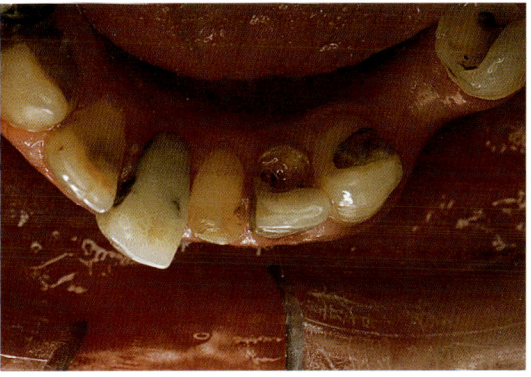

Figure 17.12

Anterior mandibular teeth—lingual view, after initial preparation

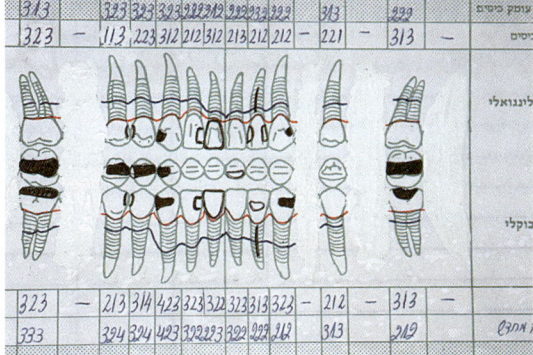

Figure 17.13

Periodontal chart—mandible, first re-evaluation

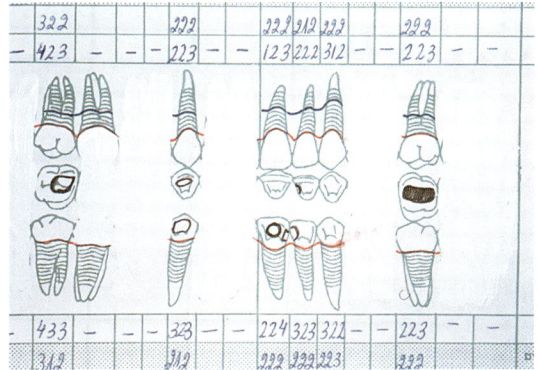

Figure 17.14

Periodontal chart—maxilla, first re-evaluation

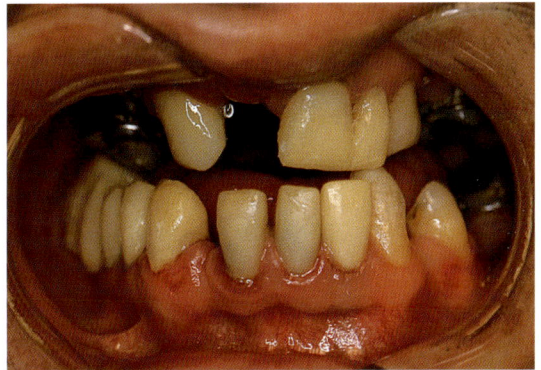

Figure 17.15

Provisional restorations—anterior view

remaining endodontically treated mandibular teeth (crown lengthening procedures). The anterior maxillary teeth were prepared for full crown restorations and temporized with provisional restorations at an increased vertical dimension (Figure 17.15).

Orthodontic treatment was planned and executed to expand the maxillary arch in order to attain an incisal tip-to-tip relationship, rather than the class III Angle that existed. The maxillary right cuspid was also treated orthodontically to bring it to a more labial position (Figure 17.16).

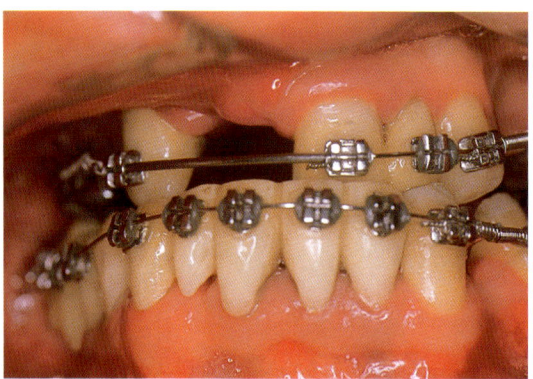

Figure 17.16

Orthodontic treatment, mandible

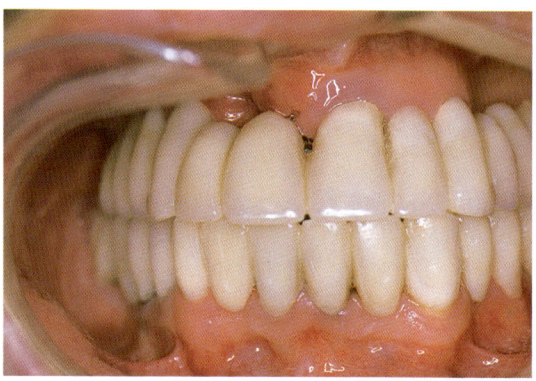

Figure 17.17

Provisional acrylic resin restorations

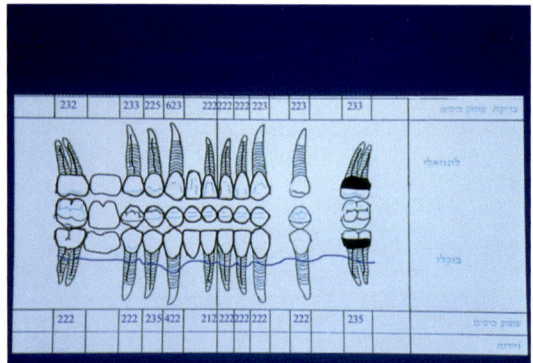

Figure 17.18

Periodontal chart—mandible, second re-evaluation

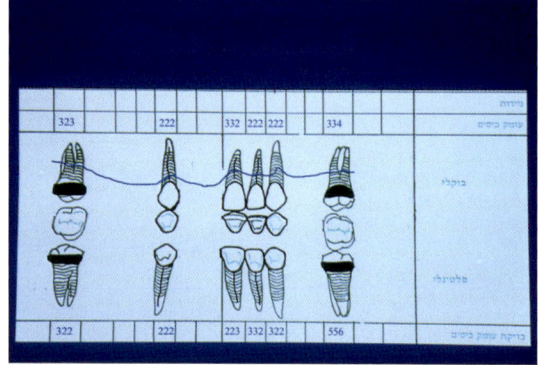

Figure 17.19

Periodontal chart—maxilla, second re-evaluation

At completion of orthodontic and periodontal treatment, the cast posts and cores were finished and cemented into place on the endodontically treated teeth. A re-evaluation regarding the final treatment plan was then carried out. New provisional restorations were made to maintain the new vertical dimension and to stabilize the teeth after the orthodontic treatment. These provisional restorations also enabled us to evaluate patient's adaptation to the new occlusal jaw relations (Figures 17.17–17.19).

After a period of 6 months with the provisional restorations at the new vertical dimension of occlusion, the patient exhibited no temporomandibular joint or muscular problems. The teeth were re-prepared (Figure 17.20), copper band elastomeric impressions were taken and the treatment was continued as outlined in the Technical Information chapter.

The treatment for the oronasal fistula was to incorporate a precision attachment on the lingual aspect of the anterior fixed prosthesis opposite the oronasal fistula. A

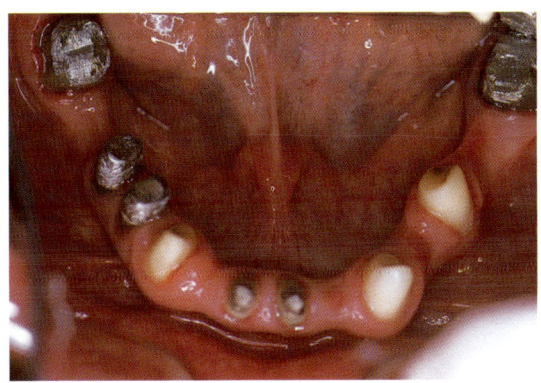

Figure 17.20

Final tooth preparation—mandible

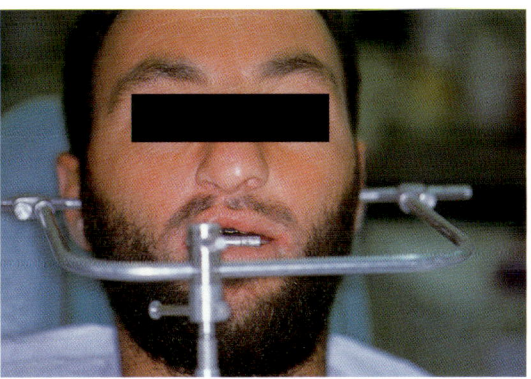

Figure 17.21

Facebow registration

removable gold foil prosthesis was then made to seal the oronasal fistula by attaching it to the fixed prosthesis by means of the precision attachment.

Full arch polyether impressions were made for tissue detail. The models were then mounted on a Hanau articulator with the aid of a facebow registration (Figure 17.21) and the porcelain was baked. The final and minute adjustments of the biscuit-bake porcelain were carried out in the mouth. The final glaze was applied to the prostheses, and they were cemented with Temp-Bond for a period of 2 weeks. They were then cemented with zinc oxyphosphate cement for permanent cementation (Figures 17.22–17.26).

SUMMARY

The patient presented with a severe problem of unilateral cleft lip and palate, remaining residual roots, caries, and malpositioned teeth. There was a pathologic occlusion with serious balancing side and protrusive premature contacts during mandibular movements. He was very concerned about esthetics. The treatment was further complicated by the severe Angle class III jaw relationships and the negative overbite and overjet. Another problem was that the patient had no understanding of good oral hygiene. Due the decision after consultation with the plastic surgery and oral and maxillofacial surgery departments, that additional surgery would not contribute to the success of the treatment and would only cause more trauma to the patient, surgery was not performed.

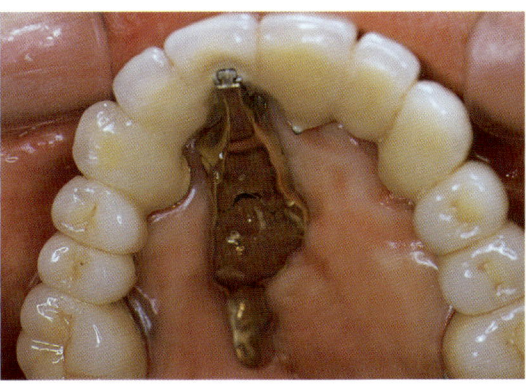

Figure 17.22

Gold foil obturator to close palatal cleft

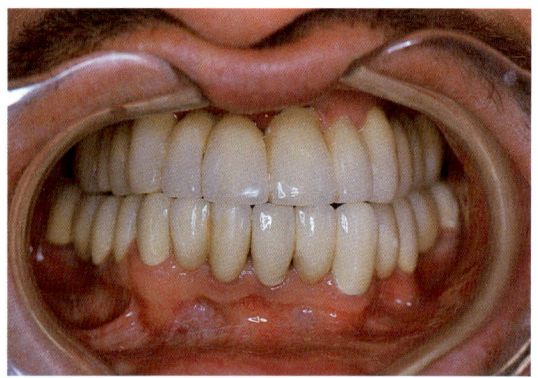

Figure 17.23

Treatment completed—anterior view

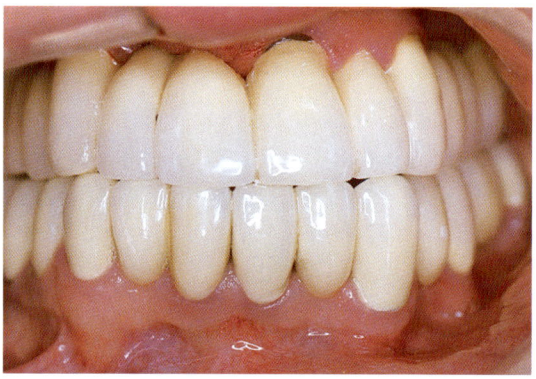

Figure 17.24

Treatment completed—anterior view, close up

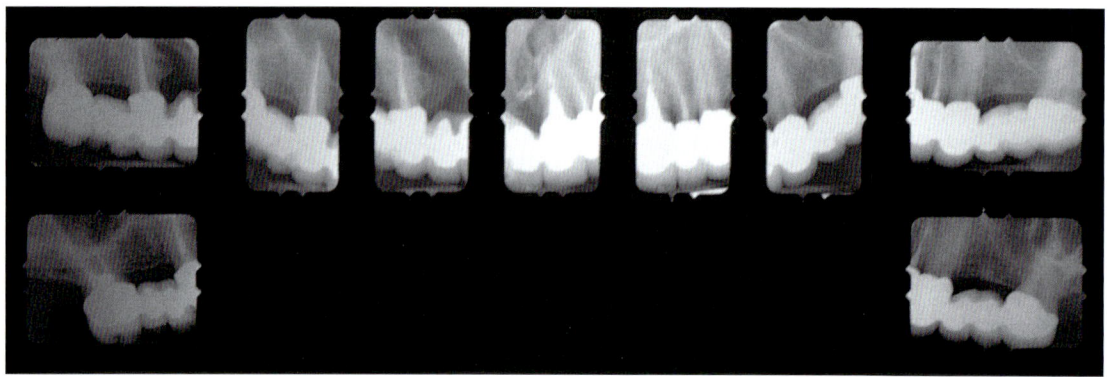

Figure 17.25

Radiographs—post-treatment, maxilla

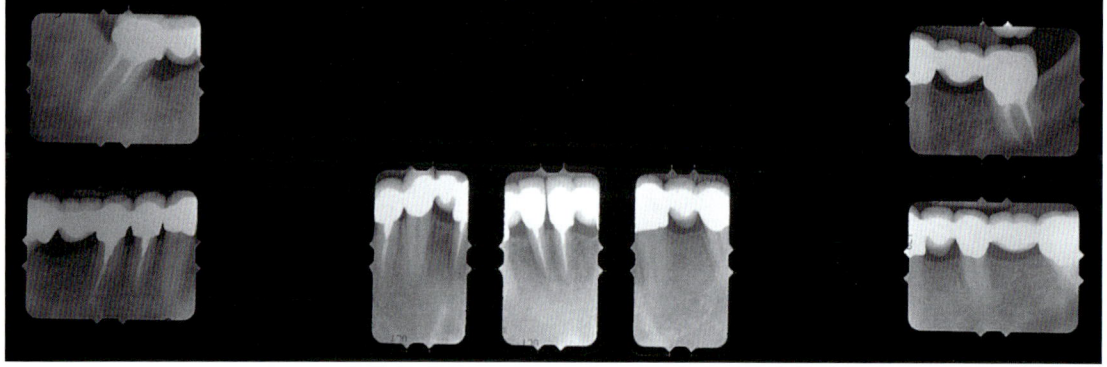

Figure 17.26

Radiographs—post-treatment, mandible

Treatment consisted of oral hygiene instruction, periodontal surgery, endodontic therapy, oral surgery, removal of caries, orthodontic treatment, and altering the vertical dimension of occlusion in order to provide a physiological occlusion and change the jaw relationship from Angle class III to that of edge-to-edge. The final restorations accomplished all of these goals as well as providing an esthetic solution to the patient's problems.

oronasal fistula. A gold foil was fabricated to seal the oronasal fistula by attaching to the fixed prosthesis by means of the precision attachment, thus providing a fixed prosthesis along with a seal of the oronasal fistula and potential access for cleaning when needed. In the execution of this treatment plan, this young patient was provided with a solution to his functional and esthetic demands, providing him with a much better quality of life.

CASE DISCUSSION
AVINOAM YAFFE

This treatment represents a prosthodontic solution to a severe unilateral cleft lip and palate, with pathologic occlusion along with interarch discrepancy. Further problems included esthetic complaints that could not be otherwise solved, due to an unsuccessful previous attempt for orthodontic treatment and limited surgical success to remedy the situation of the oronasal fistula along with the unilateral cleft lip and palate.

By using the existing small amount of intercuspal/retruded cuspal discrepancy along with optimal increase of the vertical dimension and utilizing adjunctive orthodontics, the pathologic occlusion of Angle class III was converted to an esthetically satisfactory functional physiologic occlusion with minute anterior guidance. In order to seal the oronasal fistula, and avoid a removable appliance, a precision attachment was incorporated on the lingual aspect of the anterior fixed prosthesis opposite the

CASE DISCUSSION
HAROLD PREISKEL

This patient appeared to combine a challenging cocktail of prosthodontic difficulties. Naturally, surgical closure of the naso-palatine fistula would have been preferable, but in this case had not proved feasible. The need to construct an obturator added yet one more prosthodontic difficulty. The degree of patient cooperation achieved was quite remarkable in view of the past history, and orthodontic treatment for both arches following periodontal therapy was a requirement if a good-looking outcome was to be achieved. Indeed, the maxillary orthodontic treatment involved crossing the cleft, but the subsequent construction of a fixed prosthesis should prevent any relapse. The use of transitional restorations in the evaluation of changes of a dimension of occlusion is to be recommended and the result achieved eminently satisfactory.

PATIENT 18   UNILATERAL CLEFT LIP AND PALATE AND PARTIAL ANODONTIA

Treatment by Thomas Zahavi

THE PATIENT

The patient, a 24-year-old man, came to the clinic for dental treatment. His chief complaints were (Figure 18.1):

'I want to fix my teeth.'
'My gum hurt when I eat hard food.'
'I have problems sometimes, speaking.'
'When I smile you can see that I am missing teeth.'

PAST MEDICAL HISTORY

The patient suffered from congenital unilateral cleft lip and palate and partial anodontia.

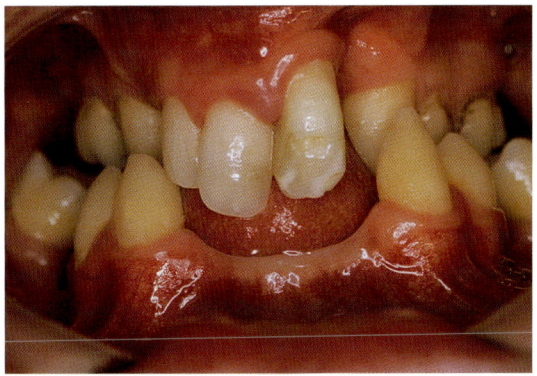

Figure 18.1

Anterior teeth—labial view

He underwent many surgical procedures when younger to close the cleft, but was left with an oro-antral fistula. At the age of 16, he underwent orthodontic treatment to expand the maxillae in order to obtain a better relationship between the posterior teeth. The treatment was unsuccessful and discontinued after one year of efforts due to the fact that the palatal scarring made tooth movement difficult.

At the age of 18, he came to Hadassah for a consultation regarding combined treatment utilizing orthodontics and surgery. Treatment was rejected because of its poor prognosis. Two years ago, the patient had plastic surgery performed in order to repair the clefts of the lip and nose and to close the oro-antral fistula. The surgery contributed to an improvement in his breathing and speech. Other than the above, his medical history was unremarkable.

PAST DENTAL HISTORY

The patient had two amalgam restorations placed a few years ago. He complained of:

- Difficulty in chewing and grinding food
- Poor esthetics

- Speech difficulty
- His front teeth are sensitive to hot and cold

EXTRA-ORAL EXAMINATION
(Figures 18.2 and 18.3)

- Asymmetrical face: non-alignment of lips, nose and eyes
- Normal profile with a sharp naso-labial angle and full lips
- Temporomandibular joint had a reciprocal click in the right joint

- Maximum opening of 46 mm without deviation (measured from the maxillary right central incisor to the mandibular anterior edentulous ridge)
- Scarred left lip

INTRA-ORAL AND FULL-MOUTH PERIAPICAL RADIOGRAPHIC EXAMINATION (Figures 18.4 and 18.5)

Maxilla (Figure 18.4):

- Narrow ridges

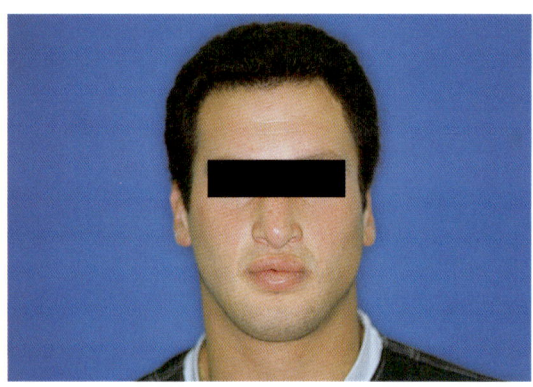

Figure 18.2

Face—frontal view

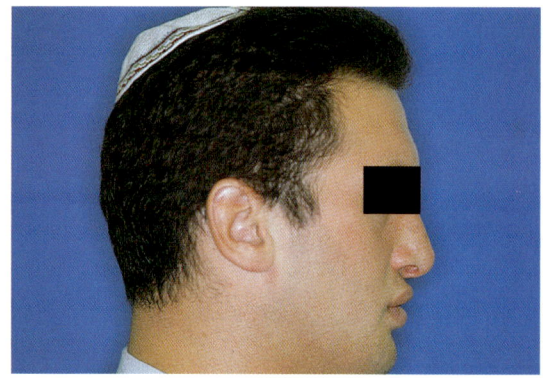

Figure 18.3

Face—side view

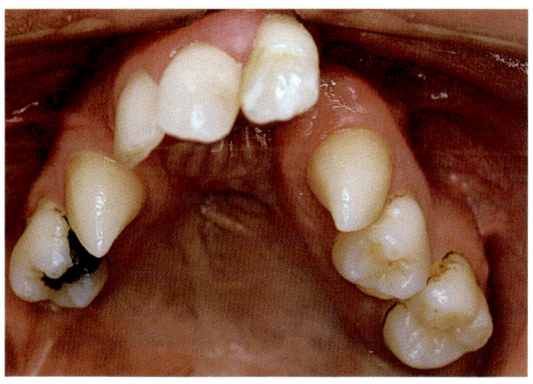

Figure 18.4

Maxillary arch—palatal view

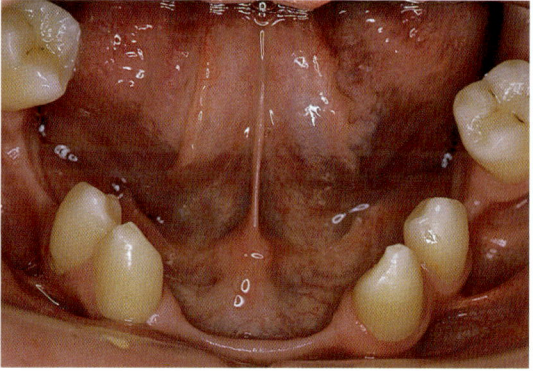

Figure 18.5

Mandibular arch—lingual view

- Triangular arch
- High palate
- Unilateral closed cleft palate
- Deciduous teeth:

$$\frac{E \mid E}{}$$

- Missing teeth:

$$\frac{8\ 7\ 6\ 5\ 4 \mid 2\ 4\ 5\ 7\ 8}{}$$

- Amalgam restorations on the right deciduous second molar
- Maxillary central incisors in labio-version
- Sharp conical-shaped cuspids
- Spacing between the right lateral incisor and right cuspid

Mandible (Figure 18.5):

- Triangular arch
- Missing teeth:

$$\frac{}{8\ 6\ 5\ 2\ 1 \mid 1\ 2\ 5\ 7\ 8}$$

- Sharp conical-shaped cuspids
- Narrow V-shaped residual ridges

Occlusal examination (Figures 18.6 and 18.7) revealed that the patient was Angle class III. The interocclusal rest space was 5.0 mm. Overjet and overbite could not be measured due to the missing anterior teeth (Figure 18.1). There was no discrepancy between centric relation and centric occlusion. Lateral jaw movements were guided only on the non-working side of the maxillary lateral incisor and the mandibular cuspid teeth on the right side, and by the maxillary central incisor and first molar and the mandibular left central incisor and first molar on the left side. Protrusive movements were guided by the left first molar maxillary and mandibular teeth.

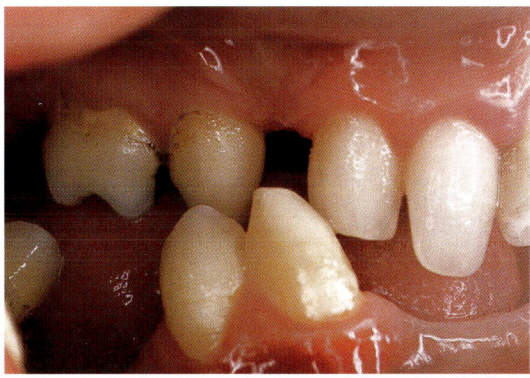

Figure 18.6

Occlusion—right side

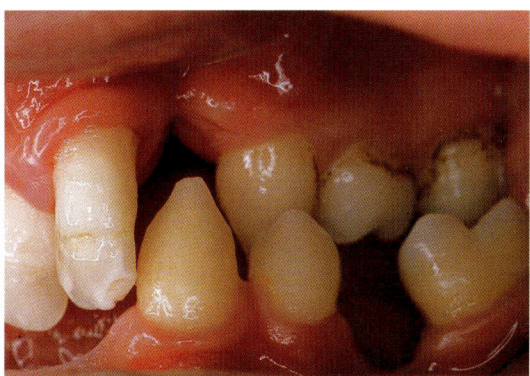

Figure 18.7

Occlusion—left side

Fremitus class 1 was noted on the maxillary right lateral incisor and the mandibular right cuspid (due to the cross-bite).

The periodontal examination (Figures 18.8 and 18.9) revealed some plaque, probing depths of up to 3.0 mm on the maxillary and mandibular teeth and bleeding (of the gingiva) on probing. There was slight gingival recession around most of the teeth and severe vertical recession on the lingual surfaces of the mandibular right second and left first molar teeth.

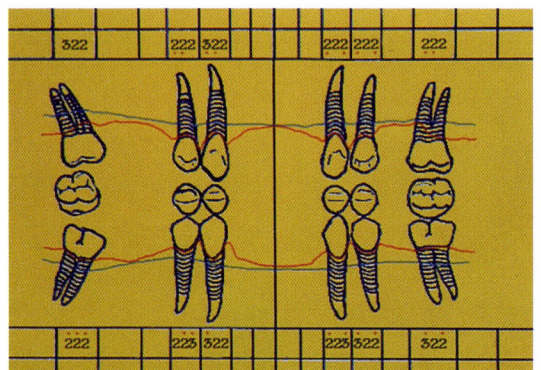

Figure 18.8

Periodontal chart—pre-treatment, mandible

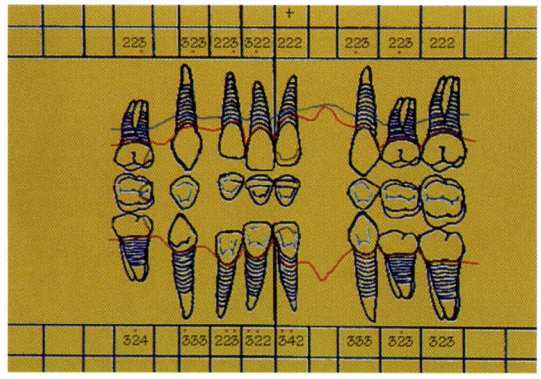

Figure 18.9

Periodontal chart—pre-treatment, maxilla

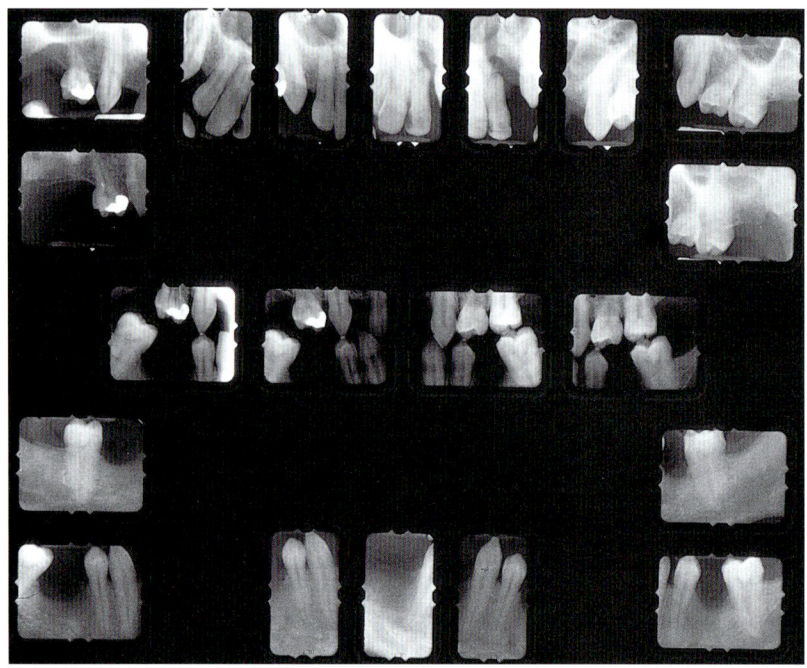

Figure 18.10

Radiographs of maxilla and mandible—pre-treatment, periapical

FULL-MOUTH PERIAPICAL SURVEY
(Figure 18.10)

- Severe bone loss around the distal surface of the maxillary left central incisor
- Vertical bone loss approximate to the areas of missing teeth

INDIVIDUAL TOOTH PROGNOSIS

- Questionable:

$$\frac{\quad 1}{\quad}$$

- Fair:

$$\frac{E \mid E}{\quad}$$

- Good:

$$\frac{3\ 2\ 1 \mid 6}{7\ 4\ 3 \mid 3\ 4\ 6}$$

SUMMARY OF FINDINGS

The 24-year-old patient, status post surgery of unilateral cleft lip and palate, came to the clinic complaining of missing teeth, difficulty when chewing food, difficulties in speaking, and esthetic problems. He presented with poor oral hygiene, plaque and calculus, and bleeding upon probing. The jaws were undeveloped in the areas where there were missing teeth. There was a discrepancy in jaw size, a significant amount of missing alveolar bone in the area of the cleft, and partial anodontia. The occlusion was cross-bite, with a scissors bite between the remaining teeth. The only teeth in occlusal contact were the left first molars and the right maxillary cuspid with the mandibular lateral incisor. There were retained deciduous teeth and sharp-pointed conical cuspids.

DIAGNOSIS

- Status post closed unilateral cleft lip and palate (left side) with scarring that resulted in a small maxilla, both antero-posteriorly and bucco-lingually
- Poor occlusal plane
- Cross-bite and scissors bite
- Partial anodontia
- Reduced occlusal support
- Primary occlusal trauma
- Decreased vertical dimension of occlusion (questionable)
- Retained deciduous teeth
- Gingivitis
- Faulty esthetics

ABOUT THE PATIENT

The patient was motivated for dental treatment in spite of his years of unsuccessful treatment. He was unaware of the importance of good oral hygiene, in particular in relation to his dental treatment. He wanted a fixed restoration, if possible.

TREATMENT POSSIBILITIES

Maxilla:

- Telescopic removable partial denture
- Overdenture
- Fixed partial prosthesis—tooth-supported

Mandible:

- Fixed prosthesis—tooth-supported
- Fixed prosthesis—tooth- and implant-supported

POTENTIAL TREATMENT PROBLEMS

- Cross-bite and missing teeth
- Difference in jaw size
- Congenital lack of many teeth
- Lack of bone support in the area of the missing teeth
- Developmental defects in the jaw
- Inability to incorporate orthodontic and surgical treatment
- Some of the supporting teeth were deciduous and their long-term prognosis was unknown

TREATMENT PLAN

PHASE 1: INITIAL PREPARATION

- Initial periodontal therapy including oral hygiene instruction, scaling and root planing

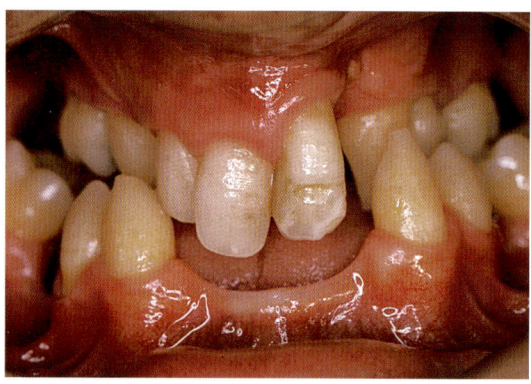

Figure 18.11

Patient after initial preparation

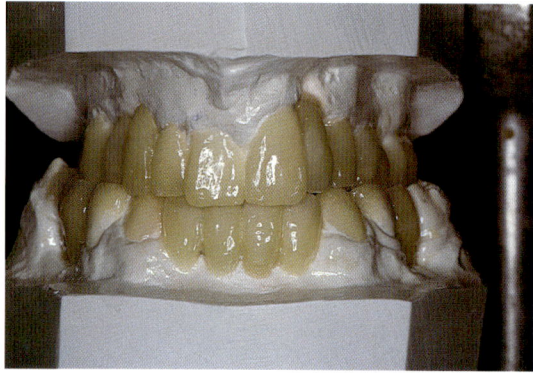

Figure 18.12

Wax-up

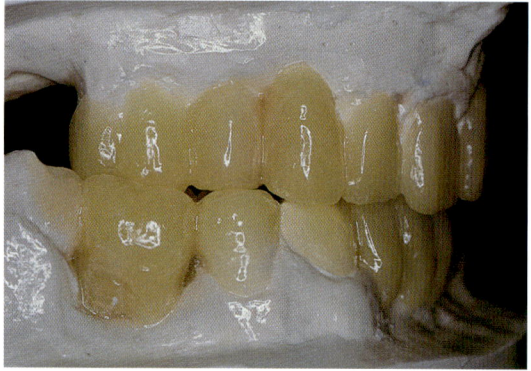

Figure 18.13

Wax-up

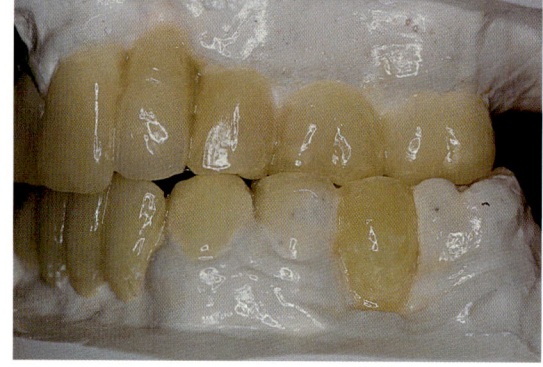

Figure 18.14

Wax-up

- Diagnostic wax-up
- Transitional restorations

PHASE 2

- Fixed restorations

TREATMENT

After a short period of initial treatment consisting of scaling, root planing, curettage, and oral hygiene instruction (Figure 18.11), study models were taken and mounted on an articulator to determine the possibility of fixed prostheses at the existing bucco-lingual jaw relationship. This was found to be impossible and a wax-up was made in which the vertical dimension was opened 5.0 mm in the incisor area (Figures 18.12–18.14).

After the wax-up on the articulator had been examined, and the amount of wax needed to build up the teeth to occlusion determined, it was decided to undertake minimal crown preparation of the teeth which were to be restored and normal crown preparation of the remaining teeth.

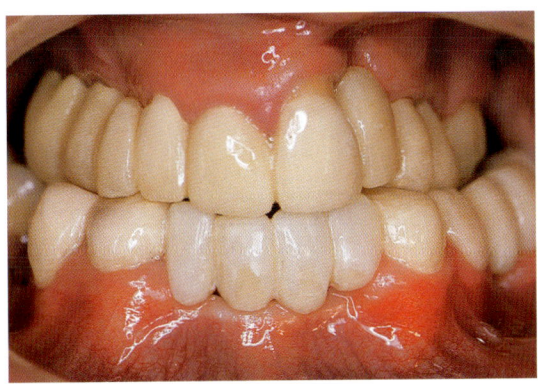

Figure 18.15

Transitional prosthesis I—anterior view

The decision to make a fixed restoration was taken with the understanding that there would be minimal tooth preparation and thus conservation of tooth structure and vitality of the teeth, thus minimizing the need for endodontic therapy.

The teeth were then prepared and the first transitional restorations were made at this new vertical dimension (Figure 18.15). At this time, endodontic treatment was undertaken on the maxillary central incisors which had pulp tested non-vital. Endodontic treatment was also carried out on the mandibular cuspids in order to improve their bucco-lingual relationships. The problem of crowding between the maxillary incisor teeth was then treated by separating them using wedges. Due to the fact that the mandibular incisors never formed, the vertical level of the soft tissue was lower than normal, thus necessitating periodontal surgery to add papillae to the mesial of the mandibular cuspid teeth. The vertical dimension of the transitional restorations was then duplicated in a second set of transitional restorations. In order to be sure that the patient adapted to the new increased vertical dimension, and that the occlusion was stable, as well as to check the vitality of the prepared teeth, the patient was maintained in these restorations for one year.

At re-evaluation one year later, the clinical situation was stable and there were no problems (Figures 18.16–18.18). The final phase of treatment was then carried out. The teeth were reprepared (slightly), and individual copper band elastomeric impressions were taken, and stone dies and Pattern resin copings made as described in the Technical Information chapter. The prostheses were then glazed and temporarily cemented in the mouth with Temp-Bond

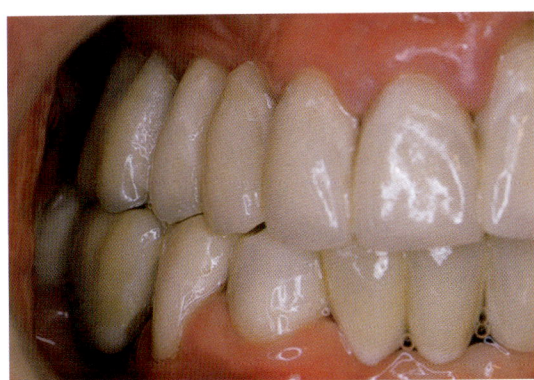

Figure 18.16

Transitional prosthesis II—right side

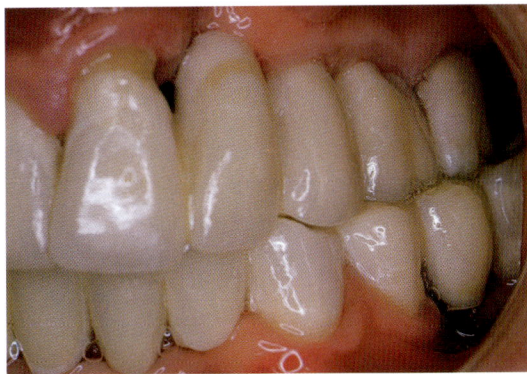

Figure 18.17

Transitional prosthesis II—left side

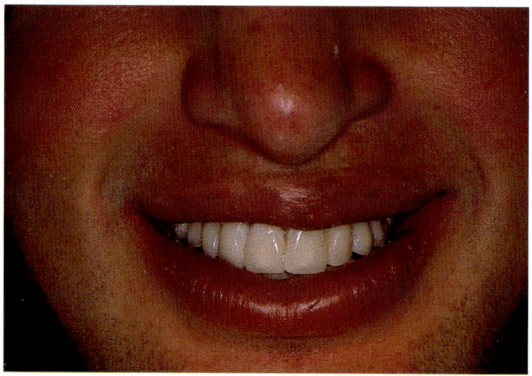

Figure 18.18

Transitional prosthesis II—patient smile

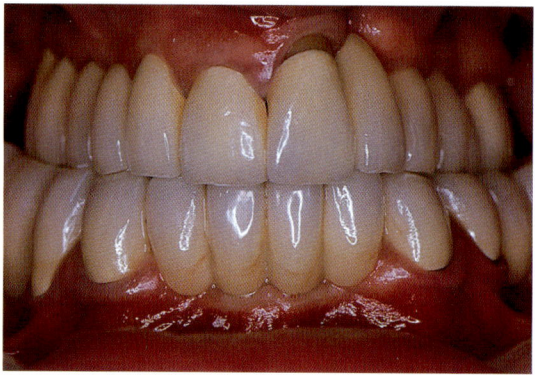

Figure 18.19

Treatment completed—anterior view

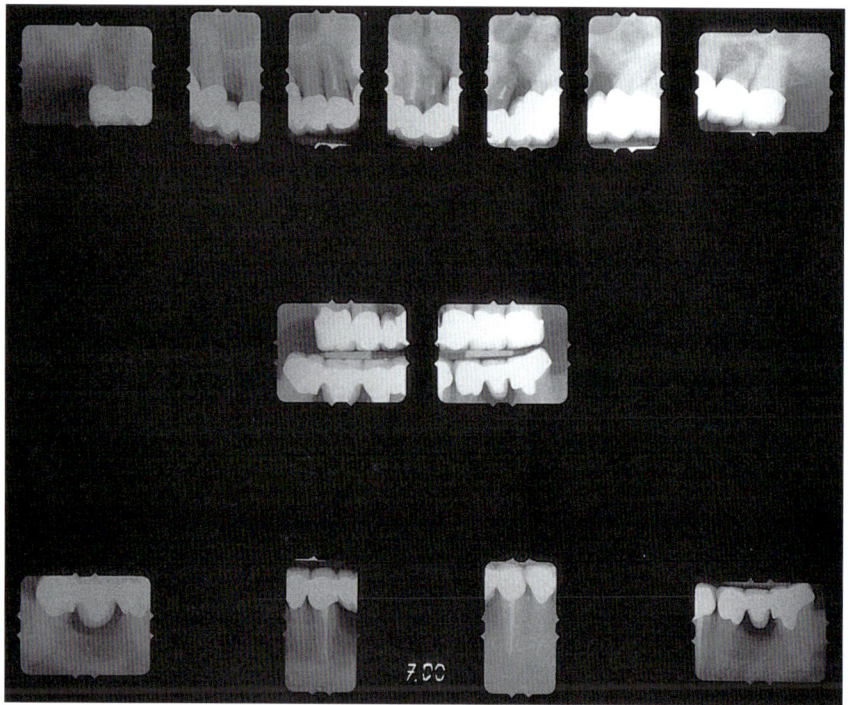

Figure 18.20

Treatment completed—
radiographs

for a period of 2 weeks. The prostheses were then cemented permanently with zinc oxyphosphate cement (Figures 18.19 and 18.20). Due to the difficulty in obtaining a parallel path of insertion in the mandible, the lower prosthesis was built in two sections.

The first bridge extended from the left mandibular first molar to the left first premolar, and the second, from the left mandibular cuspid to the right mandibular second molar. The maxillary restoration was constructed in one unit.

SUMMARY

This patient presented with severe problems. He was status post (S/P) surgery for unilateral cleft lip and palate, which left him with scarring that negated any orthodontic or surgical treatment. He had many missing teeth, mostly congenital. He had a severe cross-bite and scissor bite with a very difficult anterio-posterior and bucco-lingual jaw relationships to deal with. He wanted a fixed restoration yet was ignorant of good oral hygiene. A careful evaluation was made using mounted study models on an articulator and a tentative wax-up was done to determine whether fixed treatment was possible. The patient was then treated with transitional restorations for over one year, in order to make sure that he could adapt to the increased vertical dimension. Only then were permanent restorations made. The maxillary anterior teeth were restored esthetically in spite of the severe limitations that the patient presented. The anterior teeth were restored in a class I relationship although in the posterior region, a slight cross-bite was built in order to improve function. The cuspids guided lateral movements without any non-balancing side contacts. The maxillary left central incisor tooth was restored with supra-gingival margins in order to achieve a better path of insertion. This could be done as the patient had a high lip line and esthetics was not a problem. Total treatment time was 2 years and all the teeth remained vital, except for the four teeth that were treated endodontically at the beginning of the treatment. The treatment gave the patient esthetics and function that he had never had previously, due to his pre-existing congenital difficulties.

CASE DISCUSSION
AVINOAM YAFFE

This case represents a rather controversial treatment plan. On one hand, retained deciduous teeth served as abutment teeth for fixed partial restoration, and at the same time the vertical dimension of occlusion was increased by 5 mm. This further jeopardized the survival of the deciduous teeth. All that with the intention to facilitate, from a biomechanical aspect, fabrication of a fixed partial restoration. This case was executed with caution at each step. The team was aware of the risk, therefore the diagnostic wax-up took into account existing tooth position, and the food table was thus designed to minimize the off-center loading on the teeth. The occlusal scheme was performed with minimum rise on lateral excursions to minimize load and trauma to the teeth. At the completion of this restoration, it can be claimed that the solution provided in this case is esthetic, satisfactory from a functional standpoint, and provides the patient with a physiologic therapeutic occlusion.

CASE DISCUSSION
HAROLD PREISKEL

Treating a patient with a cleft palate and collapse of the maxillary dentition together with the associated derangement of occlusion is never straightforward. The decision to increase the vertical dimension by some 5 mm was probably correct, although the preparing of teeth at an early stage of treatment must be considered brave. A more cautious approach would have been to increase the vertical dimension using removable prostheses until the correct vertical dimension had been established, and only at this stage to undertake irreversible procedures such as tooth preparation. It is not simply the inter-arch space that poses the problem, it is the inter-abutment space and the cleansability of the resultant prosthesis that is likely to pose maintenance problems in the longer term. One can only hope that the patient's motivation is preserved, along with all the hard work that went into construction of the restoration.

PATIENT 19   GENERALIZED AMELOGENESIS IMPERFECTA

Treatment by David Lavi

THE PATIENT

The patient, a 25-year-old woman (Figure 19.1), presented herself for examination and consultation. Her complaints were as follows:

'My teeth are ugly.'
'The color of my teeth is awful.'
'My gums bleed and hurt when I brush them.'
'I feel that my mouth is one big mess.'
'Food sticks between my teeth after every meal.'
'My teeth are sensitive to anything hot or cold.'

PAST MEDICAL HISTORY

The patient had suffered some illnesses in childhood, but was currently in good health.

PAST DENTAL HISTORY

Treatment at a local dental clinic included two root canal treatments, two posts, and some amalgam restorations. Previously, because of an accident, some of her anterior maxillary teeth were extracted and a provisional fixed acrylic restoration was placed (Figure 19.2).

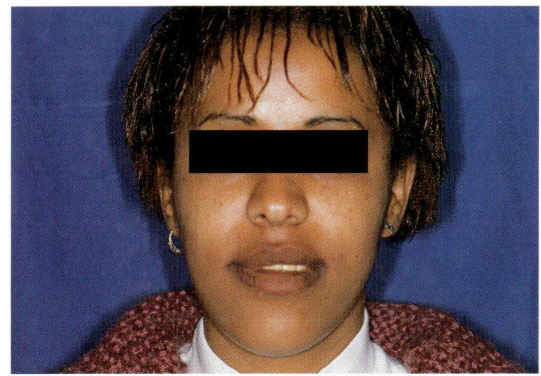

Figure 19.1

Face—frontal view

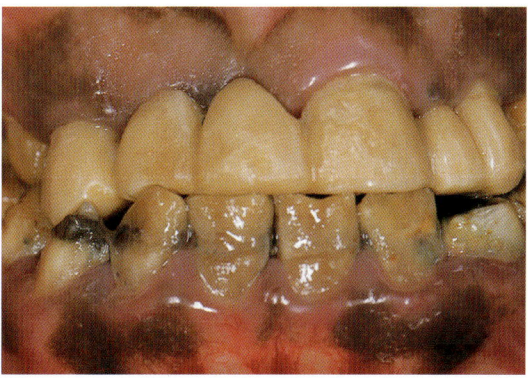

Figure 19.2

Anterior teeth—labial view

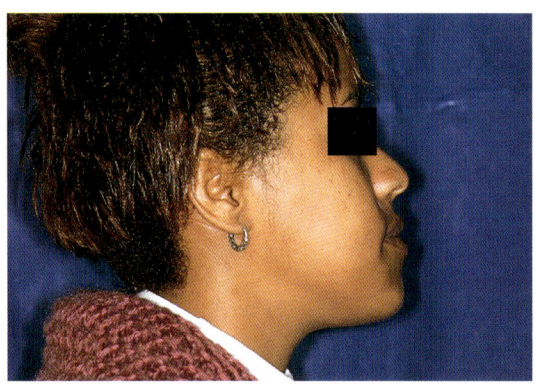

Figure 19.3

Face—profile view

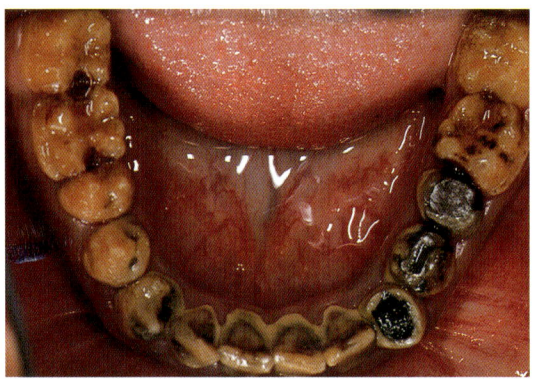

Figure 19.4

Mandibular arch

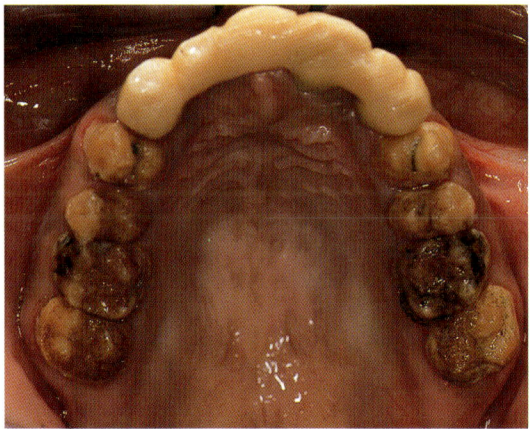

Figure 19.5

Maxillary arch

EXTRA-ORAL EXAMINATION
(Figures 19.1 and 19.3)

- Symmetrical face
- Competent lips
- Straight profile
- Normal temporomandibular joint
- Maximum opening 60 mm, with a slight deviation to the left upon opening

INTRA-ORAL EXAMINATION
(Figures 19.4 and 19.5)

- Exposed dentin
- Extensive caries
- Rounded arch form
- Wear of teeth accompanied by chipping of the enamel and cupping of the dentine
- Missing teeth:

$$\begin{array}{c|c} 8\ 2\ 1 & 1\ 2 \\ \hline 8 & 8 \end{array}$$

- Fixed provisional acrylic partial prosthesis:

$$\begin{array}{c|c} 3\text{--}X\text{--}X & 1\text{--}X\text{--}3 \\ \hline & \end{array}$$

- Irregular occlusal plane (Figures 19.6 and 19.7)

An occlusal examination revealed that the patient was Angle class III (Figures 19.6 and 19.7), with an overbite of 0.0 mm and an overjet of −1.0 to −1.5 mm. The interocclusal rest space was 2.0 mm, measured between the incisors. There was no discrepancy between centric occlusion (CO) and centric relation (CR). Balanced occlusion and anterior and bilateral posterior cross-bite were noted. There was edge to edge occlusion between the left maxillary central incisor

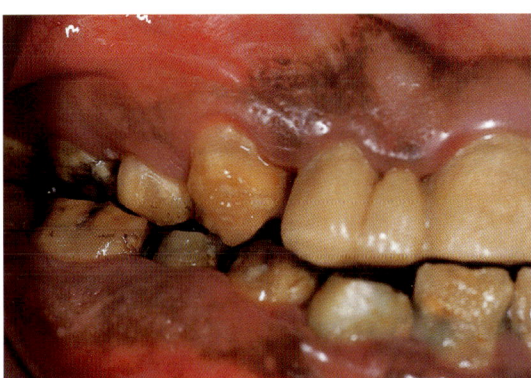

Figure 19.6

Occlusion—right side

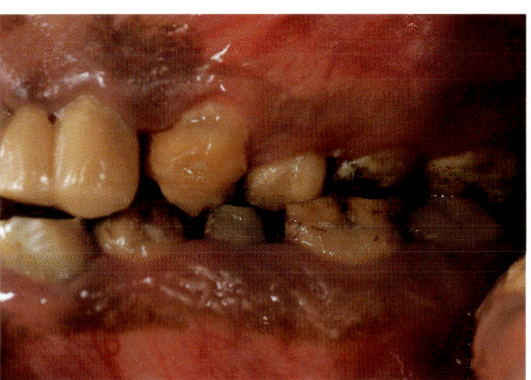

Figure 19.7

Occlusion—left side

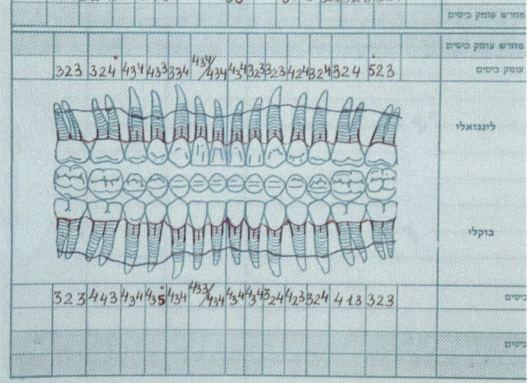

Figure 19.8

Periodontal chart—mandible

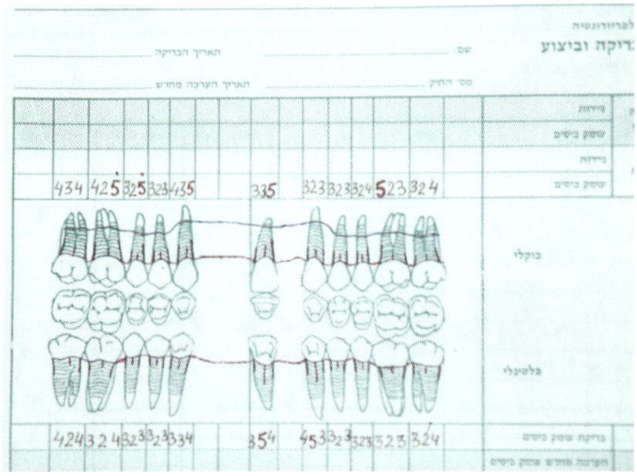

Figure 19.9

Periodontal chart—maxilla

and the left mandibular central and lateral incisor teeth (as restored by the provisional restoration).

The periodontal examination (Figures 19.8 and 19.9) showed unsatisfactory oral hygiene with large amounts of plaque and calculus. Probing depths were found of up to 5.0 mm on the maxillary teeth and up to 4.0 mm on the mandibular teeth, with bleeding on probing on some teeth. There was inflammation around most of the teeth.

FULL-MOUTH PERIAPICAL AND CEPHALOMETRIC SURVEY
(Figures 19.10 and 19.11)

- Cephalometric analysis—Angle class III
- Endodontic treatment:

$$\overline{\Big|\,3\,5}$$

- Defined radiolucent area in the right maxilla in the area of the right maxillary cuspid tooth
- Impacted maxillary left cuspid
- Caries
- Crown and root proximity

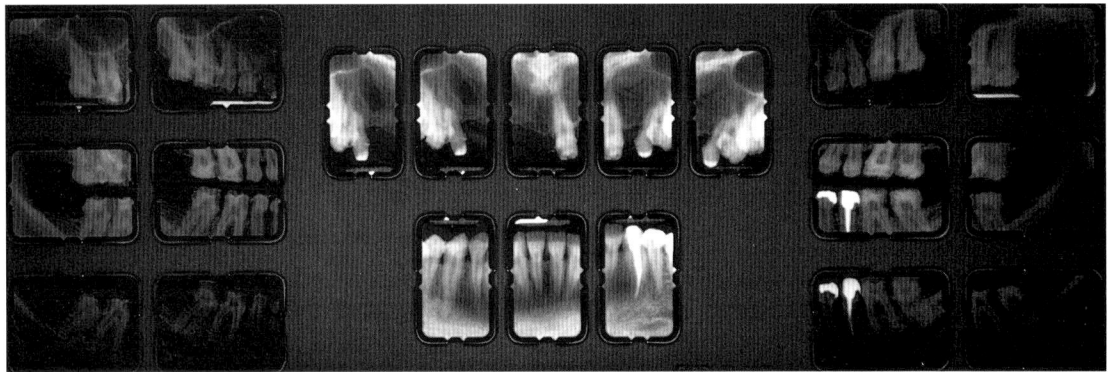

Figure 19.10

Radiographs of maxilla and mandible

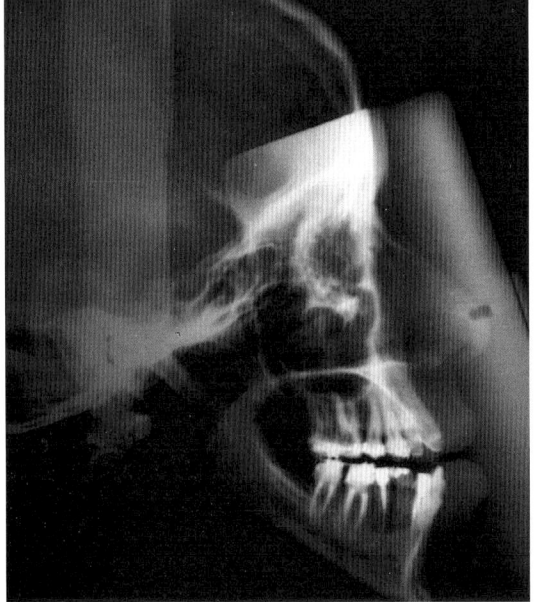

Figure 19.11

Cephalometric radiograph

INDIVIDUAL TOOTH PROGNOSIS

- Hopeless: none
- Fair:
$$\frac{2 \,\vert\, 2}{3\,5}$$
- Good: the remaining teeth

SUMMARY OF FINDINGS

The 25-year-old patient complained of poor esthetics, sensitivity in her teeth and gums, and bleeding gums on brushing. She suffered from exposed dentine, short clinical crowns, noticeable changes in the shape and color of her teeth, and root and crown proximity. She had poor oral hygiene, caries, missing anterior maxillary teeth, and faulty restorations. Probing depth was average, and there was a radiolucent area in the right maxilla.

DIAGNOSIS

- Angle class III with bilateral posterior cross-bite
- Amelogenesis imperfecta
- Multiple carious lesions
- Root and crown proximity
- Faulty restorations
- Occlusal disharmony and faulty occlusal plane
- Missing maxillary teeth
- Poor esthetics
- Gingivitis
- Radiolucent area in the right maxilla
- Impacted maxillary left cuspid

ABOUT THE PATIENT

The patient was very cooperative, and within a short period of time, her oral hygiene and her periodontal condition improved. She wanted an esthetic, fixed restoration and had high expectations of how much it would improve her appearance.

POTENTIAL TREATMENT PROBLEMS

- Amelogenesis imperfecta complicated by root and crown proximity
- Poor occlusal relationships—Angle class III with bilateral cross-bite
- Short clinical crowns that would require crown-lengthening procedures, thereby increasing the crown-to-root ratio, which might worsen the overall prognosis

TREATMENT PLAN

- Oral hygiene instruction
- Scaling and curettage
- Caries removal and endodontic therapy, where indicated
- Evaluation of patient cooperation
- Immediate provisional fixed acrylic restorations for the teeth with considerable loss of coronal tooth structure
- Orthodontic treatment to alleviate root and crown proximity
- Crown-lengthening surgery, where indicated
- Re-evaluation
- Fixed partial prostheses for both the maxilla and the mandible

TREATMENT

Initial preparation included oral hygiene instruction, scaling, and curettage. Caries removal and endodontic therapy were performed on the mandibular left first molar, second right mandibular premolar, and the right mandibular first and second molars, as indicated. The endodontically treated teeth were restored with amalgam post and cores. Full coverage provisional restorations were made serially in order to restore extensive lost tooth structure (Figure 19.12).

Orthodontic treatment was performed to alleviate root and crown proximity (Figure 19.13). At this point, after re-evaluation,

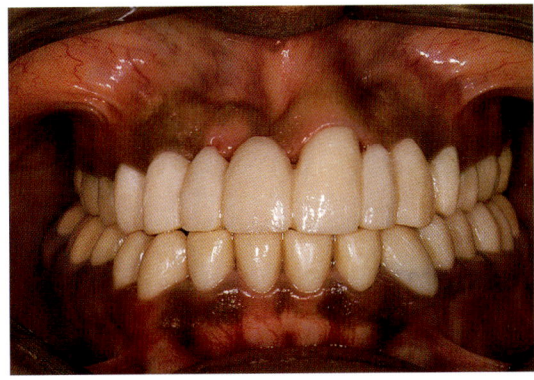

Figure 19.12

Transitional restorations

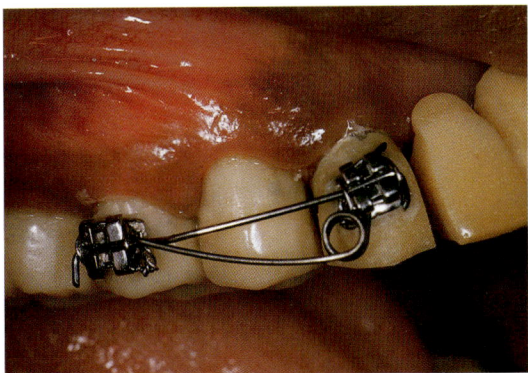

Figure 19.13

Orthodontic treatment—to alleviate root and crown proximity

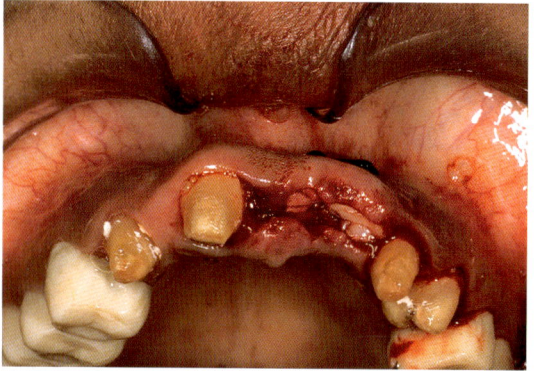

Figure 19.14

Periodontal surgery—crown lengthening procedure

localized crown lengthening was undertaken on the left maxillary and mandibular second molars. Periodontal surgery to align the gingival margins of the maxillary anterior teeth was carried out (Figure 19.14). Additional orthodontic treatment was then performed to realign the maxillary left central incisor tooth, correcting the existing midline discrepancy (Figure 19.15). At completion of orthodontic and periodontal treatment, new provisional restorations were made to maintain the newly acquired interproximal space and tissue health (Figure 19.16).

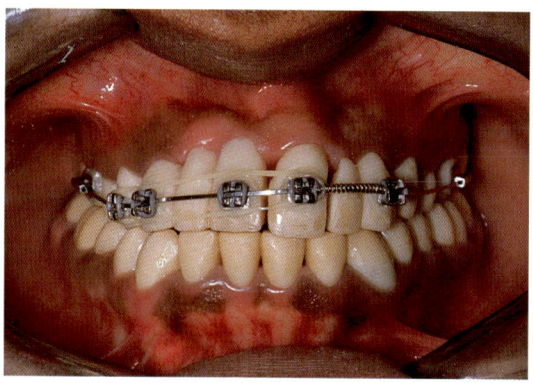

Figure 19.15

Orthodontic treatment to re-align anterior maxillary teeth

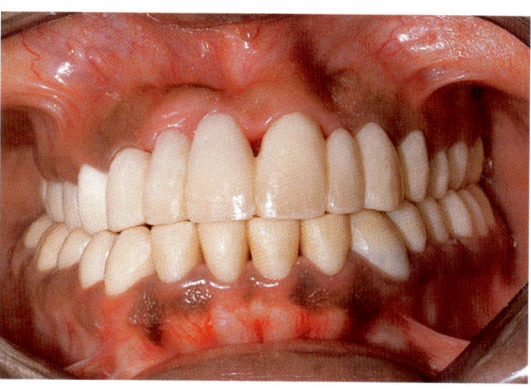

Figure 19.16

New transitional restorations after periodontal surgery

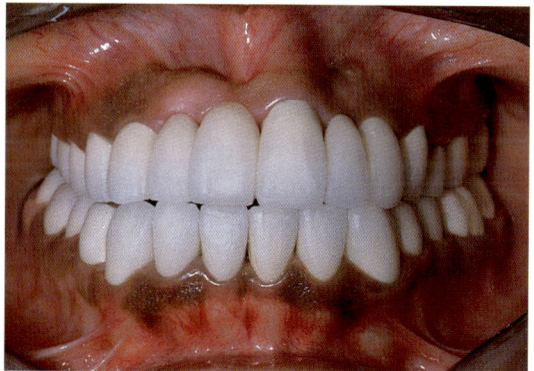

Figure 19.17

Biscuit bake porcelain try-in

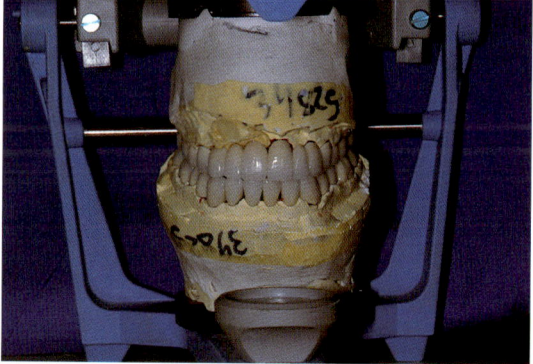

Figure 19.18

Finished restorations on Quick articulator

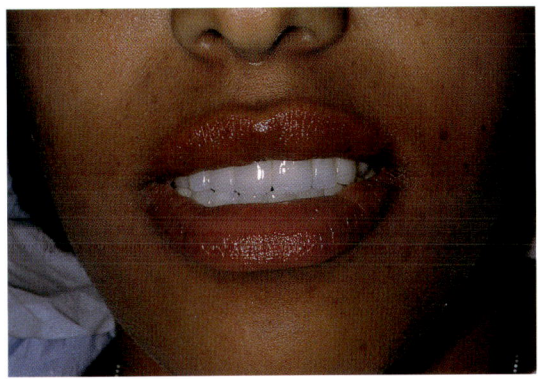

Figure 19.19

Facial view of patient's smile after treatment completion

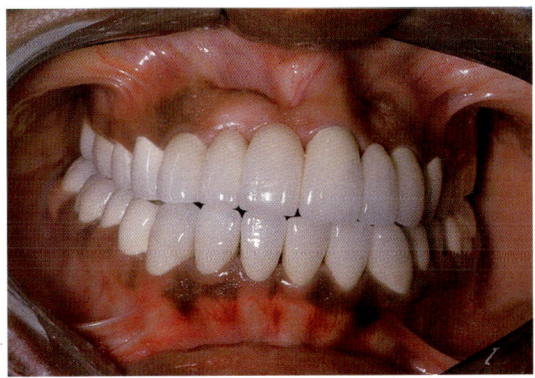

Figure 19.20

Finished restorations in mouth

Once the esthetic, physiological and functional expectations of the patient and the dentist had been attained in the transitional restorations, the teeth were reprepared, individual copper band elastomeric impressions were taken, and stone dies and Pattern resin copings made as described in the Technical Information chapter. The metal copings were fitted, connected, soldered and refitted as previously described and the porcelain biscuit bake applied. The final and minute adjustments of the biscuit bake porcelain were carried out in the mouth (Figure 19.17). The final glaze was applied to the prostheses (Figure 19.18), and the prostheses were cemented with Temp-Bond for a period of 2 weeks. They were then cemented with zinc oxyphosphate cement for permanent cementation in 1999 (Figures 19.19–19.21).

SUMMARY

The patient presented with a severe problem of enamel hypoplasia on all of her

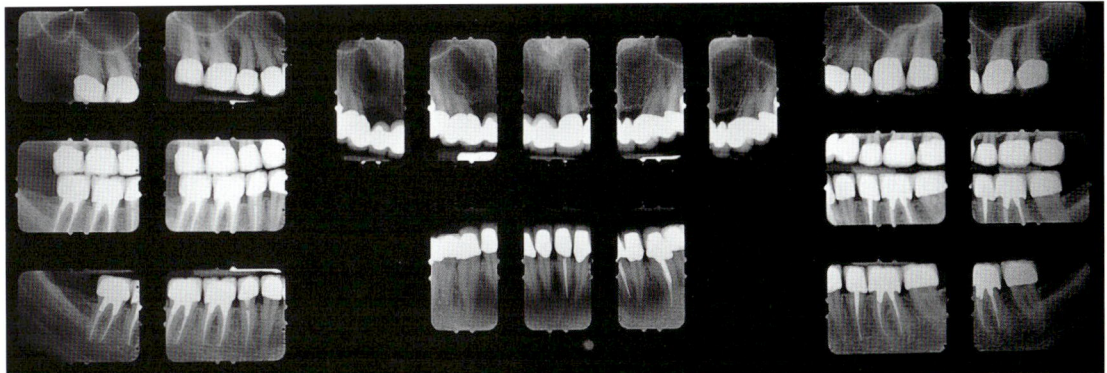

Figure 19.21

Radiographs after treatment completed

teeth, multiple carious lesions, massive loss of tooth structure, and root and crown proximity. There was a pathologic occlusion with serious non-working side and protrusive premature contacts during mandibular movements. She was very concerned about her esthetics. The treatment consisted of changing the vertical dimension of occlusion, orthodontic treatment, in order to provide a physiological occlusion and decrease the root proximity, and provide a proper foundation for the future fixed restorations. Periodontal surgery was also undertaken for crown lengthening as well as gingival alignment. The final restorations provided her with a functional, physiological, and esthetic solution.

CASE DISCUSSION
AVINOAM YAFFE

The 25-year-old patient presented to the clinic with generalized amelogenesis imperfecta complicated by multiple carious lesions with massive loss of tooth structure, and aggravated by close proximity of roots and crowns. The solution provided took into consideration all of these factors. In order to solve the problem of short crowns (retention for a fixed prosthesis) due to the loss of enamel (Amelogenesis imperfecta) the vertical dimension of occlusion was increased so that there was minimal occlusal reduction. This reduced the need for crown-lengthening procedures on one hand, and also improved the anterior–posterior occlusal relationship, gaining 1.5 mm of overjet and 1.0 mm of overbite, thus enabling a physiologic occlusion and minimally jeopardizing long-term tooth survival. At completion of the rehabilitation, all the esthetic, functional, and physiologic criteria were accomplished.

CASE DISCUSSION
HAROLD PREISKEL

This patient's treatment represents another example of what can be achieved with dedicated and skilled operators and a motivated patient. The daunting problem of amelogenesis imperfecta, malpositioned roots, caries, and active periodontal disease, were overcome in a sensible manner. It is hard to believe that little more than one practicing generation ago such a combination of problems would have been treated by the removal of the roots and the construction of complete upper and lower dentures. Nowadays, the combination of difficult root position, short clinical crowns, and caries, might have tempted operators to consider the implant approach. Indeed, this may have been a viable option, but I feel that Dr Lavi made the right decision and in the unlikely event that the restoration should not survive a reasonable period of time the implant option still remains. The periodontal care, orthodontic therapy, and restorative treatment have produced an excellent result, but one that will require unwavering enthusiasm if it is to be maintained.

PATIENT 20   BILATERAL CLEFT PALATE AND RAYNAUD'S DISEASE

Treatment by Yael Houri

THE PATIENT

The patient, a 17-year-old high school student (Figure 20.1), presented himself for examination and consultation with the following complaints:

'I have missing front teeth and the spaces are ugly.'
'I have pus coming out of my mouth.'

PAST MEDICAL HISTORY

Medical history showed a history of congenital bilateral cleft palate (Figure 20.2) and Raynaud's disease (spasm of the arterioles, usually in the digits but occasionally in the nose and tongue, with intermittent pallor or cyanosis of the skin). The cleft was familial as his sister and father both had a history of cleft palate; his sister bilateral and his father unilateral. The patient underwent many surgical procedures at an early age to close the lip and hard palate clefts, and thus exhibited much scarring. He was in orthodontic treatment until the age 13 and since then in retention with a removable retainer which also replaced the missing maxillary lateral incisor teeth (Figure 20.3). At times, food and liquids passed through the fistula from his mouth to his nose. Speech was

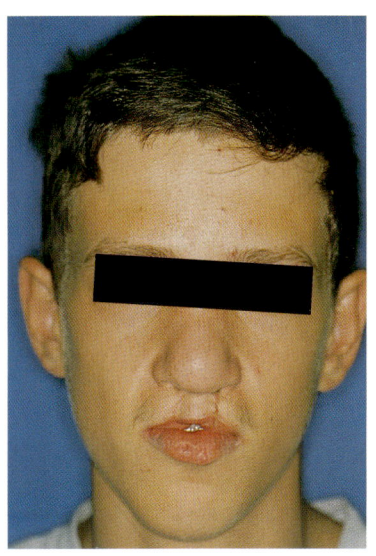

Figure 20.1

Frontal facial view

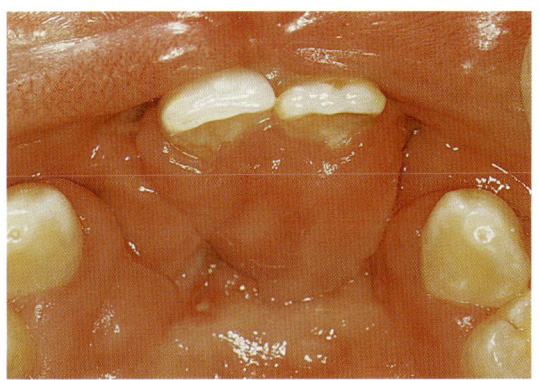

Figure 20.2

Maxillary arch—anterior palatal view

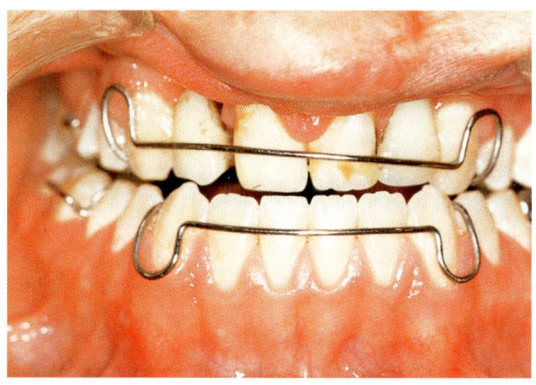

Figure 20.3

Frontal view of teeth showing orthodontic retainers

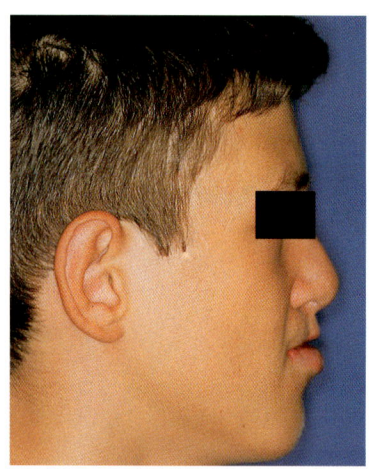

Figure 20.4

Face in profile

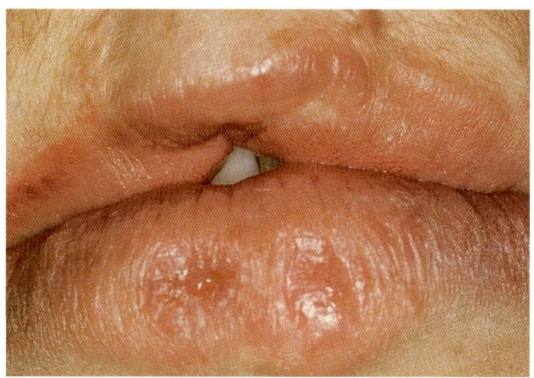

Figure 20.5

View of lips showing PITS

- Lower lip exhibited two PITS, indicative of the Raynaud's disease (Figure 20.5)
- Bridge of the nose was very wide and the nostrils were without bone support and were enlarged (Figure 20.1)
- Maximum opening was 53 mm, and there was no deviation in either opening or closing movements
- No muscle sensitivity was noted and the jaw movements were normal
- Compromised esthetics due to the bilateral lip clefts and the missing maxillary lateral incisor teeth

compromised and sometimes difficult to understand. At age 14, he underwent orthopedic surgery to build up his nose and also to close the boney hard palate clefts. There was a family history of sensitivity to Optalgin (glucose-6-phosphate dehydrogenase deficiency).

EXTRA-ORAL EXAMINATION

- Straight profile with incompetent lips (Figures 20.1 and 20.4)

INTRA-ORAL EXAMINATION

Maxilla (Figure 20.6):

- Jaw—normal size, asymmetrical, triangular, with a class 3 soft palate and shallow vestibulum
- Amalgam restorations on some of the molar teeth
- Caries on the left maxillary molars and the right maxillary first molar
- Very poor oral hygiene with inflamed gingivae accompanied by calculus and plaque

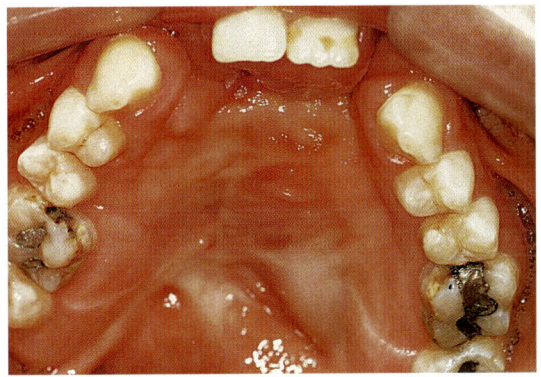

Figure 20.6

Maxillary arch

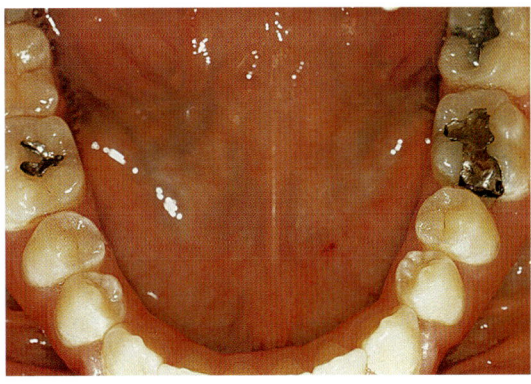

Figure 20.7

Mandibular arch

- Congenital absence of the maxillary lateral incisor teeth, an oral nasal fistula on the right side between the hard palate and the premaxilla; the pre-maxilla was slightly mobile
- Palatal scar above the left molar teeth
- Third molar teeth impacted

Mandible (Figure 20.7):

- Ovoid jaw shape
- High floor of the mouth with wide and broad muscle attachments and shallow vestibulum
- Amalgam restorations on some of the molar teeth

An occlusal examination revealed that the patient was Angle class III, with an open anterior cross-bite (Figure 20.3). The interocclusal rest space was 2.0 mm. There was no midline deviation. The posterior teeth were in an edge to edge relationship bucco-lingually. The plane of occlusion was faulty, with incomplete contacts between the maxillary and mandibular teeth (Figure 20.8). The only working side contacts in lateral jaw movements were on the second molars. There were balancing

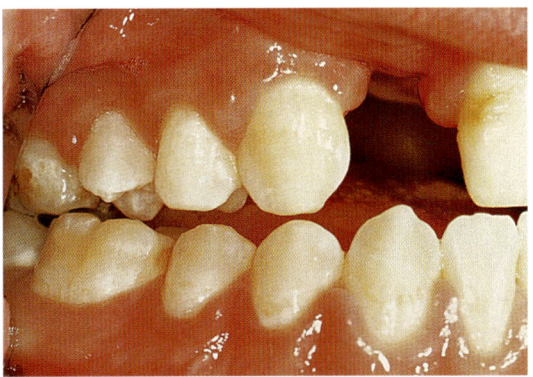

Figure 20.8

Open bite right side

side contacts between the maxillary second molars and the mandibular third molars. In protrusive movements, there was no anterior disclusion and the only contacts were on the second molars.

The periodontal examination revealed probing depths of up to 5.0 mm on the maxillary teeth and up to 4.0 mm on most of the mandibular teeth, with bleeding on probing on some teeth (Figures 20.9 and 20.10). There was slight inflammation around the maxillary and mandibular molars.

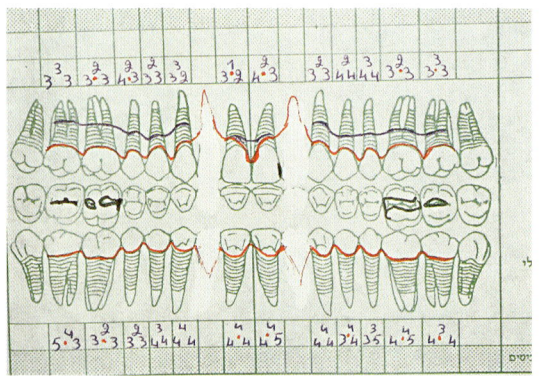

Figure 20.9

Maxillary periodontal chart

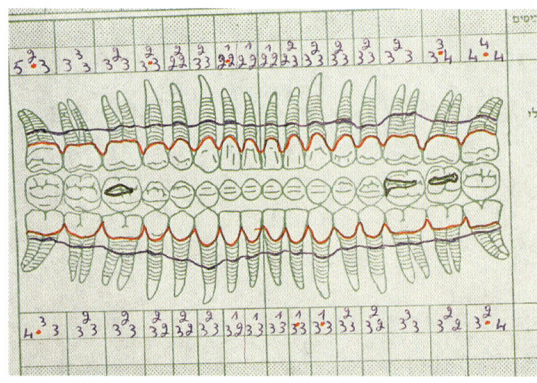

Figure 20.10

Mandibular periodontal chart

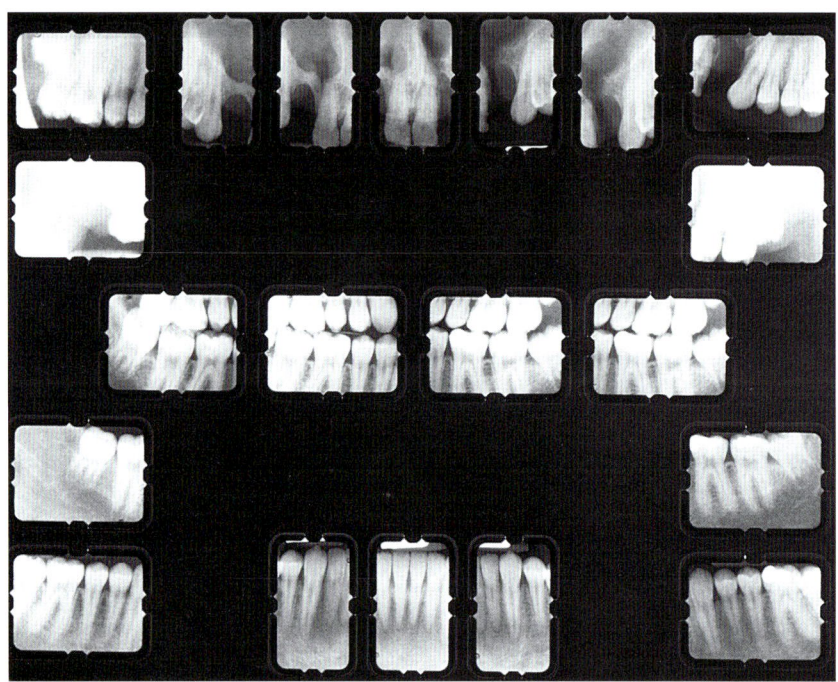

Figure 20.11

Radiographs of maxillary and mandibular anterior quadrant

FULL-MOUTH PERIAPICAL SURVEY (Figure 20.11)

A complete series of X-rays revealed the following findings:

- Missing teeth: $\dfrac{2 \mid 2}{}$

- Impacted teeth: $\dfrac{ \mid }{8 \mid 8}$

- Maxillary right first molar had an occlusal amalgam restoration with mesial caries
- Extrusion of the right mandibular third molar tooth

- Maxillary left first molar had an mesio-occlusal amalgam restoration with mesial caries
- Small distal caries in the maxillary left cuspid
- Distal caries in the right maxillary central incisor
- Occlusal amalgam restorations in the second molar teeth

INDIVIDUAL TOOTH PROGNOSIS

All the teeth had a good prognosis.

SUMMARY OF FINDINGS

The patient, a 17-year-old high school student, came to the clinic complaining of poor esthetics and missing front teeth. He was very concerned about his appearance and wanted to have a fixed prosthesis to replace his removable one.

His previous medical history consisted of congenital bilateral cleft palate and lip with many unsuccessful attempts at surgical repair, and he remained with much scarring. He suffered from Raynaud's disease. There was a lack of bone between the premaxilla and the maxilla on the left side, and on the right side there was a narrow bridge of bone connecting the premaxilla and maxilla. He had undergone orthodontic treatment and had removable maxillary and mandibular orthodontic maintainers, which also replaced the missing maxillary lateral incisor teeth. There was an oral-nasal fistula between his hard palate and premaxilla on the right side.

His oral hygiene was poor. He had large amounts of plaque and calculus causing gingivitis, but with good bone support. The maxillary lateral incisors were congenitally missing and the maxillary third molars were impacted. Some of the existing restorations were faulty and there was extrusion of the mandibular right third molar. There was caries on many teeth. He was Angle class III with an anterior cross-bite as well as an anterior open bite, with a faulty plane of occlusion.

DIAGNOSIS

- Bilateral cleft lip and palate s/p (status post) surgery
- Oral-nasal fistula
- Congenitally missing teeth
- Poor esthetics
- Anterior cross-bite
- Anterior open bite
- Gingivitis
- Caries
- Raynaud's disease
- Impacted maxillary third molars

ABOUT THE PATIENT

The young patient seemed to have no understanding of the importance of the need for his cooperation in his dental treatment. He was strongly motivated to have dental treatment for esthetic reasons, and wanted his teeth fixed before he was inducted into army service.

POTENTIAL TREATMENT PROBLEMS

The patient was a young man who had undergone multiple, extensive, but unsuccessful surgical procedures to repair a congenital condition, and was therefore wary of extensive dental treatment.

TREATMENT PLAN

Maxilla:

- Maxillofacial surgery to add needed bone in the cleft areas in order to close the oral-nasal fistula and stabilize the premaxilla, and to provide bone support for implants
- Fixed partial prosthesis to replace the missing lateral incisor teeth with a removable prosthesis to seal the oral-nasal fistula
- Removable partial denture
- Restoration of carious teeth

Mandible:

- Restoration of carious teeth

TREATMENT

Initial preparation included oral hygiene instruction, scaling, curettage, and root planing. The carious teeth were then restored. At the end of this stage, an obvious improvement in the periodontal supporting tissue could be seen, and it was observed that the pocket depths had diminished and that the bleeding on probing had disappeared.

Occlusal equilibration was performed to reduce the anterior open bite and obtain stable intercuspal position. The patient was also referred for speech therapy. Following a CT radiograph (Figure 20.12), consultation with the oral and maxillofacial surgery department revealed that the chance for successful augmentation of the cleft on the left side and closure of the fistula was almost negligible. The possibilities of treatment of the maxilla were then limited to a removable partial denture to replace the missing maxillary lateral incisor teeth and to cover the opening of the fistula, or to restore the missing lateral incisors with a fixed partial

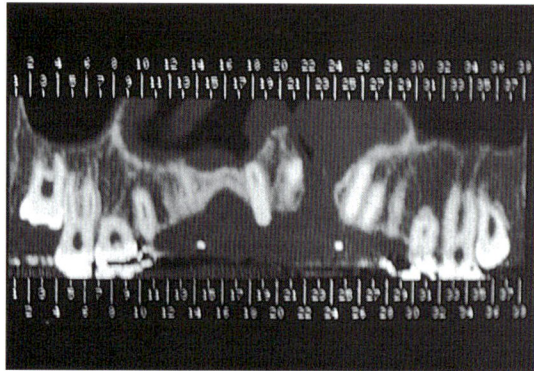

Figure 20.12

CT radiographs of the maxilla

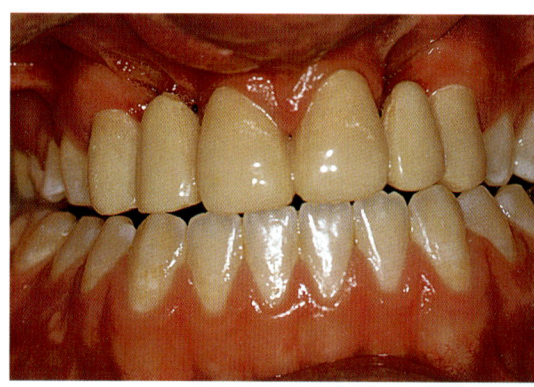

Figure 20.13

Anterior view of teeth

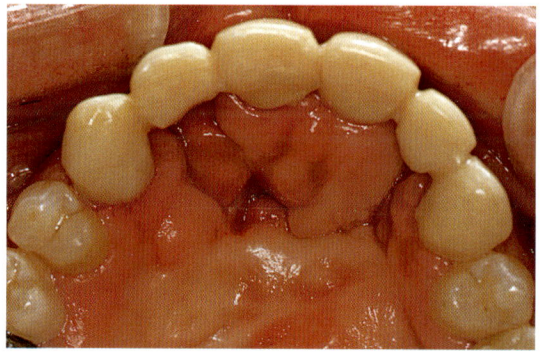

Figure 20.14

Palatal view of maxillary anterior teeth

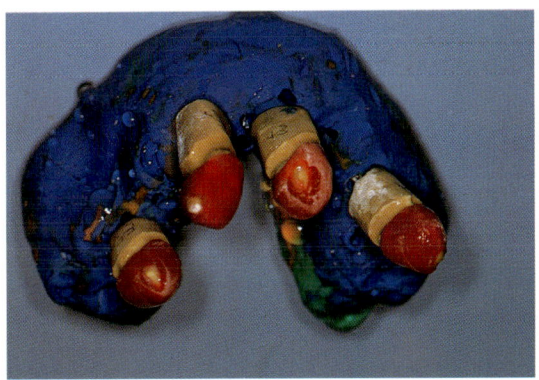

Figure 20.15

Dies and Duralay copings

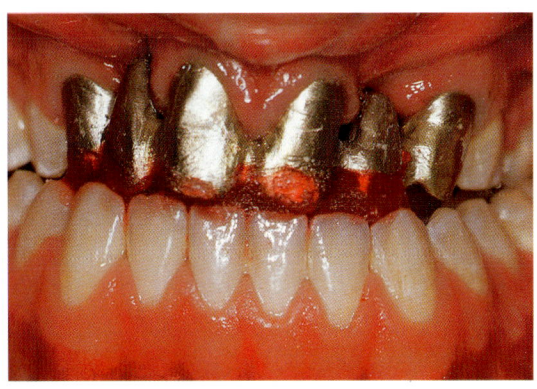

Figure 20.16

Soldered metal copings being fitted

prosthesis from the right cuspid to the left cuspid, with provision for a removable palatal attachment to cover the palatal fistula. A very accurately fitting gold palatal leaf (denture) that would seal the fistula was chosen. It would be retained by a precision attachment fitting into the maxillary right lateral incisor pontic (split lingual attachment).

The maxillary central incisor and cuspid teeth were prepared and temporized with a transitional fixed prosthesis, which also corrected the cross-bite and gave anterior contact in centric relation and anterior guidance in lateral and protrusive movements of the mandible (Figures 20.13 and 20.14). In addition, 'guided' passive eruption allowed the molars on the right side to erupt into contact. This was accomplished by building up the mandibular lingual cusps with composite resin in order to prevent lateral tongue thrust, which was preventing the teeth from erupting to contact. The composite was removed after occlusal contact had been achieved and the surfaces finely polished.

After the patient adapted to his new restorations, copper band impressions of methylmethacrylate and elastomeric impression material (Xantropen) were taken of the maxillary prepared teeth, and Duralay copings were made (Figure 20.15). These copings were used to record centric relation at the vertical dimension of occlusion as determined by the posterior teeth, and for the impression for the model to make the metal copings. The metal copings were built with a semi-precision attachment in the maxillary right lateral incisor pontic. These were then fitted and soldered and, after try-in of the soldered metal framework, a centric registration record was made in Duralay (Figure 20.16) and an elastomeric impression was made for the tissue pick-up for the master model.

The models were mounted on a semiadjustable articulator (Hanau) utilizing a facebow registration and centric records were taken at the vertical dimension of occlusion utilizing Duralay with a Neylon technique. At this point the porcelain was baked and the occlusion checked at the biscuit bake stage in the mouth and all adjustments needed were then made. A Duralay palatal attachment was fitted and relined in the mouth with Duralay (Figure 20.17). This palatal attachment was then cast in gold, with a male attachment to fit the female attachment in the right maxillary

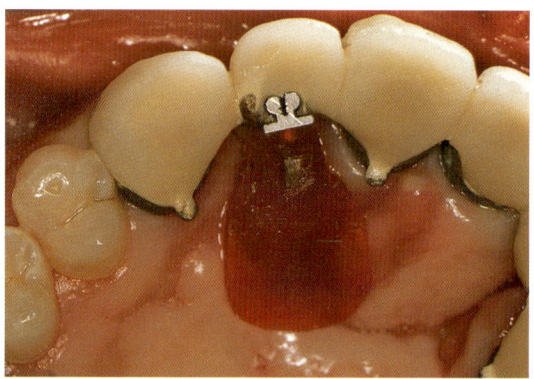

Figure 20.17

Palatal seal in Duralay

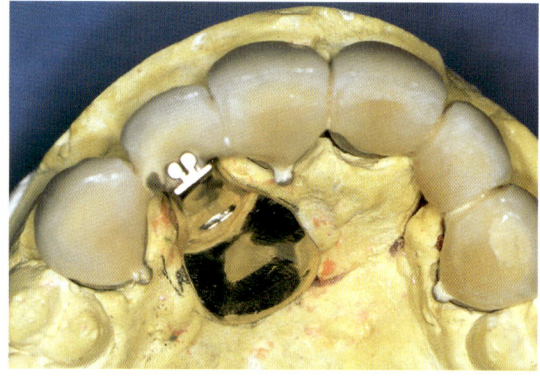

Figure 20.18

Palatal seal in gold

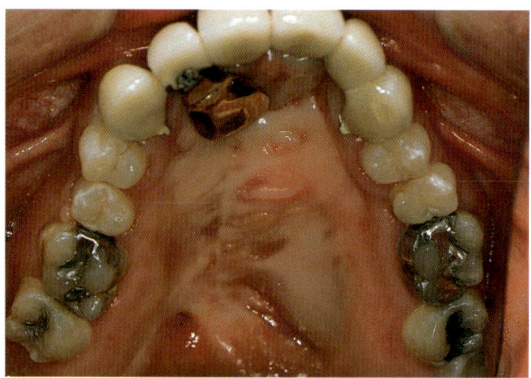

Figure 20.19

Case cemented—post-treatment anterior palatal view

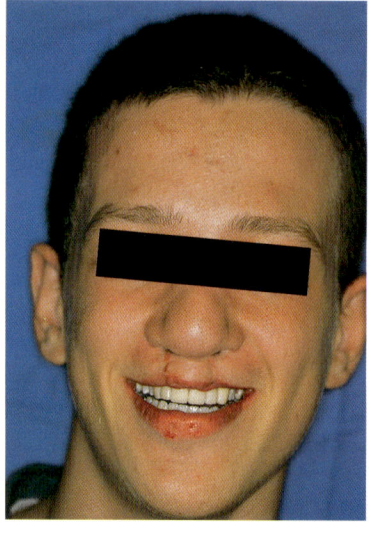

Figure 20.20

Frontal facial view of patient after treatment completion

lateral incisor pontic (Figure 20.18). The gold removable palatal attachment was fitted and checked in the mouth. The maxillary fixed prosthesis was glazed and polished, as was the gold palatal attachment. The prosthesis was cemented with Temp-Bond for a period of 2 weeks and the palatal attachment inserted (Figures 20.19 and 20.20). The patient was taught how to insert and remove the palatal attachment for cleaning purposes. The crowns and bridges were then cemented with zinc oxyphosphate cement for permanent cementation.

SUMMARY

The patient presented after many unsuccessful surgical attempts to close a bilateral congenital palate and lip cleft. He had poor oral hygiene, difficulties with speech and a very poor self-image due to severely compromised esthetics. The patient was restored to form and function with the minimal treatment necessary, which included a fixed partial prosthesis to replace the congenitally missing maxillary lateral incisor teeth, and a semi-precision gold palatal attachment to cover the existing oral-nasal fistula, thus preventing food and liquids from entering the nasal cavity.

CASE DISCUSSION
AVINOAM YAFFE

The patient, a 17-year-old high school student, presented to the clinic seeking treatment to solve esthetic and functional problems. He was anxious to get rid of his removable partial orthodontic retainer, which also restored his missing lateral incisor teeth. Once the possibility for a surgical correction of the fistula was negated, the patient, in order to prevent having a removable prosthesis, claimed that the fistula really did not bother him. However, as the fistula did create a problem, a solution was found that could satisfy the patient's wishes as well as seal the fistula. This was a fixed partial prosthesis with a small removable partial denture to cover the oral-antral fistula. Prior to fabricating the provisional prosthesis, selective grinding was performed, with the intention of obtaining a stable occlusion and freedom in mandibular movements for the

anterior fixed prosthesis. Additional occlusal support was also obtained by passive eruption of posterior teeth that formerly were not in contact.

CASE DISCUSSION
HAROLD PREISKEL

The successful outcome of this young man's treatment appears to have been achieved as a result of a team approach with successful patient motivation. As a result, the tongue thrust that was causing molar separation on the right hand side was overcome with the aid of transitional composite additions to the lower teeth and occlusal stability obtained. Missing lateral incisors were restored with fixed prostheses—something the patient had wanted from the outset—while the obturation of an oro-nasal defect was obtained by means of a very small removable device incorporating an attachment within the pontic replacing the lateral incisor. In order to obtain a perfect seal, the path of insertion of the obturator had to be carefully planned and this, in turn, was decided by the alignment of the attachment in the pontic. This highlights the importance of an overall plan of treatment, that included the path of insertion for the removable prosthesis.

INDEX